INNOVATIONS IN CLINICAL PRACTICE

A 21st Century Sourcebook

Volume 1

Edited by
JEFFERY B. ALLEN
EVE M. WOLF
LEON VANDECREEK

PROFESSIONAL RESOURCE PRESS
P.O. Box 15560
Sarasota, FL 34277-1560

Published by Professional Resource Press
(An imprint of Professional Resource Exchange, Inc.)
Post Office Box 15560
Sarasota, FL 34277-1560

Library of Congress Cataloging-in-Publication Data

Innovations in clinical practice: a 21st century sourcebook / edited by Jeffery B. Allen, Eve M. Wolf, Leon VandeCreek.
   p. cm.
Includes bibliographical references and index.
ISBN 1-56887-120-1 (978-1-56887-120-2 : alk. paper)
   1. Clinical psychology. 2. Mental health services. I. Allen, Jeffery B. II. Wolf, Eve M. III. Vandecreek, Leon.
RC467.I56 2009
616.89--dc22

2008047314

The copyeditor for this book was Patricia Rockwood and the managing editor was Laurie Girsch.

Preface

The *Innovations in Clinical Practice* series has been the go-to reference for practicing mental health professionals for 28 years. And it has evolved during its lifetime. Volumes 1 through 20 in the *Source Book* series provided a wide range of topics with no particular theme. Each volume contained new material with handouts, forms, and informal instruments as well as thought-provoking and informative articles on clinical issues and applications. Practitioners consistently praised the timeliness of the topics that we covered, the highly applied focus and usefulness of the contributions, the expertise of contributors, and the quality of our editing.

FOCUSED VOLUMES

For several years, we began to notice a shift in interest (and sales) amongst our readers that appeared to correspond to changes that had occurred in their practices; namely, readers were reporting that their practices had become more "specialized" and they were now less interested in the broad range of topics that were included in each of the earlier *Innovations in Clinical Practice: A Source Book* volumes. They were also reporting lower incomes and a desire for less expensive books and other resources. In response, we began publishing a shorter more focused version of *Innovations*. These volumes include:

- *Focus on Children & Adolescents*
- *Focus on Violence Treatment & Prevention*
- *Focus on Adults*
- *Focus on Health & Wellness*
- *Focus on Sexual Health*
- *Focus on Group, Couples, & Family Therapy*

CHANGING TRENDS

Innovations in Clinical Practice: A 21st Century Sourcebook (Vol. 1) is the first volume of this next generation of the *Innovations* series. Like the first 20 volumes of *Innovations*, it will also cover a wide range of topics.

After reviewing ongoing customer needs assessment responses, and discussing possibilities with customers and editorial staff, we made the decision to go back to our original concept and develop future volumes around broad topics of interest to practicing mental health professionals. Our customers decided that, though their practices may have narrowed, they still liked the broader array of topics that we covered in the first 20 volumes. We hope the timeliness of the topics that we cover in this and future volumes, the highly applied focus and usefulness of the contributions, the expertise of the contributors, and the quality of our editing will continue to bring praise from our readers.

A major dilemma we faced with this series was format. Our preferred version was a deluxe binder but we discovered that printing and production costs were prohibitive. Instead, we chose the more cost efficient paperbound version while still preserving the 8 1/2" x 11" format.

CREDITS

Peter A. Keller was the senior editor of *Innovations in Clinical Practice: A Source Book* through Volume 10. Lawrence G. Ritt served as coeditor of the first five volumes and continues to consult about the development of subsequent volumes. Steven R. Heyman was coeditor of Volumes 6 to 10. Beginning with the 11th volume, Leon VandeCreek assumed the position of senior editor. Samuel Knapp served as associate editor for Volumes 11 through 16. Thomas L. Jackson served as associate editor from Volume 11 through 20.

The senior and associate editors for the *Innovations in Clinical Practice: Focus* series are as follows:

- *Adults* (Leon VandeCreek, editor)
- *Children & Adolescents* (Leon VandeCreek, senior editor; Thomas L. Jackson, associate editor)
- *Group, Couples, & Family Therapy* (Leon VandeCreek, senior editor; Jeffery B. Allen, associate editor)
- *Health & Wellness* (Leon VandeCreek, senior editor; Jeffery B. Allen, associate editor)
- *Sexual Health* (Leon VandeCreek, senior editor; Frederick L. Peterson, Jr., & Jill W. Bley, associate editors)
- *Violence Treatment & Prevention* (Thomas L. Jackson, senior editor; Leon VandeCreek, associate editor)

Jeffrey B. Allen is senior editor, and Eve M. Wolf and Leon VandeCreek serve as associate editors for the *Innovations in Clinical Practice: A 21st Century Sourcebook* series.

There are several other individuals who have made important contributions to the production of the *Innovations* series. From volume 1 of *Innovations in Clinical Practice: A Source Book* through the last of the focused *Innovations* volumes, Debra Fink supervised the final production of each volume and ensured careful attention to details that others might have missed. Laurie Girsch ably assisted her beginning with Volume 8. We appreciate their thoroughness and cooperative spirit. Each year they became more important to the success of the series. In 2008, Laurie Girsch assumed the role of Managing Editor and and is solely responsible for the last several books Professional Resource Press produced. Ms. Girsch is also responsible for the production of this volume.

Other contributors to the preparation of these volumes include Patricia Rockwood and Jude Warinner, who have worked many hours copyediting and proofreading the manuscripts. Without their skilled assistance, this volume would not be a reality. We would also like to thank Jeff Klosterman for his help in preparing the current volume for distribution and Valerie Hatcher for her assistance on continuing education projects.

AN INVITATION TO SUBMIT A CONTRIBUTION

The editors are currently soliciting contributions for future volumes in the *Innovations* series. If you are doing something innovative in your work, please let us hear from you. Contact Dr. Jeffery B. Allen, ABPP-CN, Senior Editor, School of Professional Psychology, Wright State University, 3640 Colonel Glenn Highway, Dayton, OH 45435-0001, if you would like more detailed information on becoming a contributor.

CONTINUING EDUCATION

The Professional Resource Exchange is approved as a continuing education (CE) sponsor by several national and state organizations including the American Psychological Association and the National Board for Certified Counselors. CE credits are available to readers who are required to participate in CE programs, as well as by those who simply wish to validate their learning. To learn how to obtain home study continuing education credits through the *Innovations in Clinical Practice* series, please visit our website (www.prpress.com) or call 800-443-3364. These programs provide an economical means of obtaining continuing education credits while acquiring relevant clinical knowledge. Readers have been consistently positive about the experience of obtaining CE credits through this series.

COPYRIGHT POLICIES

Most of the material in this volume may be duplicated. You may photocopy materials (such as office forms and instruments) or reproduce them for use in your practice or share contributions with your students in the classroom; however, no part of this publication may be stored in a retrieval system, scanned, recorded, posted on an Internet website, or transmitted electronically by any other means or in any form. For materials on which the Professional Resource Exchange holds the copyright, no further permission is required for noncommercial, professional, or educational uses in printed formats. However, unauthorized duplication or publication for resale or large-scale distribution of any material in this volume is expressly prohibited.

Any material that you duplicate from this volume (with the exceptions mentioned below) must be acknowledged as having been reprinted from this volume and must note that copyright is held by the Professional Resource Exchange, Inc. The format and exact wording required in the acknowledgment are shown on the copyright page of this volume. The only exception to this policy is that clinical and office forms (not instruments) for use with clients in your own office may be reprinted without the acknowledgment mentioned above.

There are exceptions to our liberal copyright policy. We do not hold copyright on some of the materials included in this volume and, therefore, cannot grant permission to freely duplicate those materials. When copyright is held by another publisher or author, such copyright is noted on the appropriate page of the contribution. Unless otherwise noted in the credit and copyright citation, any reproduction or duplication of these materials is strictly and expressly forbidden without the consent of the copyright holder.

Jeffery B. Allen
Wright State University

Eve M. Wolf
Wright State University

Leon VandeCreek
Wright State University

Biographies

Jeffery B. Allen, PhD, ABPP-CN, Senior Editor, is currently a Professor in the School of Professional Psychology at Wright State University in Dayton, Ohio. Dr. Allen's professional experience includes a specialty internship in neuropsychology at Brown University and a rehabilitation focused postdoctoral fellowship at the Rehabilitation Institute of Michigan in Detroit. He is widely published in the areas of neuropsychology, head injuries, and memory in such sources as *Neuropsychologia, Brain Injuries*, and *Archives of Clinical Neuropsychology and Assessment*. His areas of teaching also include physiological psychology and clinical neuropsychology. His research interests include neurobehavioral disorders, quality of life in medical populations, cognitive and neuropsychological assessment, and outcome measurement in rehabilitation. He is Board Certified by the American Board of Professional Psychology in Clinical Neuropsychology and has recently published the text, *A General Practitioner's Guide to Neuropsychological Assessment*, through the American Psychological Association. Dr. Allen can be reached at SOPP, Wright State University, 3640 Colonel Glenn Highway, Dayton, OH 45435-0001. E-mail: jeffery.allen@wright.edu

Eve M. Wolf, PhD, is the Associate Dean for Academic Affairs at the Wright State University School of Professional Psychology in Dayton, Ohio. For over 20 years, she has been involved in clinical work and scholarship in the area of eating disorders. Currently, she supervises doctoral students in their clinical work at the university counseling center where eating problems and body image issues are common concerns. In addition, Dr. Wolf has taught doctoral courses in adult and child psychopathology, projective assessment, and the teaching of psychology. She can be reached at 117 Health Sciences Building, 3640 Colonel Glenn Highway, Dayton, OH 45435. E-mail: eve.wolf@wright.edu

Leon VandeCreek, PhD, is a licensed psychologist who is the past dean and current Professor in the School of Professional Psychology at Wright State University in Dayton, Ohio. He has been awarded the Diplomate in Clinical Psychology and he is a Fellow of several divisions of the American Psychological Association. His interests include professional training and ethical/legal issues related to professional education and practice. Dr. VandeCreek has served as President of the Pennsylvania Psychological Association, Chair of the APA Insurance Trust, Chair of the Board of Educational Affairs of the APA, and Treasurer of the Ohio Psychological Association. In 2005 he served as President of the Division of Psychotherapy of the APA. He has authored and coauthored about 150 professional presentations and publications, including 17 books. From 1992 to 2007 he served as Senior Editor of the *Innovations in Clinical Practice: A Source Book* series. Dr. VandeCreek may be contacted at the Ellis Human Development Institute, 9 N. Edwin C. Moses Boulevard, Dayton, OH 45407. E-mail: leon.vandecreek@wright.edu

Table of Contents

SECTION I:
CLINICAL ISSUES AND APPLICATIONS

Section II:
Practice Management and Professional Development

Section III:
Assessment Instruments and Client Handouts

Section IV:
Community Interventions

Section V:
Selected Topics

INNOVATIONS
IN CLINICAL PRACTICE

A 21st Century Sourcebook

Volume 1

Introduction
To the Volume

This volume of *Innovations in Clinical Practice: A 21st Century Sourcebook* is organized into five sections that reflect the diversity of contributions to the series. The subject index is contained on pages 307-316.

The first section, CLINICAL ISSUES AND APPLICATIONS, deals primarily with therapeutic concerns. The various contributions, however, go beyond traditional therapeutic issues and also address important questions of assessment, as well as treatment. Issues that relate to a number of different types of clients and situations are covered.

The second section addresses PRACTICE MANAGEMENT AND PROFESSIONAL DEVELOPMENT. This section is included because of the increasing number of clinicians who work independently and require a source of information on practice management, ethical concerns, and professional development issues. We remain in a period of dramatic changes that affect the nature of our practices. New risks as well as opportunities are constantly emerging in this era of health care reform. In this section, we try to address relevant issues that we believe will be of interest to our readers. Some of our discussions here also should be of interest to students and clinicians who practice in organizations or agencies.

The third section includes ASSESSMENT INSTRUMENTS AND CLIENT HANDOUTS. The assessment instruments are primarily informal and designed to assist clinicians in collecting information about clients. Our goal is to publish screening instruments and forms that aid in the organization of data rather than the making of formal inferences. There are some exceptions to this rule; however, we believe all fall within the bounds of accepted professional practice in the format in which they are presented. The materials presented here should be useful to psychologists and other professionals, with minimal potential for misuse. We assume that readers will be thoroughly familiar with any disorders or processes that they attempt to evaluate, and readers are advised to carefully review the introductory materials that accompany contributions to this section. We also have included in this section two handouts for use with your clients.

The fourth section on COMMUNITY INTERVENTIONS reflects our view that mental health practitioners have much to offer in the community beyond traditional clinical services. We trust that the material in this section will be of assistance to those who are interested in mental health consultation, education, prevention, and expanding their services to reach new and broader populations.

The fifth section, SELECTED TOPICS, includes a variety of contributions that do not fit neatly into one of the other sections.

Introduction to Section I: Clinical Issues and Applications

The CLINICAL ISSUES AND APPLICATIONS section includes contributions that are primarily related to new developments in theory, prevention, assessment, and treatment. This section provides a means for practitioners to access current information about new clinical techniques that might be incorporated into their practices, or to learn of new developments in specialized areas.

In the first contribution, Nicole Hunka and Alan Gilbertson highlight the significance of chronic pain as a major health problem. In contrast to traditional approaches for pain management which include pharmacological, surgical, and other medical interventions, they address psychological factors and associated psychological treatment for this serious problem. The authors provide definitions and clinical descriptions of pain, as well as address pain-related mental health diagnoses. Historic pain models are reviewed, as well as the more current biopsychosocial model. Psychosocial factors associated with pain are reviewed as well as psychological factors and comorbidities (i.e., the association between pain and depression). In addressing etiology, the authors highlight behavioral and cognitive conceptualizations of pain. A useful section summarizing psychological treatment interventions for pain management are provided at the end of the contribution.

In the second contribution to this section, Gerald J. Strauss provides useful information for the practitioner regarding pharmacological interventions for depression and anxiety. He states that regardless of whether the practitioner has aspirations to become a prescribing psychologist, it is important for all practicing psychologists to have a basic foundation and understanding of psychopharmacology. Strauss addresses key issues relating to the drug therapeutic window or level, as well as the dose-response relationship. He provides a review of various antidepressant and antianxiety medications based on class, initial dose, dosage range, peak plasma levels, elimination half-life, and potential side effects.

In the third contribution, Jennifer Goldschmied and colleagues outline key issues relating to sleep disorders in psychiatric settings. Their contribution not only addresses the prevalence and severity of common sleep disorders, but also identifies assessment tools and treatment options. They highlight problems with sleeping as a common medical complaint and note significant comorbidity between sleep disorders and common psychiatric illnesses such as depression and anxiety. The authors provide useful information regarding the diagnosis and treatment of sleep disorders including insomnia, obstructive sleep apnea, delayed/advanced sleep phase syndrome, narcolepsy, REM sleep behavior disorder, restless legs, and periodic limb movement disorder.

In the fourth contribution, Jennifer Minkin, Maurice F. Prout, and Frank Masterpasqua identify the integration of technology and psychotherapy as a promising approach for the future. More specifically, the authors highlight biofeedback instrumentation as an approach that can enhance traditional assessment and psychotherapeutic methods. Minkin and colleagues provide historical information about biofeedback as well as an overview of psychophysiology. They provide a cogent section on how the process of biofeedback works. Moreover, they provide a section on biofeedback-assisted therapy, as well as the use of biofeedback as an assessment tool. Information on psychophysiological stress profiling is addressed, as well as the clinical utility of using biofeedback in assessing the effects of cognitions on the body. The use of biofeedback to help reveal unconscious emotions is also addressed. In sum, the authors suggest that the use of biofeedback can be advantageous in the initial phase of diagnostic assessment, in ongoing assessment in order to monitor treatment progress, and in assessing treatment outcomes and efficacy.

In the fifth contribution, Carin M. Lefkowitz and Maurice F. Prout address current issues in anger management treatment. The authors begin the contribution by distinguishing between the concepts of anger, hostility, and aggression, and address the physiological, cognitive, behavioral, and social correlates of anger. Examples of cognitive distortions commonly made by chronically angry individuals are provided. In addressing the assessment of chronic anger, the authors provide examples of commonly used anger assessment tools. In addition, common physical disorders associated with chronic anger, as well as *DSM-IV* disorders correlated with anger mismanagement are addressed. Key ethical issues in working with chronically angry individuals are addressed, as well as anger management treatment considerations based on culture and gender. The authors conclude with treatment options including behavior therapy, cognitive therapy, psychopharmacology, and schema-focused therapy (SFT). In addition, they provide an outline of a nine-session treatment program, which combines empirically supported CBT interventions with key components of SFT.

In the sixth contribution, Mette Traae Brynolf addresses implications for the treatment of Anorexia Nervosa by incorporating the radical social movement of Pro-Ana (Pro-Anorexia). Dr. Traae Brynolf begins by providing the clinician with information about the Pro-Ana movement, which proposes that Anorexia Nervosa is not an illness but a lifestyle choice. She addresses how incorporating knowledge about the Pro-Ana movement can impact psychological treatment in terms of resistance and compliance. She examines resistance through Threat Rigidity theory, and addresses aspects of chaos and control through Chaos theory. In addition, readiness for change and implications for treatment are examined according to the Stages of Change model by Prochaska and DiClemente.

In the seventh contribution, Keith W. Beard addresses potential problems that mental health practitioners may encounter with clients who engage in excessive internet use. Dr. Beard provides a concise history of the internet, and addresses a number of variables which fuel the internet's appeal. He addresses the issue of "Internet Addiction," and defines problematic Internet use as one's use of the Internet that creates psychological, social, school, and/or work difficulties in a person's life. Beard and Wolf (2001) and Young (1998) have adapted *DSM-IV* criteria for pathological gambling in an effort to develop consistent criteria for diagnosing problematic Internet use.

The eighth contribution by Robert B. Denton and Richard W. Sears addresses the clinical use of mindfulness. The authors acknowledge the recent surge in mindfulness-based interventions, and aim to familiarize the clinician with the recent literature as well as mindfulness interventions and practice. They define mindfulness as a conceptual framework, rather than an isolated technique, which brings a greater awareness of thoughts, feelings, and physical sensations into the therapeutic session. The authors provide a useful overview for clinicians with little experience in mindfulness-based interventions. They address the utility of mindfulness in the treatment of depression, anxiety, and stress reduction. The authors also address ways to increase competence in mindfulness, and stress the importance of daily personal practice. The contribution ends with suggestions for practice in the form of several well-articulated meditations. In addition, two clinical case examples are provided.

In the final contribution to this section, Dennis E. O'Grady discusses the utility of communication training in clinical practice. Dr. O'Grady shares his *Talk to Me©* approach which defines two different styles of communicators: Empathizers (E-types) and Instigators (I-types). He illustrates his communication system via a series of easily readable case examples which highlight different viewpoints as a result of communication style. According to Dr. O'Grady, people assume that everyone thinks and communicates in the same way. By learning more about communication issues and practicing communication skills, individuals can increase their ability to be successful in a wide range of interpersonal events.

Psychological Influences and Interventions of Chronic Pain

Nicole Hunka and Alan Gilbertson

Chronic pain is a ubiquitous health care problem. In the United Kingdom, pain has been estimated to affect approximately 46% of the general population (Elliott et al., 1999), and, in America, pain affects more individuals than diabetes, heart disease, and cancer combined (National Institutes of Health, 2007). Relatedly, approximately 80% of all visits to a physician in the United States involve some type of pain concern (Gatchel, 2004; Stucky, Gold, & Zhang, 2001). As pain affects over 50 million Americans, it costs more than $7 billion annually in health care expenses and in lost productivity (Gatchel, 2004). Given these data, Gatchel (2004) noted that it is not surprising that the U.S. Congress designated 2001-2011 as the decade of pain control.

Traditional approaches for pain management have included pharmacological, surgical, and other medical interventions. Pharmacological interventions for chronic pain have included the use of painkillers such as Tylenol, nonsteroidal anti-inflammatory drugs, and opioids, as well as antiepileptic and psychotropic medications. Although pharmacological, surgical, and other medical interventions (i.e., nerve-blocks) can be helpful in managing pain, there are inherent problems with the use of these approaches alone. For instance, medical procedures designed to remove damage or pathology can produce further tissue damage resulting in additional pain, while medications can have side effects such as fatigue and constipation, to name only a few, that can add to a person's overall discomfort (Keefe, Abernethy, & Campbell, 2005). In addition to physical symptoms, chronic pain is associated with various comorbid psychological symptoms (Gatchel, 2004) as well as a number of personal, social, and environmental issues (Winterowd, A. T. Beck, & Gruener, 2003). Therefore, the psychosocial factors often associated with chronic pain will not be addressed by the use of pharmacological or other medical interventions alone (Keefe et al., 2005).

The purpose of this contribution is to provide a general summary of information regarding chronic pain and chronic pain management, with particular emphasis on the psychological factors and associated psychological treatment interventions for this problem. As the intent is to address chronic pain management issues from a broad perspective, interventions for the multitude of specific causes and types of pain are beyond the scope of this contribution. Therefore, in an effort to provide broad-based information, this contribution is divided into five sections that review the pertinent literature regarding chronic pain-related issues. The first section provides clinical descriptions of pain and pain-related mental health disorders. Section two reviews historic and contemporary pain models with an emphasis on the current biopsychosocial model of pain. Section three describes various psychosocial factors associated with chronic pain, while section four reviews psychological theories and how the experience of pain is conceptualized through those theories. The final section discusses the current psychological treatments considered standard in pain management, with particular detail given to cognitive-behavioral treatment interventions.

DEFINITIONS AND CLINICAL DESCRIPTIONS

What is Pain?

There is a distinction between pain and the term nociception. Nociception results from some type of injury or damage that consequently stimulates the nerves that convey information about this injury or damage to the brain (Gatchel, 2004). Therefore, nociception is purely a transmission of information which has no subjective or affective quality to the experience. The definition of pain proposed by the International Association for the Study of Pain states that pain is an unpleasant sensory and emotional experience associated with actual or potential tissue damage, or described in terms of such damage (Merskey & Bogduck, 1994). As implied in this definition, acute nociceptive stimuli are not necessarily needed to induce a perception of pain, as such things as memories have been found to elicit pain experiences (Bouckoms & Hackett, 1997).

Fordyce (1988) distinguished both pain and nociception from suffering. He noted that suffering is an emotional response in the central nervous system triggered by nociception or other aversive events such as fear, threat, or loss, and that suffering often includes an anticipatory component. Both pain and suffering are often observed in pain-related behaviors. Fordyce highlighted that pain-related behaviors, which often result from suffering, are a set of responses that blend past experiences with anticipation of perceived stimuli.

Given the above information, individual experiences of pain can be quite variable. Some individuals do not report intense pain associated with significant tissue damage, whereas others respond with extensive distress and related disability to seemingly minor damage and pain (Eccleston, 2001). This, for instance, has been observed in patient reports of intense pain where no identifiable lesions exist (Eccleston, 2001). The experience of "phantom limb pain" in amputees dramatically demonstrates the potential of perceiving pain in the absence of tissue damage. Conversely, Fordyce (1988) noted that nociception may occur without an experience of pain. He noted that this phenomenon has been illustrated in accounts of soldiers in combat who were unaware that they sustained injury or wounds for perhaps long lengths of time.

As there is variability in pain experiences, there is also variability in the categorizations of pain which have evolved. The categorizations of pain include, but are not limited to, acute, chronic, nociceptive, neuropathic, and psychogenic pain. Acute pain is recognized as a signal of potential injury or damage to muscles, tissues, or nerves; has a rather short duration (Winterowd et al., 2003); and typically resolves as injured or damaged tissue heals (Ashburn & Staats, 1999). Generally, the duration of acute pain does not exceed 3 months (see Lewandowski, 2006). Chronic pain is not just a prolonged version of acute pain (Turk & McCarberg, 2005), but is distinguished from acute pain in several ways. Chronic pain is the result of ongoing activation of pain receptors (Winterowd et al., 2003) that may persist long after tissue damage that initially triggered the onset of pain has resolved (Ashburn & Staats, 1999). Turk and McCarberg (2005) noted that as these pain signals are repeatedly generated, neural pathways undergo physiochemical changes that make them both hypersensitive to the pain signal and resistant to the body's attempts at regulation. The duration of chronic pain is typically defined as lasting longer than 3 months and interfering with daily life activities (see Lewandowski, 2006), including overall quality of life.

Nociceptive pain is defined as signals that are sent to the spinal cord and brain resulting from an injury or pathology, unaccompanied by permanent damage or alteration to the nervous system (Winterowd et al., 2003). This differs from neuropathic pain which results from damage done to the nervous system, including damage to the peripheral nerves, spinal cord, or other central nervous system regions (Gatchel et al., 2007). Each of the forms of pain described differs from psychogenic pain, which is pain defined as purely psychological in nature, with no evidence of associated physical pathology (Winterowd et al., 2003). Although pain experiences often have clear biological etiologies and associated medical diagnoses, chronic pain can also have presumed psychological components described by associated diagnostic categories. Some of these pain-related psychological classifications and disorders are outlined below.

Pain-Related Mental Health Diagnoses

The *Diagnostic and Statistical Manual of Mental Disorders* (*DSM-IV-TR*; American Psychiatric Association, 2000) classifies Pain Disorder under Somatoform Disorders. The essential feature of Pain Disorder, according to the *DSM-IV-TR*, is pain which is the predominant focus of the clinical presentation and of sufficient severity to warrant clinical attention. In addition, the *DSM-IV-TR* requires that the pain symptoms are not intentionally produced or feigned, are not better accounted for by another axis I disorder, and cause significant distress or impairment in functioning (i.e., social, academic, occupational, relational). Pain disorder can be coded under three different subtypes. According to the *DSM-IV-TR*, the subtype of Pain Disorder Associated with Psychological Factors is diagnosed when psychological factors are judged to have a major role in the onset, severity, exacerbation, or maintenance of the pain while general medical conditions play minimal or no role in onset or maintenance. The subtype of Pain Disorder Associated with Both Psychological Factors and a General Medical Condition is diagnosed when both factors are judged to play an important role in the pain experience and course. (In this case, the *DSM-IV-TR* states that the pain diagnosis is coded on axis I, while the associated medical condition is coded on axis III). A diagnosis of Pain Disorder Associated With a General Medical Condition is given when the pain is judged to result from a medical condition with psychological factors playing a limited to no role in the pain experience and course. The *DSM-IV-TR* further states that this diagnosis is not considered a mental disorder and, therefore, is coded only on axis III.

A previous edition of the *DSM* (APA, 1980) included a diagnosis of psychogenic pain which was based on the thought that pain was due to psychological causes only and was therefore not considered "real" as no specific organic causes could be found (Gatchel, 2004). The primary criteria in the *DSM-III* for psychogenic pain included the following: (a) Pain was the predominant disturbance; (b) no organic pathology, or pathophysiological mechanisms were found to account for the symptoms; (c) if organic pathology was found, the pain complaint was in gross excess of what would be expected; and (d) psychological factors were thought to be the etiology of the pain. This diagnosis has been removed from later editions of the *DSM*, as such a conceptualization of pain was thought to hinder the development of effective pain management strategies (Gatchel, 2004). It is noted that in other somatoform diagnoses, pain may be a common component but is not a required symptom (e.g., somatization) or is irrelevant to the diagnosis (e.g., hypochondriasis). Therefore, other somatoform disorders will not be further elaborated upon.

Recent editions of the *DSM* as well as the newer pain models have increasingly acknowledged the significant influence that psychological factors have on an individual's pain experience. Past and current pain models, with emphasis on the more recently accepted biopsychosocial model, are reviewed in the following section.

PAST AND CURRENT PAIN MODELS

A traditional biomedical model has dominated the modern understanding of disease and related pain (Keefe et al., 2005). During the Renaissance, the traditional dualistic view of medicine posited that the mind and body functioned independently (Gatchel, 2004; Gatchel et al., 2007). This model, therefore, did not account for the impact that psychosocial factors have more recently been recognized as having on medical disorders, symptoms, and responses to treatment (Gatchel et al., 2007). Dissatisfaction with traditional biomedical models of pain led to advances in theories during the last half of the twentieth century. One of the first of these advanced theories was the Gate Control Theory of pain proposed by Melzack and Wall (1965). This theory suggested that pain signals go though a gating system that can be opened (i.e., pain sensations being registered) or closed (i.e., pain sensations not registered) by factors associated with tissue damage as well as such factors as emotions, memory, mood, and thoughts (Lewandowski, 2006). The Gate Control theory, therefore, highlighted the potentially significant role that psychosocial factors play in perception of pain and embraced a complex multidimensional view of the pain phenomena (Gatchel, 2004). As a result of the biological and psychological connections based in this theory, the potential contribution of psychological approaches to understanding and managing pain became more recognized.

Understanding that there were various nonbiological influences to disease and pain experiences, Engel (1977) suggested a need for a new medical model and was the first to propose a biopsychosocial model to conceptualize and guide treatment of patients. Waddell (1987) specifically noted that because of the subjective nature of the pain experience, pain could not be comprehensively assessed without an understanding of the biopsychosocial context of the patient. As such, most currently accepted perspectives to understanding and treating chronic pain are grounded in the biopsychosocial model (Gatchel et al., 2007). This model views pain as the result of the interaction of physiological, psychological, and social factors which may contribute to individuals' unique perceptions of pain (Gatchel, 2004). The psychological and social factors associated with the experience and treatment of pain are outlined in more detail in the following section.

PSYCHOSOCIAL FACTORS ASSOCIATED WITH PAIN

Early theories of the psychological influences of pain suggested that there were "pain-prone patients" (e.g., Engel, 1959) and that chronic depression, guilt, and engagement in guilt-provoking situations could be expected in such patients (Adler et al., 1989). Similarly, accounts of childhood abuse and victimization had also been postulated as possible foundations for future presentations of persistent pain symptoms (Grzesiak, 2002). In addition, early theories of pain focused primarily on global factors of the individual including personality, age, and gender, while recent areas of study have developed an understanding of more specific psychological traits and specific affective states relevant to pain patients (Eccleston, 2001). The focus of this section addresses both affective states and psychological comorbidities associated with chronic pain. Particular emphasis is given to depression and anxiety as psychological comorbidities to chronic pain as well as the influence of the pain/stress cycle. Discussion of social factors that impact both mood and pain experiences will be included at the end of the section.

Psychological Factors and Comorbidities

Gatchel and colleagues (2007) stated that pain is ultimately a subjective and private experience that is described in sensory and affective properties. Persistent attempts to react and adapt to pain can result in a range of emotional concerns (Eccleston, 2001), and this affective component tends to incorporate negative emotions including depression, anxiety, and even anger (Eccleston, 2001; Winterowd et al., 2003). Bouckoms and Hackett (1997) noted that in some cases, affective disturbances, including anger, can be masked by denial or soporific medication; therefore, assessing affective disorders in patients with chronic pain can be a difficult task. This may also explain why (with the exception of depression) the associations between pain and affective states such as anger, frustration, and resentment have received less attention in the literature (Adams, Poole, & Richardson, 2006).

Past research has consistently demonstrated that chronic pain is most often associated with depressive and anxiety disorders, somatoform disorders, substance abuse, and personality disorders (Dersh, Polatin, & Gatchel, 2002; see also, McWilliams, Cox, & Enns, 2003). Furthermore, Gatchel (2004) reported that individuals with chronic pain are at an increased risk for not only depression, but also suicide. As it has become increasingly evident that chronic pain is associated with emotional distress and psychopathology (Dersh et al., 2002), if left untreated, these issues can interfere with the rehabilitation of pain conditions and may contribute to increased pain intensity and pain-related dysfunction (see Gatchel, 2006). Given the associations between pain and mood/affect, pain cannot be successfully treated without attending to patients' emotional states (Gatchel et al., 2007).

With regard to pain-related psychological comorbidities, depression has received the greatest amount of attention in the literature. Research has indicated that depressive disorders are found in approximately 40% to 50% of patients suffering from chronic pain, but the nature, including the directionality, of the relationship is controversial (Gatchel et al., 2007). Dersh et al. (2002) concluded that the answer to the question of whether chronic pain or psychopathology occurs first is that no single explanation can be generalized to all individuals; depression has been shown to be an antecedent as well as a consequence and concomitant component of chronic pain. It is not fully understood why some chronic pain patients are depressed and others are not (Keefe, Dunsmore, & Burnett, 1992).

Relative to depression, the relationship between anxiety and chronic pain has received less attention in the literature (McWilliams et al., 2003). Individuals with chronic pain may be anxious about such things as the meaning of their symptoms and their futures, possible symptom progression, whether others will believe they are suffering, and the possibility of being told that they are beyond help (Gatchel et al., 2007). In addition, it has been proposed that the tendency for health-anxious patients to misinterpret pain sensations as an indication of serious disease, or that they may have sustained serious physical damage, is likely to intensify the pain experience similar to what is found in hypochondriasis (Tang et al., 2007). As a result of anxiety and distress, autonomic arousal may be maintained, which may provoke the development of additional physical symptoms (Adams et al., 2006). This can result in an exacerbation cycle.

Noting that pain and emotional distress have a reciprocal effect on each other, Winterowd et al. (2003) described the stress-pain cycle wherein emotionally distressed patients focus on pain and negative events which exacerbate pain experiences. They further noted that this leads to increased negative thoughts resulting in tension and increased pain intensity and emotional distress. Similarly, Eccleston (2001) noted that repeated attention to the threat of pain may cause habitual worry and catastrophizing of a situation which, consequently, results in an increased stress-pain cycle. Fear of pain may also lead to avoidance of potentially healthy activities while promoting other negative pain-related behaviors. *Chronic pain* patients often avoid pain-eliciting situations, believing this avoidance to be analgesic when, in fact, such avoidance often promotes further pain (Eccleston, 2001). As such, avoidance of activities can contribute to additional problems such as fatigue, muscle atrophy, weight gain, and isolation that may actually intensify a person's overall discomfort. Hayes and Duckworth (2006) noted that avoidance is associated with higher pain intensity, more pain-related anxiety and depression, increased physical and psychosocial disability, less daily uptime, and poorer work status.

In addition to avoidance, other negative or self-defeating coping strategies that lead to increased physical and psychological distress have been observed in this population. For instance, due to unrealistic approaches to activity, some chronic pain patients may try to actually do more than their body can manage. Conversely to avoidance of activity, being overly active can not only potentially promote further injury, it can reinforce psychological problems such as denial of the chronic pain condition, perfectionism, and exaggerated independence (i.e., where asking for help may be construed as being a dependent person; Winterowd et al., 2003). This can ultimately result in frustration and intensified psychological and physical distress.

Although psychological factors including mood, affect, and coping styles can influence patients' experiences of pain, it is noteworthy that social issues can also exert influence on psychological factors. Relevant social issues that may impact chronic pain patients' mood, affect, and experience of pain are briefly reviewed below.

Social Factors

Consistent with the biopsychosocial model of pain, analyzing the social context of chronic pain patients can help to better understand overall adjustment (Keefe et al., 1992) and guide treatment. Beyond medical issues, chronic pain patients can experience various occupational, financial, family role, social/relational, and other psychosocial stressors that contribute to their overall experience of physical pain and emotional distress.

With regard to employment, pain patients may find they are unable to perform their job responsibilities, which can result in light-duty work, demotion, disability, job loss, or early retirement (Winterowd et al., 2003). Such employment issues can consequently affect an individual's financial and socioeconomical circumstances, identity (i.e., who am I and how do I contribute?), and overall adaptive functioning. Chronic pain can also dramatically influence an individual's identity and role in the family. This is evidenced in situations where a spouse/parent can no longer perform tasks necessary to fulfilling his or her expected responsibilities for the functioning of the home or family (Winterowd et al., 2003). In addition, patients with chronic pain may refrain from healthy social activities and relationships (e.g., meeting friends, attending church services or community functions) as potential pain-provoking activities may be involved (e.g., sitting uncomfortably in a car or at a table for periods of time, needing to walk, etc.). Relatedly, chronic pain patients may have negative beliefs about how others view them in light of their physical limitations. These beliefs may create emotional discomfort resulting in avoidance of social interaction. Physical limitations and avoidance behaviors associated with chronic pain can therefore, result in social isolation and reduced opportunities for support (Winterowd et al., 2003).

It is clear that the biopsychosocial challenges faced by chronic pain patients can negatively impact quality of life. In an effort to develop interventions to address these components of chronic pain, cognitive, behavioral, and other alternatives to purely medical interventions have been evaluated. Support for the efficacy of various psychological interventions for managing chronic pain are well documented in the literature (Hoffman et al., 2007). Prior to reviewing specific techniques and interventions for the management of chronic pain, background on the major theories from which these interventions emerge will be examined.

PSYCHOLOGICAL THEORIES AND CONCEPTUALIZATIONS OF PAIN

Behavioral Theory

Eysenck (1959, 1964) defined behavior therapy as the attempt to alter human behavior and emotions in a beneficial way according to the laws of modern learning theory. The assumption is that pain-related behaviors occur due to the complex synthesis of nociception, expectancies based on prior learning, and the consequences of these behaviors based on environmental contingencies (Fordyce, 1988) and can be modified through conditioning. With its roots in the various learning theories, behavioral models today utilize a variety of intervention techniques based on behavioral analysis in an attempt to modify behavior.

In the 1970s and 1980s, conceptualization of chronic pain and related treatments based on behavioral models began to emerge (Keefe, Abernethy, & Campbell, 2005). Fordyce (1976) was one of the first to explicitly apply behavioral techniques to treating chronic pain patients. He advocated using behavioral techniques to modify maladaptive pain behaviors (e.g., excessive dependence on bed rest or family members, etc.) by analyzing and changing the patient's social and environmental contingencies (Keefe, Abernethy, & Campbell, 2005). Avoidance and other related pain behaviors (e.g., behavioral responses to both nociception and related anticipated consequences of nociceptions; see Fordyce, 1988) are often targeted in behavioral treatment. Furthermore, behavioral treatment models encourage patients to plan achievable goals, as successes can then become reinforcement for more positive and healthy behaviors (Eccleston, 2001).

The cognitive revolution emerged in the 1970s and claimed that the efficacy of behavior therapy could be improved with the introduction of interventions targeting dysfunctional cognitions (Hayes et al., 2006). Background on cognitive theory and associated pain conceptualization is reviewed below.

Cognitive Theory

A. T. Beck and Weishaar (1989) noted that at its basic level, cognitive theory is based on the conceptualization that an organism needs to process information in an adaptive way in order to survive, and that much of this processing is done automatically or outside of awareness. The fundamental tenets of cognitive therapy include people's core beliefs (about themselves, others, and the world), their interpretation of events, their automatic thoughts, and how these factors influence emotions and behaviors. Judith Beck (1995) theorized that negative core beliefs are associated essentially with themes of helplessness, unlovability, or both. Negative core beliefs are usually global, overgeneralized, and absolute, and when these beliefs are activated, the person tends to easily process information that supports the negative belief but fails to accurately recognize information that is contrary to the negative belief (A. T. Beck, 1997). Thus, an individual's core beliefs and associated automatic thoughts influence his or her interpretation of situations, which consequently affects emotions and behaviors (J. Beck, 1995). The processes of cognitive therapy explore dysfunctional interpretations and distorted meanings attached to individuals' experiences and modifies unrealistic or unreasonable cognitions (A. T. Beck & Weishaar, 1989).

To summarize, the cognitive model hypothesizes that individuals' emotions and behaviors are influenced by their perception of events (J. Beck, 1995) and that dysfunctional thinking accounts for related affective and behavioral disturbances (A. T. Beck, 1997). These concepts will be further discussed in relation to the assessment and treatment of chronic pain patients.

Cognitive Conceptualization of Pain

Unrealistic cognitions about pain and related life events have a significant, negative influence on pain perceptions (Winterowd et al., 2003). In addition, chronic pain patients often come into treatment with erroneous and distorted beliefs about the cause and future course of their pain (Keefe et al., 1992). Therefore, it is concluded that when individuals think negatively about their pain and related situation, they are more likely to engage in self-defeating behaviors which can influence both pain and emotional discomfort (Winterowd et al., 2003).

In the chronic pain population, the fundamental tenets of cognitive theory (i.e., dysfunctional thinking in regard to core beliefs, automatic thoughts, and interpretation of events) are significant for global themes. These themes are primarily related to how pain has affected their lives (i.e., "I have no life because of my pain"), how they regard themselves and their relationships (i.e., "I am useless and not liked"), and how the pain will negatively affect their future (i.e., I will be pain-ridden forever"; see, e.g., Winterowd et al., 2003). Lewandowski (2006) described common thought patterns of many individuals with chronic pain that include self-blame, fear of reinjury, and catastrophizing, to name a few. These beliefs can trigger, intensify, or maintain pain while also contributing to emotional upset. As cognitions influence mood as well as pain perceptions and resulting behaviors, effort to challenge and modify maladaptive thoughts is one way of intervening in the experience of pain and the pain-stress cycle.

Separately, behavioral and cognitive conceptualizations of chronic pain guide treatment approaches to the management of chronic pain conditions. When working in tandem, these theories produce cognitive-behavioral therapy (CBT), which offers a more holistic and sophisticated approach to the treatment of chronic pain patients. CBT as an effective psychological intervention for the treatment of chronic pain is well recognized within the literature.

Cognitive-Behavioral Theory

Over the years, cognitive and behavioral therapy approaches have borrowed from each other, consequently blurring the distinction between them (Hollon & A. T. Beck, 1994). As these approaches combine cognitive and behavioral elements, both legitimately belong to the larger family of cognitive-behavioral interventions (Hollon & A. T. Beck, 1994). It is noted that CBT interventions for chronic pain have strong empirical support (Winterowd et al., 2003) and are widely used by programs within a group format, as well as by private practitioners in an individual setting, for the treatment of chronic pain patients.

The next section will review cognitive-behavioral intervention strategies commonly used in treating chronic pain. Following this review, emerging theories and interventions for chronic pain with foundations still rooted in CBT will be briefly addressed.

PSYCHOLOGICAL TREATMENT INTERVENTIONS

As noted earlier in this contribution, traditional medical approaches for chronic pain management can be helpful in abating, to some degree, the severity and duration of pain. However, these approaches alone do not address the associated psychosocial issues that often contribute to a patient's experience of chronic pain. The following section outlines specific psychological interventions to chronic pain management addressed by various authors (e.g., see J. Beck, 1995; Lewandowski, 2006; Winterowd et al., 2003) that have been guided by the cognitive, behavioral, and CBT theories previously described. Although the interventions reviewed are not an exhaustive list, the more common psychological approaches to the management of chronic pain conditions are summarized. More detailed instruction on the application of the summarized interventions can be found in the above-mentioned resources as well as in other treatment manuals (e.g., see also Turk, Meichenbaum, & Genest, 1983).

Behavioral Interventions

Winterowd et al. (2003) suggested that, during the early stages of intervention, chronic pain patients learn specific behavioral strategies to cope with their discomfort. Some of these strategies include pain monitoring, activity scheduling, relaxation training, and distraction techniques. The rationale for the use of such interventions with chronic pain patients and a basic introduction to the application of these interventions are addressed below.

Pain Monitoring/Charting

A variety of circumstances unique to each patient can trigger or exacerbate pain levels. Examples of these include strenuous exercise, drinking caffeine, bending, humidity, disrupted sleep, and stress (Winterowd et al., 2003). The purpose of pain monitoring is to help chronic pain patients identify both triggers to and patterns of pain in an effort to draw conclusions regarding what behaviors, emotions, and automatic thoughts can be modified to reduce discomfort (J. Beck, 1995). In his chronic pain workbook, Lewandowski noted that pain levels are never constant, and charting/monitoring what influences pain in any way will not only make an individual's pain more predictable, but may also give the individual some sense of control. Information gleaned from these charts can be used to break self-defeating pain cycles (see Lewandowski, 2006) and can also be used to guide symptom-focused interventions that may be targeted at a wide range of pain-exacerbating triggers. Daily pain monitoring charts can be found in various self-help workbooks, the Internet, or other references (e.g., see Lewandowski, 2006; Winterowd et al., 2003), but patients can also construct their own charts. We have included a sample Pain Monitoring Chart on page 21.

On the forms/charts used, particular information to be recorded includes times of day the pain occurred, where the pain was located on the body, and a general ranking of pain intensity. Patients are to make note of any triggers associated with the onset of pain or with an increase in pain (such as enduring a particular activity or stressor). Finally, patients are encouraged to identify ways that they positively or negatively coped with the pain (i.e., use of medications, ice/heat compresses, smoking, avoiding social contact, talking on the phone, stretching, etc.) as well as identifying any emotions that were associated with the pain. At the end of the week, individuals can review their pain chart and determine their baseline level of pain and pain exacerbations, as well as common factors and emotions associated with both the increase or relief of pain. Continued monitoring is encouraged as patients try to implement different coping strategies and track the effects of these strategies on their perceptions of pain.

Activity Monitoring and Scheduling

Activity monitoring specific to chronic pain patients is used to promote an increased awareness of activity level and choices of activities, and prepares patients for scheduling more meaningful and realistic activities that increase the sense of accomplishment and enjoyment in such endeavors (Winterowd et al., 2003). An increased sense of accomplishment and enjoyment with activity would presumably contribute to an improved quality of life, perhaps especially to patients who may have experienced significantly limited activity and avoidance of activity since the onset of their injury or condition.

An activity chart is simply a chart with the days of the week across the top and each hour of the day down the left-hand side (J. Beck, 1995). On this chart, patients are asked to record the activities they participated in throughout the day, over the course of several weeks (or months). Activities would include anything the patient participated in, including sleeping, eating, exercise, washing clothes, watching television, talking on the phone, driving, going to the mall, and so on. Patients are to indicate the level of enjoyment and accomplishment they experienced for each task. Pain monitoring can be combined with activity monitoring to help patients observe any influences or reciprocal relationships among their activities, additional triggers, emotions, and pain (Winterowd et al. 2003).We have included a sample Activity Monitoring Chart on page 22.

Activity, in the form of exercise, will be further addressed in the following section pertaining to goal setting. Before proceeding to activity goal setting, it is appropriate to repeat that limited activity/exercise has been associated with increased physical discomfort, and that physical discomfort has been associated with disrupted sleep. Both limited activity/exercise and disrupted sleep have also been associated with negative mood and affect. Therefore, monitoring exercise and sleep as part of the patient's general activity chart, or as part of a separate chart, can prove to be a beneficial task (e.g., see Lewandowski, 2006). As with any other monitoring task, patients can begin to observe self-defeating behaviors in regard to exercise and sleep that may exacerbate their pain and/or emotional discomfort. Once such awareness is achieved, patients can choose to modify their self-defeating patterns or behaviors. For instance, after charting exercise and sleep for 1 month, a patient may observe that limited activity (i.e., excessive television watching and sleeping) may be associated with the experience of generalized body aches and more disrupted sleep cycles, or that napping throughout the day is associated with poor sleep during the night. Once patients are aware of such patterns, they may then choose to generate an activity or goal schedule for more healthy activity/exercise behaviors. Many concepts associated with activity monitoring are similar to goal-setting and goal-pacing tasks which are elaborated in the following section.

Goal Setting and Pacing

As noted previously, in an effort to decrease discomfort, chronic pain patients may avoid various activities. Avoidance of activity, however, can lead to increased distress that may come in such forms as boredom, social withdrawal, depression, muscle atrophy, and loss of flexibility. In turn, each of these can potentially lead to increased maladaptive pain behaviors, physical and/or emotional discomfort, and an associated decrease in quality of life. Conversely, some patients may want to maintain the same activity level they had prior to their chronic pain condition despite their physical ability to do so. If they unrealistically push their bodies to do too much, they may put themselves at risk for additional injury or pain (Winterowd et al., 2003). Added injury and pain may not only further physically limit chronic pain patients, it could also discourage them from future engagement in healthy behaviors and exercise while promoting self-defeating behaviors such as avoidance and dependency. Therefore, setting realistic activity goals that include proper pacing is critical when attempting to manage chronic pain.

Lewandowski (2006) noted that strong, achievable goals are personally meaningful, realistic, flexible, positive, and in written form. Goals that meet these criteria, and that are both specific and measurable, are likely to be more achievable. Patients are encouraged to write down a list of what they want to achieve and, from that list, to pick one or two of those goals to begin addressing. With these factors in mind, consider an individual experiencing chronic back pain who had once enjoyed mountain bike riding on hilly and rough terrain. If this person wants to become more active, he or she would not benefit from a goal of "I will go mountain bike riding like I used to," as this goal is quite broad and likely unrealistic. The individual would be encouraged to first establish a general goal, and then document specific and realistic ways to achieve that goal. Attention to pacing and planned rest time following the activity would also be documented. Therefore, the start of an individual's goal list may begin looking like the following:

General goal: Increase my current activity level (to 3 days per week).

1. I will ride my bike on the road or other flat surface 3 days per week.
2. I will ride my bike for 10 minutes at a time on those days.

3. If I do not ride my bike on a day planned for activity, I will walk for 10 minutes.
4. I will monitor my activity over the course of the week and, if I find this activity to be tolerable (i.e., between 0 and 5 on the pain scale), I will increase by 3 to 5 minutes the following week.
5. If my pain level is above where it started before the activity (i.e., 6 to 8 on the pain scale), I will rest (lie down) for 20 minutes following this activity.
6. I will document these and other details in my daily activity and pain chart.

It is noted that goals do not have to be exclusively exercise related. Patients are encouraged to think of any goals that are meaningful to them (i.e., goals that provide a sense of accomplishment and/or enjoyment) and that may improve their overall quality of life. For instance, goals may include such activities as attending church services once per week, meeting a friend for lunch one to two times per month, making the bed daily, and so on.

Relaxation Training: Overview

The general purpose of relaxation training is to reduce anxiety, worry, and stress which often lead to muscle tension and additional physical and emotional distress. Various relaxation techniques exist, each of which is primarily aimed at redirecting an individual's focus in order to better gain a sense of control of both the body and thoughts. As previously discussed with regard to the pain-stress cycle, chronic pain patients often experience mood-related symptoms which can exacerbate their overall experience of pain. Some physical symptoms of stress and anxiety include shallow breathing and increased muscle tension, both of which can contribute to increased sensations of pain and discomfort. Specific to chronic pain patients, the purpose of relaxation training is to promote a sense of physical and emotional calmness by alleviating the tension held in the body that likely contributes to persistent pain experiences. Effective use of these techniques also promotes a sense of control and self-efficacy, which is frequently lacking in these patients. Various types of relaxation techniques are presented below.

Relaxation Training: Breathing

Breathing is the foundation of most relaxation interventions and is used for calming, focusing, and gaining a sense of control. Patients are asked to close their eyes and take notice of where their breathing occurs (i.e., through the chest or abdominal muscles). Patients are encouraged to direct their inhalations and exhalations through abdominal breathing and to keep their attention focused only on the sensation of their breathing, deflecting all other thoughts or concerns. After they have comfortably incorporated belly breathing, patients then begin to focus on the rate of their breathing with the goal of incorporating long, slow, comfortable inhalations and exhalations. Slow but comfortable breathing promotes decreased heart rate as well decreased sensations of pain, resulting in a more relaxed physical state.

Relaxation Training: Progressive Muscle Relaxation

As muscular tension can intensify pain, the progressive muscle relaxation technique is used to promote patients' awareness of the marked difference between relaxed and tensed physical states, and to teach them ways to more readily achieve a sense of relaxation. Various scripts for this task can be found on the Internet or in various workbooks and self-help guides. The process of progressive muscle relaxation typically begins with abdominal breathing that is slow and comfortable in nature. The process then includes tensing and relaxing different muscle groups (typically starting with muscles at either the very top or the very bottom of the body). Particular attention is given to the sensation of the relaxed state that follows the release of muscle tension. As this activity is not intended to induce pain, pain patients may decide which muscle groups to include or exclude, based on the location of their pain or injury (Winterowd et al., 2003). When the entire activity is completed, patients are asked to focus on the relaxed nature of their entire body and to address, with additional tension and release, any areas of their body that remain tense.

As progressive muscle relaxation is used to promote patients' awareness of physical tension and relaxation as well as their ability to readily achieve relaxed states, biofeedback provides an additional approach to achieving these goals. Biofeedback is a prominent behavioral approach to pain management in which patients learn voluntary control over their bodily reactions through the feedback of physiological processes (Nestoriuc & Martin, 2007). By monitoring physiological responses of the body (i.e., blood pressure, respirations, signaling of muscle fibers, etc.), patients can begin to learn to intervene in these responses though the implementation of different techniques (i.e., deep breathing) in an effort to abate tension and associated pain.

Relaxation Training: Guided Imagery

Chronic pain patients can experience a great deal of temporary relief by focusing on relaxing images in their mind and using these images to create a "safe haven" from their discomfort (Winterowd et al., 2003). Guided imagery, which may be facilitated through the use of audiotapes/CDs or with an individual trained in this method, typically begins with a relaxation exercise such as deep breathing to help focus attention and relieve tension (Morone & Greco, 2007). Patients are then asked to identify an image, place, or scene that represents a sense of calm and peace and to attend to all of the five senses associated with that image. For instance, patients are asked to fully attend to what sounds are heard in their image, what smells are noticed, what colors and other visuals are observed, and what the image feels like to the sense of touch (i.e., feeling the warmth from the sun, brisk breeze, etc.). As patients move through this scene deflecting all other thoughts or concerns, they are asked to reflect on the sense of relaxation and calm they are experiencing.

Hypnosis

In recent years, more controlled trials of hypnosis for chronic pain have emerged suggesting that hypnotic analgesia is consistently superior to no treatment, but equivalent to relaxation and autogenic training (e.g., Schultz & Luthe, 1959) for chronic pain conditions (Patterson & Jensen, 2003). Hypnosis is typically used to help patients achieve deeper levels of relaxation, which often leads to more peaceful sleep, increased energy, and a decreased experience of pain (Loitman, 2000). Hypnosis begins with similar relaxation techniques as outlined previously (i.e., deep breathing, muscle relaxation, etc.). Once the patient achieves a deeply relaxed state, the hypnotherapist suggests changes in behaviors, thoughts, and feelings with the underlying premise being that the patient will accept suggestions that are relevant to his or her needs and will later be able to reinforce this experience independently (Loitman, 2000).

Distraction Techniques

Distraction is a coping strategy used to help patients cope with pain by turning their attention away from their distressing bodily sensations (Winterowd et al., 2003). Although pushing thoughts out of one's mind is typically not the most therapeutic solution for long-term pain management, it is suggested that this method be used at times when cognitive restructuring is impractical or ineffective (J. Beck, 1995). Distraction can include a multitude of techniques, including interventions already described such as the various relaxation techniques. Typically, patients are asked to think about activities that have successfully distracted them from their pain in the past (i.e., listening to music, reading, playing with a pet, yoga, deep breathing exercises, imagery, talking on the phone, etc.). They are encouraged to employ these activities when necessary and to also create a list of additional activities and techniques they could engage in if needed in the future. Winterowd and colleagues (2003) noted that these and perhaps artistic types of activities (i.e., painting, various forms of media, etc.) can help patients focus on something other than themselves while promoting a sense of creativity and resourcefulness.

Positive Reinforcement for Well Behaviors

Chronic pain patients are rarely reinforced for well behaviors (Eccleston, 2001). In fact, pain patients may inadvertently receive reinforcement from their family and loved ones for self-defeating behaviors. Most family members of chronic pain patients are used to responding primarily to their loved one's needs, and lack of reinforcement for healthy behaviors may actually work to extinguish or at least diminish healthy behaviors (Eccleston, 2001). Therefore, behavioral therapists have long advocated involving spouses and family members in the treatment of chronic pain patients in an effort to teach them ways to reinforce adaptive "well" behaviors while minimizing attention to self-defeating pain behavior (Keefe et al., 1992). Family members and loved ones are encouraged to refrain from performing tasks or duties that the pain patient could in fact do on his or her own without significant risk. Family members are also encouraged to support their loved one in regard to pursuing activities that promote physical and emotional health (i.e., realistic levels of exercise and social activities, etc.) while giving minimal acknowledgment to self-defeating pain behaviors (i.e., dependency, physical expressions of discomfort that are not emergent in nature).

Cognitive Interventions

Some common cognitive strategies for pain management include education regarding both the patient's condition and associated treatment interventions, learning to identify and modify automatic thoughts and distorted beliefs, and problem solving. Each of these strategies is briefly summarized below.

Education and Empowerment

Often, the first stage of a cognitive-behavioral approach to treating chronic pain is to provide a credible rationale for the treatment (Eccleston, 2001). Helping the patient to understand that chronic pain treatment is primarily about managing symptoms rather than curing the problem promotes honest communication and realistic expectations between the patient, family, and care providers. Encouraging patients to ask questions and seek out additional information regarding their condition and treatment, as well as encouraging them to employ positive interventions and ways of coping, is a therapeutic intervention in and of itself. By seeking out information, learning to effectively communicate their concerns with their providers, and setting realistic goals, chronic pain patients can obtain some sense of control and accomplishment in their activities and lives, which can ultimately improve quality of life.

Automatic Thought Record

Individuals evaluate situations and events throughout the day. Many times they are not aware of their immediate thoughts about a situation or what may have triggered such thoughts. In regard to chronic pain patients, a variety of events or experiences such as elevations in pain, lack of a clear diagnosis, and/or financial and relationship strains can trigger negative automatic thoughts and self-talk (Winterowd et al., 2003). The use of an automatic thought record as described by Winterowd et al. can be quite helpful in teaching patients to first identify, and then evaluate and modify, their negative thoughts that are likely contributing to their emotional and physical distress.

Effective use of an automatic thought record includes first documenting the situation that occurred, followed by patients' experienced pain intensity, their associated emotions, and then the thoughts they had at that time. Winterowd and colleagues recommended documenting the information in this order, as most patients can identify pain and emotional states more readily than automatic thoughts; as a result, patients can become better primed to identify their negative self-talk. Additional examples of more generalized thought evaluation forms can be found in J. Beck (1995) and Lewandowski (2006). A sample Automatic Though Record is included on page 23.

Evaluating Cognitive Distortions

Once patients have learned to identify their automatic thoughts about pain and other distressing situations, they can then evaluate these thoughts to determine their validity and accuracy (Winterowd et al., 2003). As applied to chronic pain patients, thoughts regarding themselves and their condition are often distorted or negative in nature. These thoughts can lead to added psychological distress and maladaptive pain behaviors, resulting in increased pain intensity. Some typical distortions or errors in thinking (as outlined in A. T. Beck, 1997) include all-or-nothing thinking (i.e., see things as only "black or white"), catastrophizing (i.e., negatively predict future outcomes without considering other potential outcomes), magnification/ minimization (the tendency to magnify the negative and minimize the positive in situations), and "should" statements (i.e., unrealistic demands or expectations on self and others). An example of a patient engaging in a cognitive distortion such as all-or-nothing thinking would be: "I can't continue my construction job and I won't be able support my family." In this case, the patient's cognitive rigidity is interfering in his ability to notice any "gray area" in the situation (i.e., he does not consider how he can use his skills in construction to perhaps be a foreman or supervisor whose job may be less physically labor intensive, and/or does not consider other work options that may not be physically demanding).

The above cognitive distortion likely results in feelings of anger, guilt, anxiety, or depression. These negative feelings can then result in related maladaptive behaviors such as isolation, increased sleep, and limited exploration for other work options. In turn, these maladaptive behaviors are likely followed by negative consequences such as increased physical pain, weight gain, financial problems, and so on. Identifying and modifying the distorted thoughts that perpetuate the ongoing cycle of negative feelings, behaviors, and consequences is critical in alleviating some of this emotional and physical distress.

One way of beginning to identify distorted or negative thoughts is by giving patients a list of the common cognitive distortions and asking them to provide examples of when they recently made such an error in thinking. Keeping a written or typed record of their specific distortions and associated label (i.e., all-or-nothing thinking, magnification, etc.) is helpful in continuing to raise patients' awareness of how their thoughts are affecting their mood and pain experiences. It can also then prompt them to challenge those maladaptive thoughts and distortions.

Advantage/Disadvantage Lists

If individuals have held particular pain-related beliefs for a significant period of time, they may find difficulty in letting go of those thoughts. Therefore, it may be useful for patients to evaluate the advantages and disadvantages of continuing to hold onto their old beliefs (J. Beck, 1995).

Winterowd and colleagues (2003) noted that creating an advantage/disadvantage list of continuing to believe or ruminate on those thoughts may help patients realize the costs and benefits of thinking negatively while also helping them to evaluate their reasons for, or resistance to, changing these thoughts. Patients can evaluate this list with their therapist or physician and keep it as a reference for themselves as they work to modify such thoughts.

Problem Solving

At times, chronic pain patients' negative automatic thoughts may actually be an accurate representation of their circumstances (i.e., "My pain is going to be long term in nature, and I many no longer be able to do my current type of work"; Winterowd et al., 2003). In such cases, patients may benefit from instruction in problem solving where they learn to cope by specifying the problems, formulating a list of possible solutions, implementing those solutions, and then evaluating their effectiveness (J. Beck, 1995). Consistent with cognitive approaches, patients would be encouraged to monitor their thoughts and feelings and how those cognitions influence their efforts at the problem-solving task.

Summary of CBT Interventions

The above CBT interventions are commonly used in the treatment of chronic pain patients. It is noted that these interventions are often conducted in group settings but can also be developed within individual therapy or office sessions. Although CBT has demonstrated strong empirical support in regard to treatment of chronic pain patients, there has also been some emerging support for contextual theories and interventions for chronic pain patients that have CBT foundations. A brief review of one of these expanded CBT theories known as Acceptance and Commitment Therapy, and its relation to traditional CBT approaches to chronic pain management, is presented below.

Expanded CBT interventions

Recently, there has been rising popularity of novel behavioral approaches to therapy that deemphasize traditional cognitive interventions and instead promote behavior change through the fostering of mindfulness and acceptance of internal events (Gaudiano, 2006). These approaches have been classified as contextual forms of CBT for chronic pain (CCBT: Vowles et al., 2007). Known also as "third-wave" interventions, they focus on contextual and experimental change strategies (Hayes, 2004) through increasing psychological flexibility (McCracken & Vowles, 2007). A brief description of one third-wave therapy known as Acceptance and Commitment Therapy (ACT; Hayes, Strosahl, & Wilson, 1999) will be briefly reviewed and compared to the more traditional CBT approach.

Unlike earlier CBT approaches, ACT guides the individual to accept and mindfully defuse pain-related thoughts (Hayes & Duckworth, 2006). Hayes and colleagues (2006) outlined six core processes targeted by ACT. Those core processes include acceptance, cognitive defusion, being present, self as context, values, and committed action. Hayes and colleagues (2006) described acceptance, a key component in this model, as the alternative to avoidance involving an active embrace of events without unnecessary attempts to change their frequency or form.

In regard to pain, the goals of the contextual forms of CBT and the traditional CBT approaches are parallel in that each seeks to decrease the influence of "maladaptive thoughts" and sensations (Vowles et al., 2007). Vowles and colleagues noted that the difference between these approaches is that CBT places more emphasis on perceptions of control regarding the impact of pain, while ACT emphasizes acceptance of the uncomfortable thoughts, feelings, and sensations which reduces influences of these experiences on actions. Although there is promise in such newer theories in regard to treating chronic pain patients, ongoing research is needed to further establish their efficacy.

CONCLUSION

It is clear that the experience of chronic pain can be reciprocally influenced by a multitude of factors, including, but not limited to, social, psychological, and biological issues. Therefore, treating chronic pain conditions from a purely medical perspective is both an oversimplification of the problem and a disservice to the patient. In addition, as established theories suggest that individuals' pain-related beliefs and thoughts are influenced by their idiosyncratic perspectives of events and the world, and as maladaptive pain behaviors and cognitions are learned responses, cognitive-behavioral approaches to the psychological treatment of chronic pain conditions appear to be the most theoretically and empirically supported strategies. Consequently, addressing the biopsychosocial issues related to chronic pain with empirically validated CBT treatments, while also maintaining an openness to other potentially effective treatments, can have a positive impact on patients' management and experience of chronic pain, as well as on overall quality of life.

Sample
Pain Monitoring Chart*

Date	Location	Rate Pain 0-10	General Acties. Triggers to Pain?	Medical/Emotional Coping?	Related Thoughts and Feelings?
Sunday 8/4 8 - 9am	Lower back	4	Slept on couch.	Nothing.	"Don't sleep on couch!"
Sunday 8/4 2 - 4pm	Low back, right buttock	6	Helped mom move furniture. Lots of bending and lifting.	Ice and Aspirine. Helped.	Feel frustrated. Irritable.
Monday 8/5	N/A	1	Went to work. Took 30-minute walk after dinner.	Kept active.	Felt good to walk.
Tuesday 8/6 6 - 9pm	Low back, right buttock	5	Gardening. Lots of bending in garden.	Nothing. Watched TV. Not helpful.	"Too much bending." Feel mad at self.
Wednesday 8/7 6 - 12pm	Low back and right leg	6 to 7	Went to gym. Lifted three sets of heavier weights.	Ice and Tylenol.	Sick of taking it easy and over-did it. Frustrated with self.
Thursday 8/8	N/A	1	Went to work. Took 30-minute walk after dinner.	Kept active.	Beautiful day for a walk.
Friday 8/9 All day	Low back	3	Went to work. Very busy.	Nothing.	Very stressful day at work.
Saturday 8/10 8 - 10am	Lower back	3 to 4	Slept on couch.	Aspirine. Helped.	"When will I learn?"
Satuday 8/10 3 - 4pm	Lower back and right leg	4	Sat in car for over 1 hour on a trip.	Stretches. Not very helpful.	Irritable. Short tempered.

My observations for this week:

Sleeping on the couch and bending made pain worse, as did stress. This had a negative effect on my mood also. Positive coping seemed to include proper exercise that was not too strenuous (such as walking).

---

*From *Cognitive Therapy With Chronic Pain Patients*, by C. Winterowd, A. T. Beck, & D. Gruener, 2003, New York: Springer Publishing Company. Copyright © 2003 by Springer Publishing Company. Adapted/modified with permission.

Sample Activity Monitoring Chart*

Time	Monday 6/16		Tuesday 6/17		Wednesday 6/18		Thursday 6/19	
6:00 am	Sleeping	P0 E2	Sleeping	P0 E2	Sleeping	P0 E3	Sleeping	P0 E2
7:00 am	Wake up. Breakfast.	P1 E1	Wake up. Breakfast.	P1 E1		P0 E3	Wake up. Breakfast.	P0 E1
8:00 am	Shower. Drive.	P1 E1	Shower. Drive.	P1 E1		P0 E3		
9:00 am	Work (desk/ sitting)	P2 E2	Work (desk/ sitting)	P2 E2	Up. Off work. Breakfast.	P1 E1		
10:00 am		P2 E2		P2 E2	TV (laying)	P1 E0		
11:00 am		P2 E2	.	P3 E1	Shower. Mall trip.	P2 E2		
12:00 noon	Lunch. Sat and ate.	P1 E2	Lunch. Sat and ate.	P2 E2	Mall trip	P2 E3		
1:00 pm	Work (Gave talk. Stood.)	P2 E2	Work (desk/ sitting)	P2 E2	Lunch	P1 E2		
2:00 pm	Work (desk/ sitting)	P3 E1		P2 E1	Dr. appt.	P1 E0		
3:00 pm		P3 E1		P2 E1	Dr. appt.	P1 E0		
4:00 pm		P3 E1		P2 E1	Home. TV.	P1 E0		
5:00 pm	Drive home	P2 E1	Drive home	P2 E1	Gardening	P1 E3		
6:00 pm	Short walk	P2 E3	Softball game. Outfield.	P2 E3	Yard work	P2 E3		
7:00 pm	Dinner	P2 E2		P2 E3	Dinner	P1 E2		
8:00 pm	TV (laying)	P2 E1	Dinner	P3 E2	TV	P1 E1		
9:00 pm		P1 E0	TV (laying)	P2 E2		P1 E0		
10:00 pm	Bed/sleep	P1 E3		P2 E1		P1 E0		
11:00 pm				P1 E0		P1 E0		
12:00 am			Bed/sleep	P1 E2	Bed/sleep	P0 E2		

Key: P = pain level. E = enjoyment level.
0 = none 1 = mild 2 = moderate 3 = significant

Note: Activity monitoring charts generally contain 7 days of the week, but for demonstration purposes, this sample chart only contains 4 days.

*From *Cognitive Therapy: Basics and Beyond* by J. Beck, 1995, New York: Guilford Publications. Copyright © 1995 by Guilford Publications. Adapted/modified with permission.

Sample Automatic Thought Record*

STEP 1: Identify negative thought pattern.

An event or trigger	Automatic thoughts	Feeling based on these thoughts	Negative pain behavior	Result
Increased pain when riding bike all day.	I'll never be able to do fun things again. I'll need another surgery!	Depressed. Angry.	Significantly reduce all activities. Isolate and get others to do things I can.	Limited activity. Muscle atrophy. Bad mood.

STEP 2: Realistically challenge those thoughts.

Are those thoughts 100% true? If so, why?	If not 100% true, what are some alternative thoughts that are realistic?	Feeling based on these thoughts	Positive or negative behavior and result
Well, I can't say 100% true.	I can still ride a bike, but just not for extended amounts.	A little frustrated but not as bad as before.	+ Ice pack and feel better in a day or 2. Better mood too.
My back has hurt after other activities, then I felt better later.	I had no real injury, just a long day of biking. I'll need to rest and ice for a day. The pain does decrease.		+ Rest a bit and get back to activities, but modified.

STEP 3: Realistically ask
"What is the worst that could happen if the original automatic thoughts were true?"
Could I live with it?

The worst would be another surgery and time off to recover. I wouldn't like it, but I've been through it before and was okay. Yes, I could live with it.

STEP 4: Realistically ask
"What is the best that could happen if the original automatic thoughts were true?"

I'd rather not see surgery happen, but the purpose of surgery is to fix things or get relief. So, I guess the "best" outcome would be some relief, which is good.

STEP 5: Realistically ask
"What is the most realistic outcome here?"

Well, like I said in Step 2, I've experienced this before after a lot of activity and it has gotten better. Realistically, if I rest and ice my back for a day or 2 and be careful to ride my bike for an hour at a time rather than 3, I think I'll be fine.

STEP 6: Realistically ask
"What are the advantages and disadvantages of believing the original automatic thought?"

Advantages	Disadvantages
I may seek out medical attention . . . is that good if I really don't need it?	I'll be in a horrible mood. I may alienate myself from family and friends. Because I'm scared to injure myself more, I'll miss out on many opportunities.

*From the "Thought Evaluation Form" as it appeared in the worksheet packet from J. Beck, 1996, Bala Cynwyd, PA: Beck Institute for Cognitive Therapy and Research. Copyright © 1996 by Beck Institute for Cognitive Therapy and Research. Adapted/modified with permission. Ideas for this sample automatic thought record were also generated from J. Beck, *Cognitive Therapy: Basics and Beyond,* Guilford Publications, Inc., 1995; and C. Winterowd, A. T. Beck, & D. Gruener, *Cognitive Therapy With Chronic Pain Patients,* Springer, 2003. Adapted/modified with permissions from Guilford Publications and Springer Publishing.

CONTRIBUTORS

Nicole Hunka, MA, completed her doctoral course work in Counseling Psychology at the University of Akron. She is currently completing her doctoral dissertation and is working as a health psychology fellow at Akron General Medical Center in Akron, Ohio. Areas of research and clinical interests include health psychology broadly, with particular interest in bariatric surgery and end-of-life issues. Ms. Hunka can be reached at 400 Wabash Avenue, Akron, OH 44307. E-mail: nhunka@agmc.org

Alan Gilbertson, PhD, is currently the Chief of Psychology at Akron General Medical Center in Akron, Ohio and a Professor of Psychology in Psychiatry at the Northeastern Ohio Universities College of Medicine and Pharmacy. He received his doctorate from The Ohio State University. His research and clinical interests include health psychology and psychological assessment pertaining to clinical problems. Dr. Gilbertson may be contacted at 400 Wabash Avenue, Akron, OH 44307. E-mail: agilbertson@agmc.org

RESOURCES

Adams, N., Poole, H., & Richardson, C. (2006). Psychological approaches to chronic pain management: Part 1. *Issues in Clinical Nursing, 15,* 290-300.

Adler, R. H., Zlot, S., Hurny, D., & Minder, C. (1989). Engel's "psychogenic pain and the pain-prone patient:" A retrospective, controlled clinical study. *Psychosomatic Medicine, 51,* 87-101.

American Psychiatric Association. (1980). *Diagnostic and Statistical Manual of Mental Disorders* (*DSM-III*; 3rd ed.). Washington, DC: Author.

American Psychiatric Association. (2000). *Diagnostic and Statistical Manual of Mental Disorders* (*DSM-IV-TR*; 4th ed. text rev.). Washington, DC: Author.

Ashburn, M., & Staats, P. S. (1999). Management of chronic pain. *The Lancet, 353,* 1865-1869.

Beck, A. T. (1997). The past and future of cognitive therapy. *The Journal of Psychotherapy Practice and Research, 6,* 276-284.

Beck, A. T., & Weishaar, M. (1989). Cognitive therapy. In A. Freeman, K. M. Simon, L. E. Beutler, & H. Arkowitz (Eds.), *Comprehensive Handbook of Cognitive Therapy* (pp. 21-36). New York: Plenum Press.

Beck, J. (1995). *Cognitive Therapy: Basics and Beyond.* New York: Guilford.

Beck, J. (1996). Worksheet packet. Bala Cynwyd, PA: Beck Institute for Cognitive Therapy and Research.

Bouckoms, A. J., & Hackett, T. P. (1997). The pain patient: Evaluation and treatment. In N. Cassem (Ed.), *Massachusetts General Hospital Handbook of General Hospital Psychiatry* (4th ed., pp. 367-413). St. Louis, MO: Mosby-Yearbook.

Dersh, J., Polatin, P. B., & Gatchel. R. J. (2002). Chronic pain and psychopathology: Research findings and theoretical considerations. *Psychosomatic Medicine, 64,* 773-786.

Dixon, K., Keefe, F., Scipio, C., Perri, L. C., & Abernethy, A. (2007). Psychological interventions for arthritis pain management in adults: A meta-analysis. *Health Psychology, 26,* 241-250.

Eccleston, C. (2001). Role of psychology in pain management. *British Journal of Anesthesia, 87,* 144-152.

Elliott, A. S., Smith, B. H., Penny, K. I., Smith, W. C., & Chambers, W. A. (1999). The epidemiology of chronic pain in the community. *Lancet, 354,* 1248-1252.

Engel, G. L. (1959). Psychogenic pain and the pain-prone patient. *American Journal of Medicine, 26,* 899-918.

Engel, G. L. (1977). The need for a new medical model: A challenge for biomedicine. *Science, 196,* 129-136.

Esteve, R., Ramirez-Maestre, C., & Lopez-Martinez, A. (2007). Adjustment to chronic pain: The role of pain acceptance, coping strategies, and pain-related cognitions. *Annals in Behavioral Medicine, 33,* 179-188.

Eysenck, H. J. (1959). Learning theory and behaviour therapy. *Journal of Mental Science, 105,* 61-75.

Eysenck, H. J. (1964). Psychotherapy or behaviour therapy. *Indian Psychological Review, 1,* 33-41.

Fordyce, W. (1976). Behavioral Methods of Control of Chronic Pain and Illness. St. Louis, MO: Mosby.

Fordyce, W. (1988). Pain and suffering: A reappraisal. *American Psychologist, 43,* 276-283.

Gatchel, R. J. (2004). Comorbidity of chronic pain and mental health disorders: The biopsychosocial perspective. *American Psychologist, 59,* 795-805.

Gatchel, R. J. (2006). Psychological disorders and chronic pain: Cause and effect relationships. In R. J. Gatchel & T. C. Turk (Eds.), *Psychological Approaches to Pain Management: A Practitioner's Handbook* (pp. 33-54). New York: Guilford.

Gatchel, R. J., Bo Peng, Y., Peters, M., Fuchs, P., & Turk, D. (2007). The biopsychosocial approach to chronic pain: Scientific advances and future directions. *Psychological Bulletin, 133,* 581-624.

Gaudiano, B. A. (2006). The "third wave" behavior therapies in context: Review of Hayes et al.'s (2004) *Mindfulness and Acceptance: Expanding the Cognitive-Behavioral Tradition* and Hayes and Strosahl's (2004) *A Practical Guide to Acceptance and Commitment Therapy. Cognitive and Behavioral Practice, 13,* 101-104.

Grzesiak, R. (2002). Psychogenic pain and pain-proneness: Comments on K.G. Raphael et al. "childhood victimization and pain in adulthood." *Pain, 98,* 231-233.

Hayes, S. C. (2004). Acceptance and commitment therapy, relational frame theory, and the third wave of behavioral and cognitive therapies. *Behavior Therapy, 35,* 639-665.

Hayes, S. C., & Duckworth, M. P. (2006). Acceptance and commitment therapy and traditional cognitive behavior therapy approaches in pain. *Cognitive and Behavioral Practice, 13,* 185-187.

Hayes, S. C., Follette, V. M., & Linehan, M. M. (Eds.). (2004). *Mindfulness and Acceptance: Expanding the Cognitive-Behavioral Tradition.* New York: Guilford.

Hayes, S. C., Luoma, J. B., Bond, F. W., Masuda, A., & Lillis, J. (2006). Acceptance and commitment therapy: Model, processes and outcomes. *Behaviour Research and Therapy, 44,* 1-25.

Hayes, S. C., Strosahl, K., & Wilson, K. G. (1999). *Acceptance and Commitment Therapy: An Experimental Approach to Behavior Change.* New York: Guilford.

Hoffman, B., Papas, R., Chatkoff, D., & Kerns, R. (2007). Meta-analysis of psychological interventions for chronic low back pain. *Health Psychology, 26,* 1-9.

Hollon, S. D., & Beck, A. T. (1994). Cognitive and cognitive behavioral therapies. In A. Bergin & S. Garfield (Eds.), *Handbook of Psychotherapy and Behavior Change* (4th ed.; pp. 428-466). Oxford, England: John Wiley & Sons.

Keefe, F. J., Abernethy, A. J., & Campbell, L. C. (2005). Psychological approaches to understanding and treating disease-related pain. *Annual Review of Psychology, 56,* 601-630.

Keefe, F. J., Dunsmore, J., & Burnett, R. (1992) Behavioral and cognitive-behavioral approaches to chronic pain: Recent advances and future directions. *Journal of Consulting and Clinical Psychology, 60, 528-536.*

Lewandowski, M. (2006). *The Chronic Pain Care Workbook: A Self-Treatment Approach to Pain Relief Using the Behavioral Assessment of Pain Questionnaire.* Oakland, CA: New Harbinger Publications.

Lewandowski, W., Good, M., & Burke Draucker, C. (2005). Changes in the meaning of pain with the use of guided imagery. *Pain Management Nursing, 6,* 58-67.

Loitman, J. (2000). Pain management: Beyond pharmacology to acupuncture and hypnosis. *JAMA, 283,* 118-119.

McCracken, L., MacKichan, F., & Eccleston, C. (2007). Contextual cognitive-behavioral therapy for severely disabled chronic pain sufferers: Effectiveness and clinically significant change. *European Journal of Pain, 11,* 314-322.

McCracken, L., & Vowles, K. (2007). Psychological flexibility and traditional pain management strategies in relation to patient functioning with chronic pain: An examination of a revised instrument. *The Journal of Pain, 8,* 700-707.

McWilliams, L. A., Cox, B. J., & Enns, M. W. (2003). Mood and anxiety disorders in chronic pain: An examination in a nationally representative sample. *Pain, 106,* 127-133.

Melzack, R., & Wall, P. D. (1965). Pain mechanisms: A new theory. *Science, 150,* 971-979.

Merskey, H., & Bogduck, N. (Eds). (1994). *Classification of Chronic Pain: Descriptions of Chronic Pain Syndromes and Definitions of Pain Terms.* Report by the International Association for the Study of Pain Task Force on Taxonomy. Seattle: IASP Press.

Morone, N. E., & Greco, C. M. (2007). Mind-body interventions for chronic pain in older adults: A structured review. *Pain Medicine, 8,* 359-375.

National Institutes of Health. (2007). *Pain Management Fact Sheet.* Retrieved December 26, 2007 from http://www.nih.gov/about/researchresultsforthepublic/Pain.pdf

Nestoriuc, Y., & Martin, A. (2007). Efficacy of biofeedback for migraine: A meta-analysis. *Pain, 128,* 111-127.

Patterson, D. R., & Jensen, M. P. (2003). Hypnosis and clinical pain. *Psychological Bulletin, 129,* 495-521.

Schultz, J. H., & Luthe, W. (1959). *Autogenic Training: A Psychophysiologic Approach to Psychotherapy.* Oxford, England: Grune & Stratton.

Scott, K., Bruffaerts, R., Tsang, A., Ormel, J., Alonso, J., Angermeyer, M., Benjet, C., Bromet, E., de Girolamo, G., de Graaf, R., Gaset, I., Gureje, O., Haro, J., He, Y., Kessler, R., Levinson, D., Mneimneh, Z., Oakley Brown, M., Posada-Villa, J., Stein, D., Takeshima, T., & Von Korff, M. (2007). Depression-anxiety relationships with chronic physical pain conditions: Results from the World Mental Health Surveys. *Journal of Affective Disorders, 103,* 113-120.

Stucky, C., Gold, M., & Zhang, X. (2001). Mechanisms of pain. *Proceedings of the National Academy of Sciences of the United States of America, 98,* 11845-11846.

Tang, K. Y., Salkovskis, P., Poplavskaya, E., Wright, K. J., Hanna, M., & Hester, J. (2007). Increased use of safety-seeking behaviors in chronic back pain patients with high health anxiety. *Behaviour Research and Therapy, 45,* 2821-2835.

Thorn, B. E., Keefe, F. J., & Anderson, T. (2004). The communal coping model and interpersonal context: Problems or process? *Pain, 110,* 505-507.

Turk, D. C., & McCarberg, B. (2005). Non-pharmacological treatments for chronic pain. *Disease Management Health Outcomes, 13,* 19-30.

Turk, D. C., Meichenbaum, D., & Genest, M. (1983). *Pain and Behavioral Medicine. A Cognitive-Behavioral Perspective.* New York: Guilford.

Vowles, K. E., McCracken, L. M., & Eccleston, C. (2007). Processes of change in treatment for chronic pain: The contributions of pain, acceptance, and catastrophizing. *European Journal of Pain, 11,* 779-787.

Vowles, K. E., McNeil, D. W., Gross, R. T., McDaniel, M. A., Mouse, A., Bates, M., Gallimore, P., & McCall, C. (2007). Effects of pain acceptance and pain control strategies on physical impairment in individuals with chronic low back pain. *Behavior Therapy, 38,* 412-425.

Waddell, G. (1987). A new clinical method for the treatment of low back pain. *Spine, 12,* 632-644.

Winterowd, C., Beck, A. T., & Gruener, D. (2003). *Cognitive Therapy With Chronic Pain Patients.* New York: Springer.

Pharmacologic Interventions for Depression and Anxiety

Gerald J. Strauss

PSYCHOTHERAPY IS STILL
THE FIRST TREATMENT OF CHOICE

Despite the push toward prescriptive authority for properly trained psychologists, psychotherapy remains the mainstay of a psychologist's therapeutic armamentarium. McGrath et al. (2004) state the importance of prescribing psychologists to maintain their traditional identity as psychologists and to embrace the biopsychosocial model of practice while avoiding the medical model. Many prescribing psychologists (Wiggins & Cummings, 1998) point to their own practices as examples of how psychotherapy is the treatment of choice while pharmacotherapy is an adjunctive treatment when necessary. In fact, Cmdr. John Sexton (cited in Vedantam, 2002) stated that, compared to his psychiatric colleagues, his prescribing practices reflected significantly fewer prescriptions written. Sexton, a military psychologist who graduated from the Department of Defense Psychopharmacology Demonstration Project, found that two of his psychiatric colleagues prescribed medicines to 61% and 68% of their patients compared to Sexton who prescribed to only 13% of his patients.

Psychologists are often thrust into the position of being de facto prescribers despite not writing a single prescription. Although it is well known that primary care providers write 50% to 75% of psychotropic medications, they often ask psychologists which medication to use and at what dose. When considering this issue it is important to consider your level of competence and practice within its scope. Having said that, a number of states have explicitly identified consultation with other professionals about pharmacotherapy as part of the scope of practice for psychologists. For example, in Ohio, the Ohio Administrative Code (2004) Chapter 4732-5 (B) (13) stipulates that "psychological pharmacological consultation is allowable as a psychological procedure as defined by procedures specified in rule 4732-3-01 (C) (3)." In Chapter 4732-3-01 (3) it is stated that client supervision "may include the evaluation and management of patients and psychological effects to determine if prescribed medications might be helpful in alleviating their psychological symptoms and referring a client to a physician for prescription medication(s), . . . and when a client is on a prescribed medication, the psychologist may evaluate and monitor the psychological effects of that medication to determine the psychological effects of such medications on the patient, in a consultative relationship with the prescribing physician." At least nine jurisdictions have such rules codified.

In loving memory of Willie Carletta; he had places to go.

Thus, whether one plans (or not) to take a training course to become a prescribing (or medical) psychologist, it behooves all practicing psychologists to have a basic understanding of psychopharmacology. Lorion (1996) discussed the American Psychological Association Ad Hoc Task Force on Psychopharmacology's 1992 recommendations for training. The three levels of training were (a) Level 1: Basic Psychopharmacological Education, (b) Level 2: Collaborative Practice, and (c) Level 3: Prescription Privileges. At minimum, practicing psychologists today should be at the Level 1 basic science/clinical science level of understanding of psychotropic medications.

This contribution is one step in assisting professional psychologists to move toward Level 1 training. The contribution will not be exhaustive in its review of all psychotropic medications. Rather, it will emphasize antidepressants and anxiolytic medications. However, before delving into the medications themselves, it is important to consider some basic science issues. Psychotropic medications would have relatively little effect on targeted symptoms if the liver and other mechanisms were not available to metabolize the medications. The next section reviews hepatic processes in medication metabolism.

IMPORTANT PHYSIOLOGICAL MECHANISMS OF PHARMACOLOGY

Before a clinician decides to prescribe any medication, it is important to consider a number of physiological mechanisms pertaining to what the body does to drugs, what drugs do to the body, and the role of the liver in metabolizing the drugs. These mechanisms will be discussed in this section. There are mathematical equations related to these mechanisms. However, because this contribution is an overview, rather than an in-depth course on pharmacology, the mathematics and biochemistry of pharmacology will not be included.

Pharmacokinetics

Pharmacokinetics is the study of rates and movements of drugs through the body; essentially, what the body does to drugs. Pharmacokinetics entails absorption, distribution, metabolism, and elimination of drugs.

Drugs can be administered through a variety of routes: orally, intramuscularly, rectally, topically, and through inhalation. The rate of *absorption* of a drug into the bloodstream (regardless of the route of administration) is governed by six factors: (a) passive diffusion (no energy required), (b) concentration gradient (energy required to move the drug from a lower concentration to a higher concentration), (c) lipid solubility (lipid soluble drugs – more carbon atoms than oxygen atoms – pass easily through cell walls), (d) drug ionization (un-ionized drugs are highly lipid soluble and easily cross cell membranes; ionized drugs – those carrying an electric charge – are poorly lipid soluble and do not easily cross cell membranes), (e) molecular size of the drug (drugs with large molecules or oxygenated side chain groups are larger and absorbed more slowly), and (f) dosage form of the drug (tablets are absorbed most slowly, capsules more quickly, suspensions quicker than capsules, and solutions are absorbed most quickly) (Kester et al., 2007).

Distribution

Distribution is the process of moving a drug from the blood to the tissue where action is desired. The term describing the area of the body to which a drug is distributed is the volume of distribution (Vd). Essentially, Vd = dose (mg)/concentration (mg/L). The most important factor in determining distribution of a drug in the body is vascularity, or how much fluid is in the body. Some hydrophilic ("water-loving") drugs stay mostly in the vasculature, a compartment with a Vd of approximately 5 L (the volume of plasma in the body). Other drugs distribute to the vasculature plus the extracellular fluid compartments and have a Vd of about 15 L. Still other drugs travel to all body fluids (including the intracellular fluids) and have a Vd of 40 L. Lipid-soluble drugs have a much larger Vd compared to water-soluble drugs. Lipophilic ("fat-loving") drugs, once taken up by adipose (fat) tissue, can have a Vd of 100 L or more. Another important notion of the Vd (to be discussed later) is that it helps to determine steady-state dosing regimens (Kester et al., 2007).

Once drugs are absorbed, and while they are being distributed, they can be bound to serum protein molecules, especially albumin. While bound to serum protein, the drug is not biologically active. Nor is it able to be metabolized by the liver's Cytochrome P-450 system. The drug is gradually released from the serum protein, particularly if the drug is already on board and serum levels are dropping. Once unbound, the drug is free to distribute itself to the specific receptor where its biological effect is initiated.

Two factors related to serum albumin levels are important to mention. First, malnutrition can lower serum albumin levels. If this occurs, there may not be enough of the serum protein to bind with a drug, causing much of the drug to be "free." This large concentration of free drug can have toxic effects. Second, drugs that are highly protein bound (> 80% of the drug) can be displaced by other drugs that compete for protein binding. This is one means of leading to so-called drug-drug interaction. Again, when a highly protein-bound drug is displaced by a percent or two and becomes free, the drug effect may be toxic.

Metabolism and the Cytochrome (Microsomal) P-450 System

Kester et al. (2007) describe biotransformation as the "pharmacology language" for metabolism. The end result of metabolism is that a drug is biotransformed into a more polar, hydrophilic, and water-soluble form that is excretable by the kidney. Should drugs not be biotransformed/metabolized, almost all the drug would be reabsorbed by the body through mechanisms of the kidney.

Meanwhile, the liver is also involved in drug metabolism by zero-order or first-order kinetics. Zero-order kinetics metabolize only a few drugs, alcohol being one of them. In zero-order kinetics a drug is metabolized in a constant, linear fashion. That is, there is a fixed amount of drug that can be metabolized at one time. For example, alcohol dehydrogenase (the liver enzyme that breaks down alcohol) becomes overwhelmed if more than 10 to 14 grams of alcohol is ingested in a short period of time. Ingestion of more grams of alcohol leads to intoxication. The individual starts to sober up as the alcohol dehydrogenase metabolizes the alcohol at a rate of about 10 grams per hour.

Most drugs are metabolized by first-order kinetics. In first-order kinetics, a drug is metabolized at a constant fraction per unit of time. In other words, the greater amount of drug in the body, the faster it is metabolized. Kester et al. (2007) state that, if plotted, the first-order kinetic metabolism of a drug would be curvilinear. However, if plotted in a logarithmic fashion with drug concentration on the y-axis and time on the x-axis, the result would be a straight line. They go on to say that "since a constant fraction of a drug is metabolized per unit of time, and metabolism increases proportionally as the concentration of drug in the body increases, the time to clear the body of 50% of drug will always be constant" (p. 9). That is the definition of half-life ($T_{1/2}$): the time necessary to remove 50% of the drug from the body. They go on to cite an example of administration of 100 mg of a drug. Say it takes 4 hours to metabolize 50% of the drug; the $T_{1/2}$ is 4 hours. Knowing that, it will take 4 more hours to eliminate 25 mg, 4 more hours to eliminate 12.5 mg, and another 4 hours to eliminate 6.25 mg. Said a different way, the peak plasma concentration is reduced in half every $T_{1/2}$. Thus, it generally takes five $T_{1/2}$ to eliminate most (97%) of a drug from the body. Conversely, it will take approximately five $T_{1/2}$ of a drug to get to a peak, effective plasma concentration. This is an example why it may take weeks to get an antidepressant to an effective plasma level.

Cytochrome P-450 Isoenzymes

There are five groups of isoenzyme "families" located in the liver. The families are identified as Cytochrome (e.g., CYP prefix) and followed by their numerical designation (e.g., 1A2, 2D6, and others) (Fuller & Sajatovic, 2006). The Cytochrome P-450 isoenzymes catalyze Phase I reactions (oxidation, hydrolysis, and reduction) in the liver. These reactions add oxygen groups or remove methyl groups, thus causing drugs to become more polar and water soluble, which fosters elimination of the drug. At times, drugs cannot be fully metabolized by Phase I reactions. When that occurs, Phase II (conjugation reactions) emerges. Phase II reactions are energy-dependent, in which chemical structures are added to the drug to make it more polar and water soluble, thus excretable. The chemical structures that are added can be glycine conjugation, glutathione conjugation, sulfate formation, acetylation, methylation, or glucuronidation.

At times, certain humans may not be able to metabolize drugs as efficiently as others. These individuals are said to have genetic polymorphism. Approximately 7% to 10% of Caucasians are deficient in CYP2D6. CYP2C19 is absent in 3% of Caucasians and 20% of Asians. These individuals are said to be "poor metabolizers" of certain drugs and are at greater risk for experiencing drug reactions (Kester et al., 2007).

The Cytochrome P-450 enzymes can be *inhibited* (enzyme function is slowed) or *induced* (increased in activity or number). A *substrate* is a drug that is acted upon by a specific enzyme. Note that certain drugs may be an inhibitor to one isoenzyme while serving as a substrate for another. For example, let's examine a substrate drug of the Cytochrome P-450 1A2 family that is an antidepressant, Fluvoxamine. As the substrate drug, Fluvoxamine is the drug that is acted upon by either an inducing or inhibiting drug. Say a patient was prescribed Fluvoxamine but was also a smoker. Nicotine (in the 1A2 family) is an inducer. What this means is that the nicotine induces the P-450 1A2 enzyme system, causing the substrate drug (Fluvoxamine) to be metabolized too quickly. In doing so, the blood levels of Fluvoxamine may fall, rendering a less than adequate therapeutic effect. Conversely, say the patient had heartburn and decided to buy an over-the-counter medication, Cimetidine (an inhibitor of the 1A2 isoenzyme). Taking Cimetidine inhibits the metabolism of Fluvoxamine, which raises its level in the blood and potentially causes an adverse drug reaction. Thus, it is very important to be mindful of the various CYP isoenzymes and the substrate, inducer, and inhibitor drugs within each Cytochrome P-450 family. As a rule of thumb, Kester et al. (2007) state, "the plasma level of substrates increases with co-administration of a P-450 enzyme inhibitor and decreases with co-administration of a P-450 enzyme inducer, with varying degrees of clinical significance" (p. 10).

Elimination

Elimination is the process of excreting drug and/or metabolites from the body. This process is completed primarily by the kidneys and to a lesser degree by the liver, sweat glands, saliva, tears, and the lungs. Drugs can also be eliminated through breast milk. The kidneys filter out smaller sized molecules and those that are not bound to protein. Drugs that are not ionized and lipid soluble are reabsorbed through the kidney, while drugs that are ionized or polar are retained by the kidney and excreted in the urine. It is important to note that with advancing age, kidney disease, or competition with other drugs, the kidneys may not function effectively or efficiently. In these instances serum drug levels may be elevated to a toxic range. Lower dosages or a different drug choice may be indicated if the glomerular filtration rate of the kidney is diminished.

Drug Level

When administering a medication, the desire is to have the drug reach a therapeutic window or level. This occurs when the concentration of the drug becomes relatively constant. Essentially, the "amount of the drug administered during each $T_{1/2}$ (half-life) is equal to the amount of drug metabolized and eliminated from the body during the same time interval" (Kester et al., 2007, p. 13). If administered once per $T_{1/2}$, a drug will need 4 to 5 $T_{1/2}$ for that drug to reach a steady state of plasma concentration. Similarly, the same timing sequence occurs for elimination of a drug from the body. That is, it will take 4 to 5 $T_{1/2}$ for the drug to be eliminated from the body. For example, Paroxetine has a $T_{1/2}$ of 21 hours. Four to 5 $T_{1/2}$ will be 84 to 105 hours or approximately 3.5 to 4.5 days to reach a steady state of serum concentration; not necessarily enough time for clinical effectiveness.

Pharmacodynamics

Pharmacodynamics entails a fair amount of biochemistry. Given that the author is making the assumption that the majority of readers have not studied biochemistry, only basic concepts will be discussed.

The Dose-Response Relationship. A simple useful metaphor to understanding dose-response is a lock and key. Essentially the target (e.g., plasma membrane receptor, an enzyme, an ion channel, a transporter, etc.) is the lock in the metaphor. The key is the drug being utilized. If the key fits into the lock and opens or activates it, the drug is considered an *agonist*. However, if the key fits the lock but doesn't open it, and simply occupies the space in the lock, it is called an *antagonist* (it antagonizes the usual response of the target receptor). Other terms related to the dose-response relationship are *affinity* (the attraction or ability of a drug to interact or bind with its target; the greater the affinity, the greater the binding) and *efficacy* (the ability of a drug to interact with its target and elicit a biological response) (Kester et al., 2007).

The Time-Response Relationship. This relationship is based on three variables: (a) the time from drug dosing to the onset of action, (b) the time it takes for the peak effect to occur, and (c) the duration of the drug's action. It may be useful to think about these relationships plotted on an x- and y-axis with time on the x-axis and response or plasma concentration of the drug on the y-axis. The maximal peak response should be below the toxic dose but above the minimal effective dose.

Drugs as Agonists. Kester et al. (2007) ask the question, "How does a practitioner interpret two drugs that have equal affinities (binding) for a specific target but have different efficacies (degrees of response)" (p. 19)? The answer is, drugs that elicit a maximal response are full agonists. Partial agonists are drugs that do not elicit a maximal response. This can be important clinically, for example, when partial agonists fully saturate a receptor but the intended result is a weaker biological response.

Drugs as Antagonists. Some drugs block or compete with (a) a drug metabolite, (b) a biochemical pathway, (c) a foreign substance, or (d) another drug. Drugs that accomplish this task are called antagonists in that they block or antagonize the intended effect of the other substance, drug, or pathway. Antagonists can be reversible or irreversible.

Signaling and Receptors. This concept entails understanding of biochemistry protein synthesis and genetics. Suffice it to say that the critical points of signal transduction pathways are amplification, redundancy, cross-talk, and integration of biological signals. These concepts are beyond the scope of this contribution.

ANTIDEPRESSANT MEDICATIONS

The next section of this contribution will review various antidepressant medications. They will be described based on class (e.g., SSRI), initial dose (mg), dosage range (mg/day), peak plasma levels in hours (T_{max}), elimination half-life in hours ($T_{1/2}$), metabolizing enzymes (CYP-450), examples of CYP-450 enzyme inhibition and induction, and potential side effects. Only medications that are prescribed in the United States will be discussed. This will not be an exhaustive listing. Rather, it will include the most common antidepressants and anxiolytic medications prescribed today.

Selective Serotonin Reuptake Inhibitors (SSRIs)

Citalopram (Celexa)

Starting dose is often 20 mg q am (every morning); 10-60 mg is the range of dosages used. Citalopram peaks (T_{max}) in about 4 hours and has a half-life ($T_{1/2}$) of 23 to 45 hours. It is metabolized by CYP-450 enzymes 2D6, 2C19, and 3A4. If a patient is taking Citalopram and is also drinking grapefruit juice, the 3A4 enzyme will be inhibited and the Citalopram plasma level will rise, potentially causing adverse effects such as headache and gastrointestinal distress. If the patient had a seizure and is prescribed Phenytoin (Dilantin), the CYP-3A4 enzyme would be induced, causing the plasma levels of Citalopram to fall, which may cause an exacerbation of depression. Citalopram is FDA approved for the treatment of depression and generalized anxiety disorder (GAD). The unlabeled use of Citalopram is for the treatment of dementia, smoking cessation, ethanol abuse, obsessive-compulsive disorder (OCD) in children, and diabetic neuropathy.

Escitalopram (Lexapro)

Starting dose is often 10 mg; 5-20 mg is the range of dosages used. Escitalopram plasma levels peak in 4 to 5 hours with its metabolite in 14 hours. The $T_{1/2}$ is 27 to 32 hours. It is metabolized by CYP2D6, 3A4, and 2C19, similar to Citalopram. Therefore, the same types of drugs that cause induction or inhibition of Citalopram through the CYP-450 enzyme system will react in similar fashion for Escitalopram. Various pharmacology reference books such as Fuller and Sajatovic (2006) will list medications and which CYP-450 enzymes are induced or inhibited as additional medications are absorbed, distributed, and metabolized. Common potential side effects of SSRIs are headache, GI symptoms, and sexual dysfunction. The FDA-approved use of Escitalopram is for the treatment of depression and GAD. There are no cited off-label uses for the drug at this time.

Fluvoxamine (Luvox)

Usual starting dose is 50 mg q hs (at bed time); 50-300 mgs is the range. Fluvoxamine plasma levels (T_{max}) peak at 1.5 hours. The elimination half-life ($T_{1/2}$) is 9 to 28 hours. It is metabolized strongly by CYP-450 1A2 and 2D6. When the CYP-450 enzymes 2B6, 2D6, 3A3/4, 2C9, and 2C19 are activated by other medications such as Orphenadrine (2B6 weak), Codeine (2D6 weak), Cimetidine (3A4 weak), Fluvastatin (2C9 weak), and Topiramate (2C19 strong), among many others, there is inhibition of the CYP enzyme system that metabolizes Fluvoxamine. When inhibited, the Fluvoxamine is not readily metabolized, and the plasma levels of the drug remain high until the CYP enzymes are no longer inhibited, essentially until the second drug is discontinued. Again, the side effects for all the SSRIs are similar. The FDA-approved use of Fluvoxamine is in the treatment of OCD, including children greater than 8 years of age. The unlabeled use of Fluvoxamine is in the treatment of major depression, panic disorder, and anxiety disorders in children.

Fluoxetine (Prozac, Sarafem)

Typical starting dose is 10-20 mg q am (every morning); 10-80 mgs is the range. The T_{max} is 6 to 8 hours and the $T_{1/2}$ is very long at 24 to 144 hours for the parent drug and 200 to 330 hours for the metabolite Norfluoxetine. The CYP-450 enzymes that metabolize Fluoxetine strongly are 2C9 and 2D6 as well as 1A2, 2B6, 2C19, 2E1, and 3A4 (all weakly).Those that are inhibitors are 2D6 (strongly), 1A2 and 2C19 (moderately), and 2B6, 2C9, and 3A4 (weakly).There are no inducing CYP enzymes for Fluoxetine. The FDA-approved use of Fluoxetine is in the treatment of major depression, anorexia and bulimia, OCD, premenstrual dysphoric disorder (PMDD), and panic disorder. The unlabeled use of Fluoxetine is in the treatment of selective mutism.

Paroxetine (Paxil)

Usual starting dose for immediate-release Paroxetine is 10-20 mg, whereas 12.5 mg is the starting dose of Paroxetine CR (continuous release). The range of dosing for immediate release Paroxetine is 10-60 mg and for CR it is 12.5-75 mg. The T_{max} is 5.2 hours for immediate release and the $T_{1/2}$ is 3 to 65 hours. The metabolizing CYP-450 enzyme of Paroxetine is 2D6. The CYP-450 enzymes that inhibit Paroxetine metabolism are 2D6 (strongly), 2B6 (moderately), and 1A2, 2C9, 2C19, 3A4 (weakly). The side effects of Paroxetine are similar to the other SSRIs (headache, GI, sexual dysfunction) but have additional symptoms of minor anticholinergic side effects (dry eyes and mouth, blurred vision, constipation, dizziness) as well as drowsiness and weight gain. The FDA-approved use of Paroxetine is in the treatment of major depression, OCD, PMDD (Paxil CR), panic disorder, posttraumatic stress disorder (PTSD), social anxiety disorder, and GAD. The unlabeled uses of Paroxetine are listed for eating disorders, impulse control disorders, self-injurious behaviors, and OCD (in children).

Sertraline (Zoloft)

Usual starting dose is 25-50 mgs. The range is 25-200 mgs. The peak plasma level (T_{max}) is 6 hours; the elimination half-life ($T_{1/2}$) is 22 to 36 hours for the parent drug and 62 to 104 hours for the metabolite (N-desmethylsertraline). The CYP-450 enzymes that metabolize Sertraline are 2C19 and 2D6 (strongly) and 2B6 and 2C9 (weakly). The list of enzymes that inhibit the metabolism of Sertraline are 2B6, 2C19, 2D6, and 3A4 (moderately), and 1A2, 2C8, and 2C9 (weakly). There are no listed inducer CYP enzymes for Sertraline. Side effects are mostly gastrointestinal, headache, and sexual dysfunction. The FDA-approved uses for Sertraline are in the treatment of major depression, OCD, PMDD, panic disorder, PTSD, and social anxiety disorder. Unlabeled uses include eating disorders, GAD, and impulse control disorders.

Noradrenergic-Dopamine Reuptake Inhibitors (NDRIs)

Bupropion, Bupropion SR (Wellbutrin, Zyban)

Starting dose is 100 mg tid (three times a day) with immediate release (IR), or 150 mg for 3 to 7 days, then 150 mg bid (twice a day) for SR (sustained release; take the afternoon dose before 5:00 pm). The range of dosing is 225-450 mg/d for immediate release and 150-300 mg/d for SR. The T_{max} is 1.6 hours for IR and the $T_{1/2}$ is 10 to 14 hours for the parent drug and 20 to 27 hours for the metabolites. The most potent CYP-450 enzyme that metabolizes Bupropion is 2B6 with others (1A2, 2D6, 3A4, 2C9, 2E1) involved. Potential side effects are mild cardiac arrhythmias and GI distress. However, Bupropion should not be prescribed if a patient has a history of seizure disorder, bulimia, or anorexia as the seizure threshold is lowered with Bupropion. A reduced seizure threshold can precipitate a seizure. On the positive side, there is a low incidence of sexual dysfunction with Bupropion. The FDA-approved use of Bupropion is for the treatment of major depression, seasonal affective disorder (SAD), and adjunctly in smoking cessation. The unlabeled use is in the treatment of ADHD and depression associated with bipolar disorder.

Serotonin-Norepinephrine Reuptake Inhibitors (SNRIs)

Venlafaxine, Venlafaxine XR (Effexor, Effexor XR)

Starting dose is 25 mg bid (twice a day) or tid (three times a day) for immediate release and 37.5 mg qd (every day) for XR. Usual dose is 75-375 mg/d. The T_{max} is 2 hours for immediate release and 5.5 hours for XR. The $T_{1/2}$ is 3 to 7 hours for the parent drug and 9 to 13 hours for the metabolite. The most potent CYP-450 metabolizing enzyme is 2D6 with minor metabolizing by 3A4, 2C9, and 2C19. Example drugs that may induce metabolism of Venlafaxine are Carbamazepine and Nafcillin via the CYP3A4 system. Example drugs that inhibit the metabolism via the CYP3A4 system are Doxycycline, protease inhibitors, and Verapamil. Potential side effects of Venlafaxine are anticholinergic (dry eyes and mouth, blurred vision, urinary retention, constipation, dizziness), drowsiness, gastrointestinal (nausea), and cardiac conduction abnormalities, all to a minor degree. A higher dose of Venlafaxine is useful in treating refractory depression. Unfortunately, the frequency of hypertension increases with dosages greater than 225 mg/d. The FDA-approved use of Venlafaxine is for the treatment of major depression disorder (MDD), GAD, social anxiety and phobia disorders, and panic disorder. Unlabeled uses for which Venlafaxine has been prescribed are OCD, hot flashes, neuropathic pain, and ADHD.

Duloxetine (Cymbalta)

Starting dose can be between 40 and 60 mg/d, which is also the usual dose. The T_{max} is 6 hours and the $T_{1/2}$ is 8 to 19 hours. The most potent CYP-450 enzymes responsible for the metabolism of Duloxetine are 1A2 and 2D6. Duloxetine is also moderately inhibited by the 2D6 enzyme. Example drugs that may inhibit the metabolism of Duloxetine via the CYP2D6 pathway are Chlorpromazine, Quinidine, and Retinovir. Example drugs that induce the metabolism of Duloxetine via the CYP1A2 pathway are Carbamazepine, Phenobarbital, and Rifampin. Potential mild side effects include anticholinergic symptoms, cardiac conduction defects, and drowsiness. Gastrointestinal side effects are moderately common. Much like Venlafaxine, blood pressure should be observed when Duloxetine is prescribed because of its enhancing effects of norepinephrine (a potent vasoconstrictor causing elevated blood pressure). Duloxetine's primary treatment indication is major depression and pain associated with diabetic neuropathy. Its unlabeled use is treating urinary stress incontinence and potentially other chronic pain syndromes like fibromyalgia.

Serotonin Antagonist Reuptake Inhibitors (SARIs)

Nefazodone (Serzone)

Starting dose is 100 mg bid (twice a day) with a usual daily dose of 300-600 mg in two divided doses. The T_{max} is 2 hours and the $T_{1/2}$ is 2 to 5 hours for the parent drug and 3 to 18 hours for the metabolites. The potent metabolizing CYP-450 enzymes are 2D6 and 3A4. CYP3A4 is also a strong inhibitor of the drug as well. There are many medications that interact adversely with Nefazodone. Cases of life-threatening hepatic failure have been reported. It is a very sedating medication. Use caution in patients at risk for hypotension or with a history of previous seizure disorder. Due to these adverse side effects, extreme care is indicated in deciding to use the medication. Nefazodone has a low incidence of sexual side effects. The indication for use is depression with an unlabeled use for PTSD.

Trazodone (Desyrel)

Starting dose is 50 mg tid (three times a day) with a usual daily dose of 150-600 mg in three divided doses. The T_{max} is 2 hours and the $T_{1/2}$ is 4 to 9 hours. CYP-450 3A4 is the major metabolizing enzyme, with 2D6 having minor metabolizing properties with Trazodone as the substrate. CYP2D6 moderately inhibits substrate medications such as amphetamines; beta blockers; many antidepressants, such as Fluoxetine, Mirtazapine, and Venlafaxine; and tricyclic antidepressants among other medications when combined with Trazodone. Adverse side effects are dizziness, headache, sedation, nausea, and blurred vision. The indicated use of Trazodone is depression. However, it is rarely used these days as a first-line agent to treat depression. The unlabeled use is potential augmentation of antidepressant medications or sedation at bedtime for improving sleep. However, as stated above, Trazodone inhibits the 2D6 enzyme when combined with various antidepressants. Therefore, if Trazodone is combined with antidepressants for augmentation of the antidepressant effects or for sedation, the dose of Trazodone should be the lowest possible and judiciously titrated upward if necessary.

Noradrenergic Serotonin Antagonist (NaSA)

Mirtazapine (Remeron)

Starting dose is 15 mg q hs (at bed time) with a usual dose of 15-45 mg/day. The dose increase should not occur more frequently than every 1 to 2 weeks. Initially, Mirtazapine is quite sedating; however, there is an inverse relationship between increasing dose and sedation. The T_{max} is 2 hours and the $T_{1/2}$ is 20 to 40 hours. When Mirtazapine is the substrate drug, the metabolizing CYP-450 enzymes are 1A2 and 2D6. An adverse interaction may occur when a patient is taking Mirtazapine with the antihypertensive medication Clonidine. This occurs because Mirtazapine is metabolized by CYP1A2, which is a potent inhibitor of Clonidine. When inhibited by the 1A2 enzyme, the lower blood levels of Clonidine may lead to elevated blood pressure. Mirtazapine should not be prescribed to patients who are taking Clonidine to control their blood pressure. Example drugs that induce CYP1A2, thus reducing the serum level of Mirtazapine, are Carbamazepine and Phenobarbital. Example drugs that inhibit CYP1A2, thus increasing the serum level of Mirtazapine, are Ciprofloxacin, Fluvoxamine, and Ketoconazole. Adverse side effects are somnolence, increased cholesterol, constipation, and increased appetite and weight; the latter two are sometimes desired side effects for patients who may have lost their appetites due to depression. Patients should be monitored for a sore throat early on in pharmacotherapy as this may be a sign of agranulocytosis, a potentially life-threatening immunosuppressing condition. Mirtazapine has a low incidence of sexual side effects.

Tricyclic Antidepressants (TCAs)

Amitriptyline (Elavil)

Starting dose is 25-75 mg q hs (at bed time) with a usual dose of 100-300 mg. The T_{max} of Amitriptyline is 2 to 8 hours with the $T_{1/2}$ of 10 to 46 hours. When Amitriptyline is the substrate drug, the major CYP-450 enzyme is 2D6 with a number of other enzymes playing a minor role. There are many medications that inhibit the enzymes responsible for the metabolism of Amitriptyline, thus increasing the serum level of the drug. Adverse drug effects may consist of significant anticholinergic side effects (blurred vision, dry mouth, constipation) and sedation. There may be cardiac conduction defects noted on electrocardiogram (ECG), particularly prolongation of QTc intervals. (The QT interval is the measured distance [on an ECG] from the Q-wave to the T-wave. Functionally, it is the time from onset of ventricular depolarization [contraction] to completion of ventricular repolarization [relaxation]. The QTc is the corrected QT interval. Prolongation of the QTc has been associated with sudden cardiac death [Straus, Kors, DeBruin, 2006]). This can lead to life-threatening arrhythmias, particularly in higher dosages. In fact, suicide attempts can be successful if a 1-week supply of a TCA is taken in a single dose. The use of TCAs as primary drugs of choice for the treatment of depression has fallen off over the past 10 years. Tricyclic drugs have been relegated to the management of other syndromes and symptoms. Generally, Amitriptyline is used for the treatment of chronic pain syndromes (particularly neuropathies) and has been the gold standard against which most nonopioid pain medications have been measured. It has also been used in the treatment of migraine headaches and as a hypnotic for improved sleep.

There are other TCAs of note (Nortriptyline, Desipramine, and Doxepin, among others). However, because of the relatively infrequent use of these agents in the treatment of depression, they will not be discussed further.

Monoamine Oxidase Inhibitors (MAOIs)

Selegiline (EmSam) Transdermal

Initial dose is 6 mg/day per transdermal patch with usual daily dose range of 6-12 mg qd (every day). The T_{max} of Selegiline is 25% to 30% of the total Selegiline content over 24 hours. The oral form is within 1 hour. The $T_{1/2}$ is 18 to 25 hours for transdermal and 10 hours for oral preparations. Selegiline is metabolized mostly by the CYP-450 2B6 enzyme although 1A2, 2A6, 2C8 2C19, 2D6, and 3A4 play minor roles. Selegiline is inhibited weakly by most of the same CYP enzymes. For example, if Paroxetine or Sertraline were prescribed to a patient already taking Selegiline, the CYP2B6 enzyme would inhibit the metabolism of Selegiline, resulting in an increased serum level of the drug. Conversely, if a patient taking Selegiline was prescribed Carbamazepine, Phenobarbital, or Phenytoin, the CYP2B6 enzyme induction would sharply metabolize the Selegiline resulting in a reduction of serum level and potentially lessened clinical effectiveness. Adverse side effects may include headache, insomnia, nausea, and irritation of the patch site. There are many contraindications of concomitant drug use with Selegiline. A short list consists of dextromethorphan, methadone, propoxyphene, tramadol, other MAOIs, SSRIs, SNRI, TCAs, buspirone, mirtaxapine, cyclobenzaprine, and St. John's Wort, among others. Generally, a diet low in tyrosine (no wine, beer, smoked products, etc.) is required when taking an MAOI. However, the transdermal preparation of Selegiline reportedly does not require the low tyrosine diet. That remains to be seen, as the medication is prescribed more frequently in clinical settings. The oral preparation of Selegiline (and the other MAOIs) does require a low tyrosine diet; otherwise, a hypertensive crisis may ensue. The approved use of the drug in its transdermal form is for depression. It is used in Parkinson's disease (oral product only) as an adjunct when levodopa/carbidopa therapy is no longer effective. An unlabeled use of Selegiline is seen in the treatment of ADHD, negative symptoms of schizophrenia, extrapyramidal symptoms, and Alzheimer's disease (to improve cognitive and behavioral performance). If there is to be a switch to another form of antidepressant, a minimum of 2 weeks washout of the MAOI medication is required. If switching from Fluoxetine to Selegiline, a 5-week washout is required due to the long half-life of Fluoxetine.

Isocarboxazid (Marplan), Phenelzine (Nardil), and Tranylcypromine (Parnate) are the other MAOIs on the market. They are rarely used these days due to the cumbersome diet requirements and significant drug/drug interactions. Therefore, these MAOIs will not be discussed further in this contribution.

Additional Considerations When Prescribing Antidepressants

It is important to note that all antidepressants come with a warning that the various medications increase the risk of suicidal thinking and behavior in children and adolescents with major depression disorder and other depressive disorders. As such, some of the antidepressant medications (e.g., Citalopram, Sertraline) are not FDA approved for the treatment of depression in children. However, some of the medications (e.g., Sertraline, Fluoxetine) are FDA approved for the treatment of OCD in children above certain ages (e.g., greater than 6 or 7 years of age). Various pharmacotherapy reference texts (e.g., Fuller & Sajatovic, 2007) cite the warning and limits of medication uses.

Dosage considerations must be addressed in many situations. For example, lower than usual starting dosages should be considered in children/adolescents (if the medication may be used at all), geriatric populations, and those with impaired liver and renal functioning. Similarly, as indicated in the above discussions about the CYP-450 enzymes, an antidepressant's metabolism that is inhibited by a concomitantly prescribed medication necessitates starting the antidepressant at a lower dose. For example, when considering starting Fluvoxamine, start at a lower dose, because the Cimetidine inhibits the CYP1A2 enzyme that metabolizes Fluvoxamine when it is the substrate. So, even starting Fluvoxamine at a lower dose will result in a serum level that may rival the usual higher starting dose.

Benzodiazepine and Other Antianxiety Medications

Alprazolam (Xanax)

Initial dose is 0.25-0.5 mg tid (three times a day). Adult oral dosage range is 0.75-4 mg/day. The peak plasma level (T_{max}) of Alprazolam is 1 to 2 hours with half-life ($T_{1/2}$) of 12 to 14 hours. Alprazolam is metabolized in the liver by the CYP3A4 enzyme. When Alprazolam is combined with certain SSRIs (Fluoxetine, Fluvoxamine, and Sertraline), some TCAs, and an SARI (Nefazodone), the Alprazolam plasma levels rise (by as much as 100% when combined with Fluvoxamine) due to the inhibited metabolism of the Alprazolam via the CYP3A4 enzyme. Thus, caution in combining these medications is advised. Alprazolam has an intermediate onset of clinical effectiveness. Side effects can include ataxia, cognitive slowing, depression (or mania in some depressed patients), drowsiness, fatigue, memory impairment, and sedation. Combining alcohol with any benzodiazepine may result in coma and death. Smoking tobacco may decrease Alprazolam serum concentrations by 50%. Any benzodiazepine use in the elderly should be judicious and prescribed at the lowest possible dose to avoid side effects. It is FDA approved for the treatment of anxiety, anxiety associated with depression, and panic disorder.

Chlordiazepoxide (Librium)

Initial dosing is 5-25 mg tid (three times a day) or qid (four times a day). The usual adult dosage range is 15-100 mg/day. The T_{max} is 2 to 4 hours with a much longer $T_{1/2}$ of 5 to 30 hours for the parent drug and 24 to 96 hours for the active metabolite. Thus, the effects of the medication are long lasting. Chlordiazepoxide is metabolized in the liver via the CYP3A4 enzyme. So, any medication that inhibits the metabolism of Chlordiazepoxide via CYP3A4 will result in even longer lasting effects and possible adverse effects due to higher serum levels. It has an intermediate onset of action. FDA-approved uses of the medication are for anxiety, alcohol withdrawal, and an adjunct to anesthesia when used intravenously.

Diazepam (Valium)

Initial dosing is 2 to 10 mg bid (twice a day) or qid (four times a day). The usual daily adult dose range is 4-40 mg/day. The T_{max} is 0.5-2 hours with a $T_{1/2}$ of 20 to 80 hours for the parent drug and 50 to 100 hours for the active metabolite. Diazepam is metabolized in the liver by the CYP2C19 and 3A4 enzymes. Example drugs that inhibit 2C19 (thus increasing serum levels of Diazepam) are Fluvoxamine, Fluconazole, and Omeprazole. Example drugs that inhibit 3A4 are Clarithromycine, Nefazodone, protease inhibitors (for the treatment of HIV), and Verapamil. Diazepam has a rapid onset of action. It has FDA approval for the treatment of anxiety, alcohol withdrawal, an adjunct to anesthesia when used I.V., anxiety/amnestic effect when used in cardioversion and endoscopic procedures (I.V.), convulsions/status epilepticus (I.V.), adjunct in epilepsy, and skeletal muscle spasms.

Lorazepam (Ativan)

Initial dosing is 0.5-2 mg tid (three times a day) or qid (four times a day). The usual daily adult dose range is 2-4 mg/day. The T_{max} is 1 to 6 hours and the $T_{1/2}$ is 10 to 20 hours with no active metabolite. Lorazepam is metabolized in the liver. However, it is not metabolized by Phase I reactions which consist of the CYP-450 System. Instead, Lorazepam is metabolized by Phase II reactions in the liver. Phase II reactions cause drugs to be inactivated as well as increase the inactivated drug's polarity so that it can be easily excreted in the urine. This type of metabolism makes Lorazepam somewhat unique and safe in prevention of delirium tremens during hospitalization. Alcoholics often have liver damage, and use of other benzodiazepines that require the CYP-450 system to metabolize the benzodiazepine may result in much longer half-life simply because the liver can't do the job of metabolizing the drug. In that Lorazepam is metabolized by a different mechanism, the half-life is not extended and the medication is used effectively and efficiently. The onset of action of Lorazepam is intermediate. The FDA-approved uses of the medication are anxiety, anxiety associated with depression, adjunct to anesthesia (I.V.), and convulsions/status epilepticus (I.V.). Using Lorazepam for alcohol detoxification is an unlabeled, but common, use of the drug.

Oxazepam (Serax)

Initial adult dosing is 10 to 30 mg tid (three times a day) or qid (four times a day) with adult oral dosage range of 30-120 mg/day. The T_{max} is 2 to 4 hours and the $T_{1/2}$ is 5 to 20 hours with no active metabolites. Oxazepam is metabolized by the Phase II mechanism (rather the CYP-450) being conjugated to oxazepam glucuronide. This metabolite is not active pharmacologically. Oxazepam has a slow onset of action. It has no metabolic interactions with other drugs. Its FDA-approved use is for the treatment of anxiety and alcohol withdrawal. Its unlabeled use is for the treatment of partial complex seizures and as a hypnotic.

Clonazepam (Klonapin)

The initial adult dosing is 0.5 mg tid (three times a day) with a usual oral dosing range of 1.5-20 mg/day. The T_{max} is 1 to 2 hours and the $T_{1/2}$ is 18 to 50 hours with no metabolites. The metabolism of Clonazepam is through the Phase II mechanism in the liver via glucuronide and sulfate conjugation. Clonazepam serum levels may rise if the CYP3A4 enzyme is inhibited by combined use of other medications such as azole antifungals, Clarithromycine, Nefazodone, protease inhibitors, Quinidine, and Verapamil, among others. Clonazepam has an intermediate onset of action. The FDA-approved uses of Clonazepam are as a solo or adjunct treatment of petit mal (Lennon-Gastaut), akinetic, and myoclonic seizures, petit mal (absent) seizures unresponsive to succimides, and panic disorder with or with agoraphobia. Unlabeled uses of Clonazepam are anxiety disorders, restless leg syndrome, multifocal tic disorder, parkinsonian dysarthria, bipolar disorder, and adjunctive therapy for schizophrenia.

Clorazepate (Tranxene)

The initial adult dosing is 7.5-15 mg bid (twice a day) or qid (four times a day) with the oral dosing range of 15-60 mg/day. The T_{max} is 1 to 2 hours and $T_{1/2}$ is not significant. However, the half life of the metabolite (desmethyldiazepam) is long at 50 to 100 hours. Clorazepate is broken down in the stomach by the acid environment prior to absorption, then metabolized in the liver by the CYP3A4 enzyme. Clorazepate induction and inhibition by concurrent use of other medications (listed above) is the same method of induction and inhibition for other benzodiazepines that are metabolized by the CYP3A4 enzyme. The onset of action is rapid. Approved FDA uses of the medication are in the treatment of GAD, management of alcohol withdrawal, and as an adjunct anticonvulsant in the management of partial seizures.

Midazolam (Versed)

There is no oral dosing of this medication; it is injectable only. The T_{max} is 0.4 to 0.7 hours and the $T_{1/2}$ is 2 to 5 hours with no metabolites. Midazolam is metabolized in the liver by the CYP3A4 enzyme and is induced and inhibited by the concomitant use of other medications that induce or inhibit the CYP3A4 enzyme when Midazolam is the substrate drug. The onset of action is rapid if not immediate. The FDA-approved use of the medication is as an adjunct to anesthesia and an antianxiety/amnestic agent during medical procedures like endoscopy and cardioversion.

Non-Benzodiazepine Antianxiety Medication

Buspirone (Buspar)

Initial dosing is 7.5 mg bid (twice a day) with a range of oral dosing up to 60 mg/day. Dosing may be increased from the 7.5 mg bid by increments of 5 mg/day every 2 to 4 days, up to the maximum of 60 mg/day (divided dosing). Target dosing for most adults is 30 mg/day (15 mg bid). The T_{max} is 0.7 to 1.5 hours with a $T_{1/2}$ of 2 to 11 hours. Buspirone is metabolized in the liver by the CYP3A4 enzyme. Although not a benzodiazepine, Buspirone interacts with the same drugs that induce and inhibit it and benzodiazepines via the CYP3A4 enzyme when those drugs (e.g., inducers such as Carbamazepine and Phenytoin, and inhibitors such as azole antifungals, Clarithromycin, and protease inhibitors) are prescribed concomitantly. The FDA-approved use of Buspirone is in the treatment of GAD. However, the off-label use is for the management of aggression in mental retardation and secondary mental disorders, major depression, potential augmentation of antidepressants, and premenstrual syndrome. Buspirone reduces anxiety and worry without having sedating, muscle relaxing, or dependency or abuse potential, unlike benzodiazepines. Also unlike benzodiazepines, Buspirone cannot be used to prevent alcohol withdrawal or treat seizure disorders. Additional disadvantages of Buspirone are that it takes weeks to have a therapeutic effect, requires multiple daily dosing, and cannot be used in a prn (as needed) dosing.

Sedative/Hypnotic Medications

Sedative/Hypnotics like Estazolam (ProSom), Flurazepam (Dalmane), Quazepam (Doral), Temazepam (Restoril), and Triazolam (Halcion) are benzodiazepines. However, they are used in the treatment of insomnia, not anxiety, and therefore will not be discussed in this contribution.

CONCLUSION

All antidepressant medications are equally effective in treating depression. Often it is a particular desired side effect of the medication that leads a clinician to choose one antidepressant over another. For example, Mirtazapine may be chosen not only to treat the depression, but also to enhance appetite and weight gain in a patient who has anorexia secondary to depression. Antidepressant medications may also be useful in the treatment of anxiety. However, generally the dosage of the antidepressant must be raised to levels above the usual dose needed to effectively treat depression in order to ameliorate the anxiety. Once an effective dose of antidepressant is achieved, the patient should be maintained on the medication for 6 to 12 months. If the dose of the antidepressant is higher than an initial starting dose, the medication should be tapered down before complete discontinuation to avoid withdrawal symptoms.

All benzodiazepines are DEA (U.S. Drug Enforcement Administration) Schedule IV controlled substances. Short-term use of the medications can be quite beneficial in the treatment of anxiety disorders as the primary concern or as a secondary disorder associated with depression, schizophrenia, or dementias. Benzodiazepines act, in part, on the gamma-aminobutyric (GABA) receptors in the brain. Specifically, it is the GABA-A receptors that respond to benzodiazepines.

When the benzodiazepine has been used for maintenance purposes but will be discontinued, it should be slowly tapered down over 8 to 12 weeks in order to avoid withdrawal symptoms of anxiety, tremor, autonomic arousal, and GI disturbances. Abrupt discontinuation of short-acting benzodiazepines, like Alprazolam, has been associated with psychosis and seizures. It is best to switch patients from short-acting to long-acting (e.g., Clonazepam) benzodiazepines if tapering to discontinuation is planned. Benzodiazepines should not generally be prescribed to patients with a history of alcohol or other substance abuse problems.

In the event of overdose, patients may experience both cognitive and respiratory suppression. The benzodiazepine antagonist, Flumazenil, will reverse the cognitive suppression but not the respiratory suppression. Patients will still need ventilator support until stable. All anxiolytic medications should be used with caution in patients with any pulmonary disease (e.g., chronic obstructive pulmonary disease, and sleep apnea, among others).

CONTRIBUTOR

Gerald J. Strauss, PhD, is Section Chief of Health Psychology at the Cleveland VA Medical Center. He is a Clinical Assistant Professor of Medicine at the CWRU School of Medicine, a Past-President of the Ohio Psychological Association, and was OPA's first Chair of the Prescriptive Authority Task Force. In 2001 he was awarded Clinician of the Year by Division 18 of the American Psychological Association. He is widely published in the areas of shared medical appointments and improving quality of life in prostate surgery patients. Dr. Strauss may be contacted through the VA at 10701 East Boulevard (Firm A), Cleveland, OH 44106. E-mail: gerald.strauss@med.va.gov

RESOURCES

Bezchlibnyk-Butler, K. Z., & Jeffries, J. J. (2006). *Clinical Handbook of Psychotropic Drugs (16ᵗʰ ed.).* Toronto: Hogrefe & Huber.

Fuller, M. A., & Sajatovic, M. (2006). *Drug Information Handbook for Psychiatry: A Comprehensive Reference of Psychotropic, Nonpsychotropic, and Herbal Agents (6ᵗʰ ed.).* Hudson, OH: Lexi-Comp.

Kester, M., Vrana, K. E., Quraishi, S. A., & Karpa, K. D. (2007). *Elsevier's Integrated Pharmacology.* Philadelphia: Mosby.

Lorion, R. P. (1996). Applying our medicine to the psychopharmacological debate. *American Psychologist, 51,* 219-224.

McGrath, R. E., Wiggins, J. G., Sammons, M. T., Levant, R. F., Brown, A., & Stock, W. (2004). Professional issues in pharmacotherapy for psychologists. *Professional Psychology: Research and Practice, 15,* 158-163.

Ohio Administrative Code, 4732-50-01 (B) (13) and 4732-3-01 (3), (2004). Retrieved November 4, 2007, from http://codes.ohio.gov/oac/4732-5 and http://codes.ohio.gov/oac/4732-3

Straus, S. M., Kors, J. A., DeBruin, M. L. (2006). Prolonged QTc interval and risk of sudden cardiac death in a population of older adults. *Journal of the American College of Cardiology, 47,* 362-367.

Vedantam, S. (2002, July 1). For psychiatrists, a bitter pill in New Mexico; Law giving psychologists right to prescribe medications spurs a battle with MDs. *The Washington Post.* Retrieved July 7, 2008 from http://vedantam.com/rxrights07-2002.html

Wiggins, J. G., & Cummings, N. A. (1998). National study of the experience of psychologists with psychotropic medication and psychotherapy. *Professional Psychology: Research and Practice, 29,* 549-552.

Sleep Disorders: An Overview of Conditions, Assessment, and Treatment Options

Jennifer Goldschmied, Ryan Asherin,
Christopher E. Knoepke, and Mark S. Aloia

INTRODUCTION

Trouble with sleeping has silently become one of America's most common medical complaints. Many Americans suffer from one or more symptoms of a sleep disorder several days a week. A nationwide poll constructed by the National Sleep Foundation (NSF; 2002) indicated just how profound sleep disorders have become, reporting that "74% of respondents in the 2002 study experienced at least one symptom of a sleep disorder a few nights a week or more" (p. 9). The NSF recommends an average of 7 to 9 hours of sleep each night for most adults and even more for children and adolescents. Yet, nearly 25% of adults in America (47 million people) do not even get the minimum amount of sleep they need to be fully alert the next day.

In this contribution we are going to analyze the prevalence and severity of common sleep disorders, assessment tools used to identify these disorders, and the options commonly used for treatment. The goal of the contribution is to serve as a primer for those working in the field of mental health. It is not intended to be exhaustive, but rather to provide the basic tools needed to consider sleep disorders in patients, assess in a cursory manner, and refer for additional assessment and treatment.

Individuals who currently report a sleep disturbance are significantly more likely to develop a psychiatric illness in their lifetime. In 1989, Ford and Kamerow demonstrated that 40% of respondents with a sleep disorder had an additional psychiatric disorder, compared to 16.4% of individuals with no sleep complaints. The frequency of the comorbidity between sleep disorders and common psychiatric illnesses is recognized when one looks at the etiology of the various pathologies. According to the *Diagnostic and Statistical Manual of Mental Disorders* (*DSM-IV*; APA, 1994), sleep disturbances are a diagnostic criterion for many psychiatric disorders, including mood disorders, anxiety, and psychosis. In this first section we will be identifying the comorbidity between common psychiatric disorders and sleep disturbances.

MOOD DISORDERS

A direct link between sleep disturbance and clinical depression has long been recognized in psychiatry. Subjective feelings of anhedonia, fatigue, psychomotor retardation, or agitation are all common symptoms experienced by those with various sleep disturbances. Similarly, these symptoms are a key component of the diagnostic criteria that define Bipolar Disorder and Depression. In both clinical (Benca et al., 1992) and epidemiological (Ford & Cooper-Patrick, 2001) studies it has been shown that difficulties with sleep are among the most common complaints reported by depressed patients. Eaton, Badawi, & Melton (1995) stated that difficulties with sleep identify 47% of new major depressive cases that will occur in the next year. Additionally, the onset of sleep-related problems is tracked as a measure of the patients' response to treatment.

Insomnia

Insomnia is often the chief complaint of depressed patients who are seeking help (Ford & Cooper-Patrick, 2001). Insomnia can be characterized as initiation insomnia (trouble falling asleep), maintenance insomnia (trouble staying asleep), or terminal insomnia (waking too early). Although terminal insomnia is most commonly related to depression, any form of insomnia, or combination of forms, could be seen as comorbid. Some estimates of insomnia go as high as two thirds of individuals reporting to a sleep disorders center; a comorbid mood disorder is expected in almost half of those with insomnia (Tan et al., 1984). Clinically diagnosed cases of mood disorders almost always identify prodromal symptoms of insomnia. Insomniacs are far more likely to develop a new mood disorder within the following 3.5 years: 4 times and 2.9 times respectively (Breslau, Kilbey, & Andreski, 1991). In a 2000 study it was seen that 93% of depressed patients complained of insomnia (McCall, Reboussin, & Cohen, 2000). Furthermore, these sleep disturbances often contribute to the indication of the mood disorder episode. Even more powerful is the role that sleep architecture might play in heralding the onset of depression. Giles et al. (1989) found that first-degree relatives of people with depression, despite having not themselves been depressed, were 4 times as likely to develop a future major depressive episode if they demonstrated a short latency to their first Rapid Eye Movement (REM) sleep period. This study represents the power that sleep may play in comorbid mental illness.

Sleep Apnea

Although obstructive sleep apnea (OSA) is primarily seen as a respiratory condition, it has been reported that OSA can be linked to increased levels of depression (Andrew & Oei, 2004). Up to 41% of patients with obstructive sleep apnea display significantly higher scores of depression when compared to healthy controls (Aikens & Mendleson, 1999; Vandeputte & de Weerd, 2003). These higher rates of depression remain present for OSA patients, even after controlling for obesity and hypertension (Ohayon, 2003). Aloia et al. (2004) found that 33% of individuals with moderate to severe OSA and screened for untreated depression continued to report significant depressive symptoms. Interestingly, somatic symptoms were most related to apnea severity in men, while cognitive symptoms of depression were related to obesity in women. The complicated part of this relation lies in the multitude of comorbid conditions that present with OSA including obesity, diabetes, and cardiovascular disease, all of which have been related to depressed mood.

Other Disorders

There are many other forms of sleep disorders that also present a significant increase in comorbidity with a mood disorder. Subjective feeling of symptoms associated with various mood disorders is significantly increased in patients with a primary sleep disorder. Associated symptoms of depression have been found in patients with narcolepsy (37%), restless leg syndrome (53%), delayed sleep phase syndrome (41%), advanced sleep phase syndrome (83%), and parasomnias (29%) (Vandeputte & de Weerd, 2003). When diagnostically evaluating a patient for a sleep disorder, it is important to consider the comorbidity of associated mood disorders and plan for their assessment and treatment when yielding a primary diagnosis.

ANXIETY DISORDERS

Some levels of stress and anxiety are a very natural part of life that affects everyone. However, significant levels of stress and anxiety are quite common. A recent study found that anxiety disorders affect 19.1 million adults; anxiety is considered the most common psychiatric illness in America, affecting 13.3% of adults (National Institute of Mental Health [NIMH], 2001). Anxiety generally refers to a patient's subjective feeling of nervousness, fear, apprehension, or worry. Frequently, feelings of anxiety can be accompanied by a multitude of physical complaints including chest pain, shortness of breath, and gastrointestinal systems. Research has shown a relation between chronic sleep problems and anxiety (Breslau et al., 1991). The directionality of the relation, however, is not fully understood.

Insomnia/Hypersomnia

It is not surprising that anxiety disorders have a high rate of comorbidity with sleep disorders when you consider that anxiety disorders are the most common psychiatric illness affecting adults (NIMH, 2001). Anxiety disorders have been found to be the most common mental disorder faced by patients with either insomnia (23.9%) or hypersomnia (27.6%) (Ford & Kamerow, 1989). In 1996, Breslau et al. reported that individuals with a diagnosis of insomnia are 35.9% more likely to have a comorbid anxiety diagnosis, whereas the risk of developing a comorbid anxiety disorder is increased to 42.2% for individuals diagnosed with hypersomnia (see Table 1 below).

TABLE 1: Lifetime Prevalence of Psychiatric Disorders at Baseline (per 100) by Type of Sleep Disturbance (*n* = 1007)

	Insomnia only (*n* = 167)	Hypersomnia only (*n* = 83)	Insomnia plus Hyper-somnia (*n* = 81)	Neither Insomnia nor Hypersomnia (*n* = 676)
Major Depression	31.1	25.3	54.3	2.7
GAD	7.8	4.8	6.2	1.2
Panic Disorder	6	4.8	9.9	1.2
OCD	5.4	1.2	12.4	1
Phobia	25.2	37.4	48.2	17.8
Any Anxiety*	35.9	42.4	53.1	19.1
Alcohol A/D	30	36.1	34.6	16.7
Drug A/D	14.4	22.9	27.2	7.7
Nicotine Dependence	31.1	30.1	39.5	13.8
Any Disorder**	70.7	78.3	88.9	40.8
Multiple Disorders (≥3)	24.6	24.1	43.2	4.4

* Any anxiety includes GAD, panic disorder, OCD, and any phobia.

** Any Disorder includes any anxiety, major depression, alcohol abuse or dependence, illicit drug abuse or dependence, and nicotine dependence.

Many insomnia specialists actually view chronic insomnia as being on the spectrum of anxiety disorders. Insomnia is thought to begin acutely by some precipitating event (e.g., illness, excessive stress, a change in lifestyle, etc.). Precipitating events for insomnia affect some people more than others, suggesting a predisposition toward insomnia. As the insomnia persists, the individual often attempts to gain control over the situation and, in so doing, develops maladaptive sleep habits (e.g., going to bed too early to try to catch up on sleep). These habits often develop into perpetuating factors for the insomnia, making the insomnia behaviorally maintained. One example of this is the conditioning that occurs with the bed. The individual goes through a nightly struggle for sleep, eventually entraining his or her body to "struggle" in bed at night. These individuals often report having little to no trouble sleeping in a hotel. They also report being "wide awake when my head hits the pillow" despite being sleepy just prior. These are hallmark signs of a conditioned insomnia. Behavioral treatments, discussed later in this contribution, are then thought to be most helpful, as could be argued for any anxiety-related disorder.

Sleep Apnea

The presence of anxiety in sleep apnea is well recognized, however still not fully understood. The National Institutes of Health lists anxiety as one of the many symptoms of sleep apnea (Tasali & Van Cauter, 2002). However, the relationship between the two disorders has been difficult to separate. Reviews have noted that the rates of comorbidity between sleep apnea and anxiety disorders fluctuated greatly between published manuscripts (Kryger, Walid, & Manfreda, 2002). Prevalence figures ranged from 11% to 70% (B. Sadock & V. Sadock, 2000). Still, it has been noted that adherence to continuous positive airway pressure (PAP), a common form of treatment for OSA, may allay subjective feelings of anxiety (Schroder & O'Hara, 2005). Hypoxemia and presumably concomitant hypercapnia, caused by sleep apnea, have been thought to have anxiogenic properties or may even induce panic attacks (National Institutes of Heath [NIH], 2007; Griez et al., 1987; Papp, Klein, & Gorman, 1993). Youakim, Doghramji, and Schutte (1998) posited that a desaturation of high CO_2 levels through CPAP treatment, effectively treating hypercapnia, may explain the decrease in anxiety symptoms. Additionally, complaints of posttraumatic stress disorder (PTSD) have also been seen to be highly associated with individuals who are suffering from sleep apnea (Ohayon & Shapiro, 2000). It has been shown that CPAP adherence can dramatically improve symptoms of PTSD, with notable improvements in sleep continuity and diminished experiences of intrusive nightmares (Hurwitz et al., 1997). These findings all illustrate a substantial link between sleep apnea and anxiety disorders, but it is imperative that future research studies explore the comorbidity of the etiologies to further our knowledge in this area.

Other Disorders

Nightmares are consistently seen in individuals who suffer from PTSD, which ultimately affects the individual's subjective feelings of sleep quality and may increase their overall level of anxiety (Germain et al., 2007). A recent report identified a significant relation between anxiety and narcolepsy, circadian rhythm complaints, and sleepwalking (Spoormaker & van den Bout, 2005). A high level of nightmares and restless leg syndrome/periodic limb movement has also been found to be associated with anxiety disorders (Spoormaker & van den Bout, 2005).

PSYCHOSIS

Although a direct pathophysiological link has not been identified, sleep disturbances have been linked with various psychopathologies since the last century. The renowned English neurologist Hughlings Jackson stated, "Find out about dreams and you will find out about psychosis." In the early 1900s, Sigmund Freud popularized the use of dream analysis as a tool of psychoanalysis, and beginning in the 1960s sleep architecture was analyzed to learn more about mental illness, most commonly in patients with schizophrenia (Gierz, Campbell, & Gillin, 1987). A recent study demonstrated that nearly half of the hallucinations reported in the general population occurred at sleep onset (i.e., hypnagogic hallucinations) (Ohayon, 2000). However, it is important to note that psychosis symptoms can manifest in many different pathologies (e.g., Bipolar Disorder, Major Depression, and PTSD) (APA, 1994). Additionally, sleep disturbances have been shown to be reduced by patients being treated on antipsychotics, particularly newer atypical antipsychotics.

Insomnia

Psychosis, and specifically schizophrenia, has a strong link to insomnia. The prevalence of sleep disturbance in patients with schizophrenia has been reported to be at 90% (Szuba, Dinges, & Kloss, 2003). However, there is much debate as to whether insomnia exacerbates psychosis, or whether the psychosis causes the sleep disturbance. Schizophrenia patients report a notable increase in sleep disturbances, including insomnia, during a psychotic episode (Szuba et al., 2003). It is possible that the overactivity of the dopaminergic system plays a role in insomnia in this population, but this, as yet, remains unclear (J. Monti & D. Monti, 2005).

Sleep Apnea

Similar to insomnia, sleep apnea significantly reduces an individual's sleep quality, which can ultimately exacerbate psychosis. Recent correlational studies have identified a common comorbidity between psychosis and sleep apnea. It was found that 5.1% of individuals with obstructive sleep apnea also report suffering from psychosis (Sharafkhaneh et al., 2005). The comorbid prevalence of sleep apnea and psychosis is a great illustration of how a physical illness can have grossly negative repercussions on an individual's psyche. This work is only now being investigated and has been limited to a number of laboratories.

Other Disorders

Since the 1960s, studies have been carried out by sleep researchers and psychiatrists testing the hypothesis that hallucinations might correspond with waking dreams or some derangement of REM sleep. Most commonly electroencephalography (EEG) is used to explore the sleep cycles of individuals diagnosed with schizophrenia. It has been shown that prolonged sleep latency, decreased sleep continuity, decreased total sleep time, reduced slow wave sleep, short REM latency, increased REM sleep, increased REM sleep density, and loss of stages 3 and 4 sleep are the most frequently reported abnormalities in schizophrenia (Gierz et al., 1987; Kryger et al., 2002). Psychosis also presents with narcolepsy. Hypnagogic hallucinations, meaning that the hallucinations occur at the onset of sleep, have been seen as a frequent complaint of narcoleptic patients (Germain et al., 2007). The intensity and frequency of these hallucinations can result in the patient being diagnosed with a psychotic disorder.

Summary of Comorbidity of Mental Illness and Sleep Disorders

Links between sleep and psychiatric disorders have been reinforced by modern findings in psychiatry and neurobiology. It is well documented that sleep is critical for optimal cognitive functioning; when sleep is disturbed, individuals are not able to function effectively (Coleman et al., 1982). Poor cognitive function additionally impacts one's mood or affect. Additionally, secondary sleep disorders are common in the mentally ill population, as many psychiatric illnesses can impede sleep quantity and quality. Most recently studies have identified a role that sleep length and quality potentially plays in the development of diabetes and obesity, both of which could affect mood (Tasali & Van Cauter, 2002). Further research is needed to continue to identify the comorbidity of the over 90 sleep pathologies that have been identified by the International Classification of Sleep Disorders (ICSD) as associated with mental illnesses (American Academy of Sleep Medicine, 2005). Additionally, future research studies can continue to explore the possibility of a biological link to psychopathology.

Because it is common for most patients to discuss their sleep disturbances with their primary care physician, it is increasingly important that physicians understand how to best assess, treat, or triage complaints of disturbed sleep (APA, 1994). There are many different options that primary care physicians may utilize to best assess the severity and comorbidity of their patients' sleep disturbances. After thorough assessment, one may then consider the various options of treatment that are currently available.

DIAGNOSING SLEEP DISORDERS

Insomnia

Insomnia is the most commonly reported sleep complaint (Vgontzas & Kales, 1999), and because of this, many other sleep disorders present initially as insomnia. A clinician should recognize that daytime sleepiness is much less often seen as a problem than is insomnia. Individuals generally feel as though their sleep is fine if they can fall asleep quickly, but rarely see daytime sleepiness as a sign of a disorder.

Psychophysiologic insomnia, as defined by the ICSD, is a disorder of somatisized tension and learned sleep-preventing associations that results in a complaint of insomnia and perceived decreased functioning during wakefulness. Insomnia can be divided into two main categories. Whereas *initiation insomnia* is characterized by a difficulty falling asleep, those suffering from *maintenance insomnia* can usually fall asleep in under 30 minutes, but report waking up frequently throughout the course of a night or waking too early in the morning without being able to fall back asleep (also referred to as *terminal insomnia*). The signs and symptoms of insomnia generally include daytime sleepiness, difficulty concentrating, and memory problems, though many of these symptoms may not be present in any given individual. Prolonged insomnia commonly leads to feelings of anxiety, depressed mood, and irritability (National Heart Lung and Blood Institute [NHLBI], 2006a).

There are many tools that can be used to assess for insomnia; however, it is beneficial to keep in mind that complaints of insomnia may actually represent a different sleep disorder. One example of this lies in the patient with sleep-onset apnea, in which apnea events early in the night maintain wakefulness and present as insomnia. Referrals to a sleep clinician should always be considered for reasons such as this.

The *Structured Interview for Sleep Disorders (SIS-D*; Schramm et al., 1993) is a 20- to 30-minute clinical interview, which is used to help the clinician in the diagnostic process. This tool includes a complete sleep, medical, psychiatric, and medication history and uses the format of the Structured Clinical Interview for the *DSM*. The reliability of the SIS-D has been evaluated to illustrate a kappa coefficient mean of .77 with a range of .49 for other dysomnias to .91 for all insomnias. Validity of the SIS-D was high, with 90% of patients diagnosed with insomnia by the SIS-D having confirmed reports by polysomnography (PSG) as well (Schramm et al., 1993).

Informant reports may also be helpful in differentiating among sleep disorders. They can assist in identifying concerns such as periodic limb movements, cessation of breathing, acts of violence during sleep, and periods of time spent awake for which the patient may have limited awareness (Vgontzas & Kales, 1999).

Sleep diaries are an important piece of assessing the severity of insomnia (Buysse et al., 2006). Although there is no set form for a sleep diary, the average log is 1 week long, as anything below 7 days is viewed as not clinically valuable. Diaries collect data on nightly bedtimes, wake times, perceived time to sleep onset, number of nocturnal awakenings, and perceived amount of time up in the night. Times are estimates, as patients are not encouraged to track times during the night. Total sleep time and sleep efficiency (amount of time asleep divided by the amount of time lying in bed) are calculated by the clinician from these data. The general targets for insomnia treatment are sleep onset latency and sleep efficiency. Total sleep time is not a typical target, as there is significant interindividual variability on this measure. Wrist actigraphy is another method of establishing sleep/wake patterns in a behavioral context by monitoring the intensity and frequency of wrist movements across time. These movements have been validated against the gold standard for sleep measurement, PSG, to provide confidence in the general judgment of sleep versus wake (Sadeh et al., 1995). Actigraphs are seen as more reliable and objective, but it should always be remembered that insomnia is a subjective complaint.

There are also certain instruments that can be used to assess the symptoms associated with insomnia such as daytime sleepiness. The MSLT, or multiple sleep latency test, measures how quickly one can fall asleep under permitting conditions and is a valuable tool to assess excessive sleepiness (Carskadon et al., 1986). There are also self-report questionnaires of sleepiness and sleep quality that are common in sleep settings and are well understood by physicians receiving sleep referrals (Weaver, 2001). The *Epworth Sleepiness Scale* is an 8-item questionnaire on a 4-point scale about the likelihood of falling asleep in common situations. A score of 10 or more is considered sleepy, and a score over 18 is very sleepy (Johns, 1991). *The Pittsburgh Sleep Quality Index* measures sleep quality over 1 month. On the 21-point scale, a score over 6 indicates a poor level of sleep quality (Buysse et al., 1989). The *Insomnia Severity Index* is a 7-item questionnaire on a 5-point scale, which evaluates insomnia severity on the basis of multiple sleep complaints, with a maximum score of 28. A score under 14 is not considered to be clinically significant, whereas scores between 15 and 21 are considered to be a sign of moderate insomnia, and scores above 22, severe clinical insomnia (Bastien, Vallieres, & Morin, 2001).

PSG is not needed to diagnose insomnia. However, it may be needed to rule out other disorders that may present as insomnia.

Obstructive Sleep Apnea

According to the National Heart Lung and Blood Institute (2008), over 12 million Americans suffer from Obstructive Sleep Apnea (OSA), which is characterized by repetitive episodes of upper airway obstruction that occur during sleep, usually associated with a reduction in blood oxygen saturation.

The signs that a patient may be suffering from OSA include repetitive episodes of cessation of breathing, loud snoring, and choking or gasping during sleep that can lead to reduced blood oxygen saturation. There are many symptoms with OSA that can grossly affect the patient. These symptoms include excessive daytime sleepiness; morning headaches; poor memory; poor concentration; learning problems; mood swings or personality changes; feelings of anxiety, depression, and irritability; and dry throat upon waking (NHLBI, 2008). Approximately 67% of OSA patients will also suffer from high blood pressure (Young et al., 1997).

PSG, which is a method of monitoring breathing as well as brain and muscle activity during sleep (Man, 1996), can be performed in a laboratory setting or with ambulatory monitoring in the home, and reveals the number and type of breathing interruptions during sleep.

The apnea hypopnea index (AHI) is the most often reported metric. This metric describes the number of apneas (complete breathing cessation) and hypopneas (partial cessations of breathing with accompanying drops in blood oxygenation) per hour of sleep. As a general rule, an AHI below 5 is normal, while mild OSA falls between 5 and 15 events per hour, moderate falls between 15 and 30 events per hour, and severe is above 30 events per hour. Severe apnea would, therefore, involve a breathing episode every other minute of sleep. Although it is not possible to accurately diagnose OSA without overnight PSG, many physicians and researchers gather valuable information in the clinic as well. In addition to the clinical interview, a thorough clinical examination can be extremely revealing. Studies have reported that a high body mass index (BMI) can be an indication of an increased risk for OSA (Hoffstein & Szalai, 1993). Additionally, a neck circumference greater than 17 inches has also been shown to be indicative of OSA (Davies & Stradling, 1990). And, although the validity has been questioned, many physicians and researchers have used overnight oximetry, the measurement of blood oxygenation, to assess for OSA (Deegan & McNicholas, 1996).

One self-report measure, the Berlin Questionnaire, is a 10-item measure that has been developed in order to screen for the most common risk factors of OSA. These risk factors include weight change, snoring, pauses in breathing during sleep, daytime sleepiness, and high blood pressure. Netzer et al. (1999) have reported internal consistency with Cronbach correlations from 0.86 to 0.92.

Clinical measures of sleepiness can be utilized to assess for severe daytime sleepiness, a cardinal symptom of OSA, as well. Objective measures such as the MSLT, in addition to subjective measures such as the *Epworth Sleepiness Scale* (Johns, 1991), the *Karolinska Sleepiness Scale* (Gillberg, Kecklund, & Akerstedt, 1994), and the *Stanford Sleepiness Scale* (Hoddes et al., 1973), have shown to accurately measure severe sleepiness.

Delayed/Advanced Sleep Phase Syndrome

Phase disorders are more common than previously realized. Patients with phase disorders report getting a normal amount of sleep (7-8 hours per night), but their sleep/wake schedule is many hours either ahead of or behind the average person (e.g., advanced or delayed, respectively). ICSD defines delayed sleep-phase syndrome as a disorder in which the major sleep episode is delayed in relation to the desired clock time, resulting in symptoms of sleep-onset insomnia, or difficulty in awakening at the desired time. Advanced sleep-phase syndrome, on the other hand, is a disorder in which the major sleep episode is advanced in relation to the desired clock time, resulting in symptoms of compelling evening sleepiness, an early sleep onset, and an awakening that is earlier than desired.

For patients suffering from either delayed or advanced sleep-phase disorders, some signs must be present to be diagnosed. Sleep onset times must occur at nearly the same daily clock hour each day, the pattern must be present for 3 months, and there must be little or no reported difficulty in maintaining sleep once sleep has begun. Specifically, signs of delayed sleep-phase disorder include sleep-onset insomnia, not being able to fall asleep at a conventional hour, and difficulty waking in the morning. Signs of advanced sleep-phase disorder include the inability to stay awake until the desired bedtime or inability to remain asleep until the desired time of awakening (e.g., early morning awakening).

In order to accurately assess for delayed or advanced sleep-phase disorder, a physician would require the use of a sleep diary. There must be evidence of at least a month where sleep length and quality are normal but where the sleep phase is either advanced or delayed. In addition to the sleep diary, actigraphy can be an important component of the assessment. Temperature monitoring can also be a valuable method to assess for circadian rhythm disorders, as our body temperature typically decreases throughout the night while we sleep, to reach a minimum around 4 a.m. The temperature cycle of a person suffering from delayed or advanced sleep phase would also advance or be delayed and could then be detected by temperature monitoring (Ozaki et al., 1996).

The Morningness-Eveningness Questionnaire by Horne and Östberg (1976) is a 7-item, self-report measure of circadian preference that can be used to determine if a patient identifies himself or herself as a morning or evening type. With delayed and advanced sleep-phase disorder, as with insomnia, PSG is necessary only to rule out other sleep disorders.

Narcolepsy

Narcolepsy is a disorder of unknown etiology that is characterized by excessive sleepiness that typically is associated with cataplexy and other REM-sleep phenomena, such as sleep paralysis and hypnagogic hallucinations (American Academy of Sleep Medicine, 2005).

The signs and symptoms of narcolepsy include excessive daytime sleepiness, cataplexy (the sudden loss of muscle tone or weakness usually triggered by strong emotion, such as laughter, fear, or surprise), sleep paralysis, and hypnagogic hallucinations (NHLBI, 2006b). These symptoms can also result in fragmented nighttime sleep. Although many patients with narcolepsy will experience all of the above-mentioned symptoms, it is not necessary to manifest all of the symptoms to be diagnosed with narcolepsy. The ICSD recognizes narcolepsy in multiple forms: narcolepsy with cataplexy, narcolepsy without cataplexy, narcolepsy due to a medical condition, and narcolepsy unspecified.

Diagnosis of narcolepsy must include a full PSG to document rapid onset of REM sleep (Aldrich, 1998). During the PSG, a narcoleptic will notably fall asleep quickly and usually lapse into the REM period early in the sleep cycle. The MSLT is another useful measure of narcolepsy. Narcoleptics will usually present an MSLT with a mean sleep latency of less than 8 minutes and two or more sleep onset REM periods (Moscovitch, Partinen, & Guilleminault, 1993).

REM Sleep Behavior Disorder

Most commonly observed in males over the age of 60, REM sleep behavior disorder (RBD), as defined by the ICSD, is characterized by the intermittent loss of REM sleep electromyographic (EMG) atonia during sleep and by the appearance of elaborate motor activity associated with dream mentation. RBD will present itself as dream-enacting behaviors occurring most often during the second half of the night, during the REM cycle of sleep. These behaviors are sometimes violent, causing self-injury or injury to the bed partner.

Because RBD behaviors occur during sleep, bed partners are typically more likely to express concern than the patient. In order to accurately assess the patient, a comprehensive clinical interview and sleep history from both the patient and the bed partner must be completed. PSG including EMG and EEG to monitor muscle tone during REM, in addition to time-synchronized videotaping to observe the behavior during sleep, must also be carried out (Schenck & Mahowald, 1996).

RBD has also recently been associated with the increase in likelihood of developing Parkinson's disease, Parkinson-related dementias, and Lewy Body dementia (Boeve et al., 1998). To that end, a psychiatric and neurologic interview should also be conducted in order to rule out other psychiatric or neurological disorders that may be present.

Restless Leg Syndrome and Periodic Limb Movement Disorder

There are two sleep disorders that affect the limbs of the body: restless leg syndrome (RLS) and periodic limb movement disorder (PLMD). Both disorders disturb sleep by agitating the legs, which either prevents the patient from falling asleep, in the case of RLS, or arouses the patient from sleep, in the case of PLMD.

The ICSD defines RLS as a disorder characterized by disagreeable leg sensations that usually occur prior to sleep onset and that cause an almost irresistible urge to move the legs. Patients experience an irritating sensation in the legs and an irresistible urge to move them. These symptoms worsen at rest or closer to bedtime, which results in difficulty falling asleep or staying asleep (Allen & Earley, 2001). Sensations dissipate with movement. In the morning, most people suffer from excessive daytime sleepiness from a lack of restful sleep. PSG is not required to assess for RLS (Stiasny, Oertel, & Trenkwalder, 2002). A full clinical interview, including medical and family history, should be conducted, in addition to a sleep diary for at least 2 weeks.

The *Suggested Immobilization Test* (SIT) is a method to assess for RLS. During this test, a patient's muscular activity in the anterior tibialis of the leg is recorded using an electromyogram (EMG) for 1 hour while the patient is sitting in a bed. A study by Montplaisir et al. (1997) found that an SIT index greater than 40 was found to discriminate patients with RLS from control subjects.

The ICSD defines PLMD as periodic episodes of repetitive and highly stereotyped limb movement that occur during sleep. These involuntary limb movements can occur in the knee, ankle, or big toe joints, and can last about 2 seconds and occur every 20 to 40 seconds. The movements can result in sleep disruption, with people suffering from PLMD usually reporting their covers being all over the bed upon waking in the morning. These ongoing disruptions of sleep can lead to excessive daytime sleepiness. An accurate diagnosis of PLMD relies upon the results of overnight PSG with time-synchronized videotaping (Stiasny et al., 2002). A full clinical interview should also be conducted. Additional self-report measures, such as the *Epworth Sleepiness Scale*, can be utilized to reveal symptoms of PLMD such as excessive daytime sleepiness.

COMMON TREATMENTS FOR COMMON SLEEP DISORDERS

Insomnia

Popular treatments for this common complaint include both pharmacological and behavioral treatments. Once the differential diagnosis is complete and the decision has been made that the patient's sleep problems are not secondary to another condition, treatments can be prescribed. In instances where insomnia is believed to be symptomatic of a medical or psychiatric condition, the primary condition should be addressed first. Psychotherapy may be indicated as a primary intervention or in instances where it facilitates primary medical treatments or addresses stress associated with excessive daytime sleepiness (Morin et al., 2006; Seligman, 1998).

Pharmacological therapies for insomnia include traditional benzodiazepines and nonbenzodiazepine hypnotics as well as antidepressants and antihistamines. Each of these medication classes has its own strengths and limitations, as well as indications for their use over other treatment modalities.

Traditional benzodiazepines and other GABA-ergic agents are among the most commonly prescribed medications for insomnia. They include clonazepam, lorazepam, oxazepam, zaleplon, zolpidem, and others, as well as their brand-name equivalents. Many of these medications are marketed specifically for use in the treatment of sleep disorders, while others are marketed as anxiolytics and prescribed off-label in these circumstances. These medications represent improvement on older pharmacotherapies in their more selective hypnotic effects and decreased risk of dependence. For instance, newer benzodiazepines have pharmacokinetic properties that allow them to reach peak plasma levels within very short periods of time, often in 2 hours or less (Mendelson, 2005; Morin & Espie, 2003). One potential patient benefit of frontloading the drug's effects in this way is that sleep latency can be decreased while holding risk of daytime residual sedation, or any other side effect, to a minimum.

Antidepressive serotinergic agents have also been used extensively, often off-label, as a first-line treatment for insomnia. Most research addressing this use has been conducted on doxepin, amitryptyline, trimipramine, trazodone, nefazodone, and mirtazapine. Studies assessing the validity of this approach have typically analyzed these drugs' effects on sleep in depressed patients (Mendelson, 2005). These limitations notwithstanding, many of these drugs have consistently illustrated a strong ability to decrease sleep latency and increase sleep continuity while having a negligible effect on percentage of time spent in Stage 3 or 4 non-REM sleep (Mendelson, 2005).

First-generation antihistamines, which can typically be purchased over the counter and have either diphenhydramine or doxylamine as their active ingredients, can also be used to affect patients' subjective assessment of their own drowsiness and quality of sleep, but are not an empirically derived intervention for any sleep disorder. Aside from Central Nervous System (CNS) depression and the ensuing hypnotic effect, studies investigating the utility of these drugs as a sleep aid have not analyzed their effect on sleep architecture, but have rather focused on daytime sleepiness (Mendelson, 2005). The issue with these results is that, although daytime sleepiness is often a useful outcome variable, it can often be experienced as a side effect of these medications. In practice, many individuals have attempted using these medications as hypnotics to little or no avail prior to seeking care for their sleep problems. This alone should effectively negate them as a first-line treatment.

Cognitive Behavioral Therapy (CBT) for insomnia is the most well-supported psychotherapeutic intervention for this disorder. In a manner similar to other CBT protocols, this treatment calls for careful analysis of counterproductive sleep behaviors and cognitions. Frequently, short-term bouts of difficulty sleeping (which happen to everyone) have distressed the insomnia sufferer. The ensuing cycle of worrying about and excessive effort devoted to sleeping, as well as adoption of sleep-incompatible behaviors, leads to further sleep difficulty. Cognitive factors that frequently have a deleterious effect on sleep include unrealistic expectations about sleep, misunderstanding of the relationship between sleep, cognitive performance, and health and safety, and faulty attributions of causality. The behavioral aspects of CBT for insomnia typically include sleep restriction, where clients are instructed to restrict the amount of time they are in bed to the amount of time they need to sleep, and stimulus control (Morin, 2006). Practices such as meditation, positive imagery, and mindfulness can enhance the effectiveness of behavioral interventions. The use of paradoxical intention, whereby a patient who is having difficulty falling sleep attempts to stay awake, can also be used as an adjunctive practice (Morin, 2006; Seligman, 1998). Recent studies have found that CBT treatment of insomnia is associated with significant improvement in sleep-onset latency, maintenance, and sleep efficiency. Also, the format in which the intervention is delivered – individual, group, or over the phone – has no significant effect on its efficacy (Bastien et al., 2004). Although CBT may have limited usefulness in populations with comorbid psychosocial or medical conditions, gains made in terms of insomnia symptom reduction are typically well sustained in all client groups (Morin et al., 2006). Psychotherapy, and particularly CBT for insomnia, is recommended as a first-line treatment based on these data and without the risk of dependence and side effects common among pharmacological insomnia treatments.

Obstructive Sleep Apnea

Treatment strategies for Obstructive Sleep Apnea are threefold: surgical, behavioral, and mechanical. Methods are often employed alone, but can be used in combination as well. Early interventions tended to be surgical in nature, but more recent advances have favored behavioral and mechanical methods. It should be noted that although many different pharmacological agents have been tested as potential therapies, none have illustrated efficacy in treating apnea. Provigil (modafinil), however, has been identified as an effective treatment of daytime sleepiness accompanying OSA or as an adjunct to other therapies when sleepiness persists despite decrease in apneic events (Morgenthaler, Kapen, et al., 2006). Physiological factors with a provocative effect on apnea symptoms should be assessed before a treatment plan is designed. Specifically, nasal reconstruction may be a viable option for individuals whose apnea would be positively affected by decreased effort necessary to breathe through the nose and subsequent mouth breathing.

Surgery

When treatment first originated for OSA, most patients with moderate to severe OSA were offered surgery as a primary treatment. Uvulopalatopharyngeoplasty (UPPP) is the primary surgery offered today for the disorder. UPPP is designed to reduce potential obstruction of the patient's upper airway by removing excess of the soft palate, tonsils, and other tissues. Until the early 1990s, UPPP surgery was originally an inpatient procedure requiring at least one night of overnight observation. Recent advances, however, have made the procedure less intrusive, thereby eliminating the need for extended observation and greatly reducing the amount of pain experienced during recovery. The success rate of this procedure, however, has been called into question. A 1996 meta-analysis of UPPP efficacy studies found only a 40% rate of response (Sher, Schechtman, & Piccirillo, 1996). Variability in the response to this procedure is thought to be due to the high degree of physiological variability between patients as well as the experience of surgeons conducting UPPP procedures. This success rate, coupled with the discomfort and inconvenience associated with the procedure, have combined to decrease UPPP's popularity as a first-line treatment for OSA.

Radio frequency ablation (RFA) and injection snoreplasty are two other medical procedures that have shown efficacy with some OSA patients. In these procedures, radio waves or chemicals are injected into the formations of the soft palate involved in snoring, stiffening them and reducing the likelihood of obstruction in the upper airway during atonia. Although these methods are far less invasive than UPPP surgery, their efficacy has only been observed in patients with mild OSA. Another similar surgical procedure is palatal implants. This surgery involves placing several small cylindrical pieces of porous fiber into the palate, causing it to stiffen. The few studies investigating this procedure have found that it is generally well accepted by patients, has a low rate of complications, and dramatically reduces bed partners' perceptions of snoring (Romanow & Catalano, 2006). Positive effects on AHI and daytime sleepiness are less impressive, however, and these drawbacks should be discussed with any patient considering this procedure (Nordgard et al., 2007).

Oral Appliances

Oral appliances have gained popularity as a treatment for mild to moderate OSA. These devices either hold the patient's tongue forward (out of the airway) or force the lower jaw forward slightly. By virtue of stiffening the tongue muscle and opening the upper airway, many patients see marked improvement in their apnea symptoms. These appliances are most successful with individuals whose apnea is worse when sleeping in the supine position (on their back). Walker-Engstrom and her colleagues (2002) found that, over a 4-year period, dental appliances illustrated more drastic improvement in AHI in patients with mild to moderate apnea than UPPP surgery with a low rate of adjustments or necessary repairs. Adherence to these devices remains a largely unanswered question. In the same study, 82% of participants were compliant with dental device usage after 1 year and 78% used the device without significant breaks for 4 years. Another study found that more severe apnea can be treated with roughly the same efficacy with increased advancement of the mandible: 75% advancement versus the more typical 50% (Walker-Engstrom et al., 2003). More studies with greater statistical power are necessary, however, to determine whether dental appliances meet both the efficacy and adherence thresholds necessary to recommend them for widespread clinical use.

Positive Airway Pressure (PAP)

By far, the most commonly prescribed treatment for OSA is positive air pressure, or PAP. In this treatment, patients wear a mask that delivers pressurized air through their nose and down the upper airway, acting as a pneumatic splint during sleep. PAP treatment is currently the most efficacious treatment for OSA. Patients at all levels of apnea severity can expect an immediate reduction of symptoms to subclinical levels upon initiation of PAP treatment. The secondary advantages to PAP treatment are also impressive. Studies have shown PAP treatment to coincide with decreases in daytime blood pressure, even in nonhypotensive patients (Faccenda et al., 2001). The observed decreases in both systolic and diastolic pressure were most pronounced in patients with good compliance with PAP treatment and frequent blood oxygen desaturations.

PAP's greatest downfall, however, is low adherence. Recent data suggest that only 70% of patients prescribed PAP use their devices for 4 or more hours a night on 70% of nights, far below the optimal standard of all night, every night use. Common complaints about the device include general discomfort, noise, increased nasal congestion, a feeling of being "closed in," and concerns about attractiveness when wearing the PAP mask. Despite enormous improvements to the machines since the introduction of PAP in the early 1980s, PAP adherence continues to be poor. A number of psychosocial modalities are being investigated as possible moderators of PAP adherence, including patient education (both delivered by healthcare professionals and bibliotherapy), systematic desensitization to PAP's side effects, and a motivational enhancement intervention built upon the same theoretical foundation as Motivational Interviewing (Aloia et al., 2004).

Behavioral Techniques

Behavioral interventions in the treatment of OSA, except in the case of sleep position training, tend to mirror health behavior interventions used in the treatment of numerous medical conditions. Smoking and obesity, both factors which also have a provocative effect on the severity of OSA, are the targets of numerous treatments. This may be a significant proportion of apnea sufferers, because excess weight has a provocative effect on OSA, affecting 41% to 58% of patients (Young, Peppard, & Taheri, 2005). A more extensive review of these treatments, however, is beyond the scope of this contribution.

Sleep position training operates on the principle that sleeping in the supine position increases the likelihood of upper airway collapse and subsequent apneic events. Strategies ranging from simple education about sleep position to the use of specialized sleeping shirts forcing nonsupine positioning have shown modest ability to reduce apneas and daytime sleepiness. A number of studies have examined the efficacy of positional sleep devices, including posture alarms and specially designed pillows. Both modalities illustrated an ability to improve AHI in mild to moderate apnea sufferers, although more dramatically in the case of the pillows with a reduction of 17 events per hour compared to 5 (Cartwright et al., 1991; Zuberi, Rekab, & Nguyen, 2004). A follow-up trial conducted by Kushida and his colleagues replicated these changes observed in patients with mild apnea, but did not observe similar changes in patients suffering from severe OSA (Kushida et al., 1999). Although these strategies are valuable in that they target behaviors that are likely to moderate the severity of apnea with low risk of side effects, they fall short in their ability to mitigate daytime sleepiness and cognitive effects in clinically significant ways (Veasey et al., 2006).

Alternative Therapies

A relatively new and unorthodox treatment method for snoring and sleep apnea is didgeridoo training. Playing the didgeridoo, a wooden trumpet invented by indigenous Australians, requires exceptional strength and tone of upper airway muscles. Thus, by practicing and playing the instrument, patients strengthen the areas of their airway most likely to collapse during sleep. A 2005 study published in the *British Medical Journal* found that participants with moderate apnea assigned to a group receiving didgeridoo lessons experienced significant reductions in AHI, sleep disturbance, and daytime sleepiness after daily practice for 4 months (Puhan et al., 2005).

Another unconventional approach to apnea treatment is acupuncture. Friere and her colleagues (2007) completed a randomized trial of both manual and electronic acupuncture stimulation of posterior areas of the neck. The authors note that both forms of acupuncture corresponded with immediate reductions in AHI, microarousals, and respiratory events. The authors are currently investigating different methods of acupuncture delivery, the sustainability of clinical gains, and the relationship between treatment and endothelial factors.

These unconventional therapies have obviously not gained a level of support and clinical consensus comparable to PAP treatment or behavioral health interventions. Intuitively, didgeridoo training would be most effective in patients with apnea and snoring that is solely due to excessive softness in the palate and upper airway, not those many apnea sufferers for whom weight loss would mitigate their symptoms. If an individual is sufficiently motivated to engage in activity as frequently as the didgeridoo lessons described in the aforementioned study, they are likely to benefit from either an exercise and nutrition regimen, PAP treatment, or both. Exercise and weight loss, as well as increased oxygen saturation in the blood, would positively affect other health factors in addition to apnea.

Circadian Sleep Disorders

Circadian Sleep Disorders can be exceptionally receptive to behavioral therapies and other nonpharmacological or medical techniques. "Lifestyle modification" (Seligman, 1998) techniques are often sufficient to treat the most common etiological factors contributing to these disorders. Basic fundamentals of sleep hygiene, relaxation training, exercise, stress management, and avoidance of caffeine, alcohol, and afternoon naps can be a successful treatment regimen with these disorders.

Chronotherapy, whereby the body's rhythm is reset to match a desirable sleep/wake pattern, can be effective in treating sleep phase disorders or jet lag. Delayed Sleep Phase Disorder can also be treated through progressive phase advancement, whereby a patient's time in bed is scheduled and his or her bedtime is moved earlier in increments of 15 to 30 minutes (Seligman, 1998).

Narcolepsy

Narcolepsy management strategies have consisted, by and large, of strictly pharmacological regimens. The only exception to this rule is that practitioners have long recognized the benefits patients seem to experience from having two to three scheduled naps of 20 to 30 minutes daily (B. Sadock & V. Sadock, 2000; Anders, 1996, cited in Seligman, 1998). In some instances, planned napping is a sufficient treatment on its own. When additional treatments are deemed necessary, stimulants are normally prescribed in an attempt to manage daytime sleep attacks. Typically, these have included amphetamine, dextroamphetamine, and methylphenidate. Newer adrenergic receptor agonists, particularly Modafinil, have illustrated similar efficacy to their older counterparts with lower instances of side effects and tolerance (B. Sadock & V. Sadock, 2000).

The other major treatment consideration is the presence or absence of cataplexy in patients' presentation. Additional medications, including GHB (sodium oxybate) and tricyclic antidepressants, may be considered when cataplexy is a focus of clinical attention. It should be noted that, out of these drugs, only GHB has gained FDA approval for treatment of cataplexy in narcolepsy despite the fact that its mechanism of action is presently unknown (Epocrates, 2007; Guilliminault & Fromherz, 2005).

REM Sleep Behavior Disorder

REM sleep behavior disorder (RBD) management strategies are also typically pharmacological, but commonsense behavioral approaches can help reduce the risk of injury to both the patient and the bed partner. These include covering of doors or windows, surrounding the patient with pillows, and, in severe cases, tethering the individual to the bed or placing the mattress on the floor. In practice, however, many patients and their families try these methods on their own prior to seeking treatment.

Clonazepam has long been the most commonly prescribed medication in the management of RBD. Its efficacy has been illustrated in as many as 90% of patients without the potential for abuse and tolerance observed in other benzodiazepine preparations (Schenck & Mahowald, 1990). Continued treatment adherence is critical with benzodiazepine treatment, however, as relapse is reliably predicted by discontinuation.

Few other medications have received the same level of empirical support, but one of those is melatonin, which may be used as a stand-alone or adjunctive treatment in patients with clonazepam-refractory RBD (Boeve, Silber, & Ferman, 2003). Other medications with lesser levels of support include levodopa, carbamazepine, and MAO-I agents. Tricyclic antidepressants have been used in patients with RBD associated with narcolepsy. These myriad treatments are thought to represent the equally disparate proposed neurological mechanisms that play a role in RBD's etiology (Mahowald & Schenck, 2005).

Restless Leg/PLMD

A number of pharmacological treatments have been used in the treatment of Restless Leg Syndrome and Periodic Limb Movement Disorder with safety and efficacy. Primary among these drugs are dopaminergic agents, benzodiazepines, opioids, and anticonvulsants. Pharmacological treatments are generally not advised for the treatment of perinatal PLMD as it most often subsides a few weeks postpartum. Additionally, many mild sufferers of Restless Leg Syndrome or PLMD may not require treatment, especially in cases where microarousals are not present or infrequent.

Perhaps the greatest amount of evidence supports the use of dopamine agonists and precursors as they seem most able to reduce the number of observed PLMs and increase subjective sleep quality (Edinger, 2003) with lower risk of dependence commonly seen in benzodiazepines and opioids. Pramipexole is currently the only dopamine agonist FDA approved for treatment of PLMD, but bromocriptine has also been reviewed as an effective treatment (Edinger, 2003; Littner et al., 2004).

Opioids and anticonvulsants have also been used extensively as an off-label treatment for PLMD. Although they represent a relatively effective treatment of the symptoms of PLMD, caution is advised regarding their use. Specifically, the risk of dependency or crossover addiction in opioids is well known. Treatment with anticonvulsants also has its drawbacks, as many patients experience daytime somnolence, and a lesser number have decreased liver function (Epocrates, 2007).

Behavioral interventions for PLMD and Restless Leg Syndrome are unique to sleep medicine in that they target sleep quality as both a symptom and an etiological factor. Some therapies have attempted to affect the physiological etiology of PLMs without medication with mixed results. Thermal biofeedback, which teaches patients how to regulate the temperature of their limbs, showed ability to teach those skills without appreciable improvement in PLMs (Ancoli-Israel, Seifert, & Lemon, 1986), while Kovacevic-Ristanovic, Cartwright, and Lloyd (1991) were able to dramatically reduce incidence of limb movements through the use of a muscle stimulator. This technique was not able to improve sleep continuity, however.

Some techniques derived from those used to treat insomnia, such as CBT, sleep restriction, and avoidance of alcohol, caffeine, and nicotine have been used with moderate efficacy in some clients. The theory driving this practice came from Coleman, Pollack, and Weitzman's (1980) early work on the sequelae of PLMs within sleep disturbance. They posited that PLMs were actually consequent to disturbance, rather than the cause. In this sense, PLMD sufferers experience the same disruptions common among insomnia sufferers, but differently manifest. Indeed, a few studies seem to suggest that behavioral management strategies for insomnia increase sleep efficiency and decrease daytime sleepiness and napping in patients with PLMD. These studies are limited either by small sample sizes or the fact that they did not use PSG-assessed PLMs as an outcome variable. It is not currently known whether increasing PLM severity will decrease patients' response to behavioral interventions or whether there exists an ideal balance between these interventions and pharmacological therapies for any set of PLMD patients.

CONTRIBUTORS

Jennifer Goldschmied, BA, is currently a Behavioral Health Researcher at National Jewish Medical and Research Center in Denver, Colorado, investigating treatment methods for Obstructive Sleep Apnea Syndrome. Prior to assuming this position, she was a student research assistant at the Unit for Experimental Psychiatry at the University of Pennsylvania, studying the effects of chronic sleep deprivation. Her research experience includes work in neuroimaging and depression. Ms. Goldschmied may be contacted at 1400 Jackson Street B113, Denver, CO 80206. E-mail: j.goldschmied@gmail.com

Ryan Asherin, BA, is currently a Research Assistant for the Department of Psychiatry at The Children's Hospital in Aurora, Colorado. Prior to assuming this position, he was a Research Coordinator at the Department of Psychiatry at the University of Colorado Health and Science Center. He has been involved in various levels of psychiatric research relating to severe mental illness, neuroimaging, clinical drug trials, and early childhood intervention. He has been a contributing author on several articles, abstracts, and presentations regarding these topics. Mr. Asherin may be contacted at 11845 S.W. Walker Road, Portland, OR 97005. E-mail: ryan.asherin@gmail.com

Christopher E. Knoepke, MSW, is currently a Behavioral Researcher at National Jewish Medical & Research Center in Denver, Colorado. Prior to this position, he worked at the Center for Mental Health Services Research at Washington University in St. Louis investigating factors affecting mental health evaluation and medication management for children in the child welfare system. His clinical training and experience include outpatient community mental health, treatment of anxiety disorders, crisis assessment, psychosocial evaluation of correctional inmates, and sex offender treatment. Mr. Knoepke may be contacted at 1400 Jackson Street, B113, Denver, CO 80206. E-mail: cknoepke@gmail.com

Mark S. Aloia, PhD, is currently an Associate Professor of Medicine and the Director of Sleep Research at National Jewish Medical and Research Center in Denver, Colorado. Prior to assuming this position, he was an Assistant Professor of Psychiatry at Brown University in Providence, Rhode Island. Dr. Aloia's degree is in Clinical Psychology with specializations in Neuropsychology and Sleep. He is board certified in Behavioral Sleep Medicine and has received over $10 million in grant funding to pursue his research interests. He has authored numerous peer-reviewed papers focusing on findings methods to improve treatment response in patients with chronic sleep disorders. Dr. Aloia may be contacted at National Jewish Medical and Research Center, Denver, CO 80206. E-mail: aloiam@njc.org

RESOURCES

Aikens, J. E., & Mendleson, W. B. (1999). MMPI correlates of sleep and respiratory disturbances in obstructive sleep apnea. *Sleep, 22*(3), 362-369.

Aldrich, M. (1998). Diagnostic aspects of narcolepsy. *Neurology, 50*(Suppl. 1), S2-S7.

Allen, R., & Earley, C. (2001). Restless Legs Syndrome: A review of clinical and pathophysiologic features. *Journal of Clinical Neurophysiology, 18*(2), 128-147.

Aloia, M. S., Arnedt, J. T., Riggs, R. L., Hecht, J., & Borrelli, B. (2004). Clinical management of poor adherence to CPAP: Motivational enhancement. *Behavioral Sleep Medicine, 2*(4), 205-222.

Aloia, M. S., Arnedt, J. T., Smith, L., Skrekas, J., Stanchina, M., & Millman, R. P. (2005). Examining the construct of depression in obstructive sleep apnea syndrome. *Sleep Medicine, 6*(2), 115-121.

American Academy of Sleep Medicine. (2005). *International Classification of Sleep Disorders* (2nd ed.) Westchester, IL: Author.

American Psychiatric Association. (1994). *Diagnostic and Statistical Manual of Mental Disorders* (4th ed.). Washington, DC: Author.

Ancoli-Israel, S., Seifert, A. R., & Lemon, M. (1986). Thermal biofeedback and periodic movements in sleep: Patients' subjective reports and a case study. *Applied Psychophysiology and Biofeedback, 11*(3), 177-188.

Andrew, J. G., & Oei, T. P. S. (2004). The roles of depression and anxiety in the understanding and treatment of Obstructive Sleep Apnea Syndrome. *Clinical Psychology Review, 24,* 1031-1049.

Bastien, C. H., Morin, C. M., Ouellet, M. C., Blais, F. C., & Bouchard, S. (2004). Cognitive-behavioral therapy for insomnia: Comparison of individual therapy, group therapy, and telephone consultations. *Journal of Consulting and Clinical Psychology, 72*(4), 653-659.

Bastien, C., Vallieres, A., & Morin, C. (2001). Validation of the Insomnia Severity Index as an outcome measure for insomnia research. *Sleep Medicine, 2,* 297-307.

Benca, R. M., Obermeyer, W. H., Thisted, R. A., & Gilpen, J. C. (1992). Sleep and psychiatric disorders: A meta-analysis. *Archives of General Psychiatry, 49,* 651-668.

Boeve, B. F., Silber, M. H., & Ferman, T. J. (2003). Melatonin for treatment of REM sleep behavior disorder in neurologic disorders: Results in 14 patients. *Sleep Medicine, 4*(4), 281-284.

Boeve, B. F., Silber, M. H., Ferman, T. J., Kokmen, E., Smith, G. E., Ivnik, R. J., et al. (1998). REM sleep behavior disorder and degenerative dementia: An association likely reflecting Lewy body disease. *Neurology, 51*(2), 363-370.

Breslau, N., Kilbey, M. M., & Andreski, P. (1991). Nicotine dependence, major depression, and anxiety in young adults. *Archives of General Psychiatry, 48,* 1069-1074.

Breslau, N., Roth, T., Rosenthal, L., & Andreski, P. (1996). Sleep disturbance and psychiatric disorders: A longitudinal epidemiological study of young adults. *Biological Psychiatry, 39,* 411-418.

Buysse, D., Ancoli-Israel, S., Edinger, J., Lichstein, K., & Morin, C. (2006). Recommendations for a standard research assessment of insomnia. *Sleep, 29*(9), 1155–1173.

Buysse, D., Reynolds, C., Monk, T., Berman, S., & Kupfer, D. (1989). The Pittsburgh Sleep Quality Index: A new instrument for psychiatric practice and research. *Psychiatry Research, 28,* 193-213.

Carskadon, M., Dement, W., Mitler, M., Roth, T., Westbrook, P., & Keenan, S. (1986). Guidelines for the multiple sleep latency test (MSLT): A standard measure of sleepiness. *Sleep, 9*(4), 519-524.

Cartwright, R., Ruzicka-Ristanociv, F. D., Caldarelli, D., & Adler, G. (1991). A comparative study of treatments for positional sleep apnea. *Sleep, 14,* 546-552.

Coleman, R. M., Pollack, C. P., & Weitzman, E. D. (1980). Periodic movements in sleep (nocturnal myoclonus): Relation to sleep disorders. *Annals of Neurology, 8,* 416-421.

Coleman, R. M., Roffwarg, H. P., Kennedy, S. J., Guilleminault, C., Cinque, J., Cohn, M. A., et al. (1982). Sleep-wake disorders based on polysomnography diagnosis. A National Cooperative Study. *JAMA, 247,* 997-1003.

Davies, R., & Stradling, J. (1990). The relationship between neck circumference, radiographic pharyngeal anatomy, and the obstructive sleep apnoea syndrome. *European Respiratory Journal, 3,* 509-514.

Deegan, P., & McNicholas, W. (1996). Predictive value of clinical features for the obstructive sleep apnoea syndrome. *European Respiratory Journal, 9,* 117-124.

Eaton, W. W., Badawi, M., & Melton, B. (1995). Prodromes and precursors: Epidemiologic data for primary prevention of disorders with slow onset. *American Journal of Psychiatry, 152,* 967-972.

Edinger, J. D. (2003). Periodic limb movements: Assessment and management strategies. In M. L. Perlis & K. L. Lichstein, (Eds.), *Treating Sleep Disorders: Principles and Practice of Behavioral Sleep Medicine* (pp. 100-117). Hoboken, NJ: John Wiley & Sons.

Epocrates Rx Online (Web-based database on the Internet; continuous content updates). (2007). Retrieved November 15, 2007 from http://www.epocrates.com

Faccenda, J. F., Mackay, T. W., Boon, N. A., & Douglas, N. J. (2001). Randomized placebo-controlled trial of continuous positive airway pressure on blood pressure in the sleep apnea-hypopnea syndrome. *American Journal of Respiratory Critical Care, 163,* 344-348.

Ford, D. E., & Cooper-Patrick, L. (2001). Sleep disturbances and mood disorders: An epidemiologic perspective. *Depression and Anxiety, 14,* 3-6.

Ford, D. E., & Kamerow, D. B. (1989). Epidemiologic study of sleep disturbances and psychiatric disorders. An opportunity for prevention? *JAMA, 262,* 1479-1484.

Friere, A. O., Sugai, G. C., Chrispin, F. S., Togeiro, S. M., Yamamura, Y., Mello, L. E., & Tufik, S. (2007). Treatment of moderate obstructive sleep apnea syndrome with acupuncture: A randomized, placebo-controlled pilot trial. *Sleep Medicine, 8*(1), 43-50.

Germain, A., Shear, M. K., Hall, M., & Buysse, D. J. (2007). Effects of a brief behavioral treatment for PTSD-related sleep disturbances: A pilot study. *Behaviour Research and Therapy, 45,* 627-632.

Gierz, M., Campbell, S., & Gillin, J. C. (1987). Sleep disturbances in various nonaffective psychiatric disorders. *Psychiatric Clinics of North America, 10*(4), 565-581.

Giles, D. E., Jarrett, R. B., Biggs, M. M., Guzick, D. S., & Rush, A. J. (1989). Clinical predictors of recurrence in depression. *American Journal of Psychiatry, 146,* 764-767.

Gillberg, M., Kecklund, G., & Akerstedt, T. (1994). Relations between performance and subjective ratings of sleepiness during a night awake. *Sleep, 17,* 236-241.

Griez, E. J. L., Lousberg, H., van den Hout, M. A., & van der Molen, G. M. (1987). CO_2 vulnerability in panic disorder. *Psychiatry Research, 20,* 87-95.

Guilliminault, C., & Fromherz, S. (2005). Narcolepsy: Diagnosis and management. In M. H. Kryger, T. Roth, & W. C. Dement (Eds.), *Principles and Practice of Sleep Medicine* (pp. 780-790). Philadelphia: Elsevier Saunders.

Hoddes, E., Zarcone, V., Smythe, H., Phillips, R., & Dement, W. C. (1973). Quantification of sleepiness: A new approach. *Psychophysiology, 10,* 431-436.

Hoffstein, V., & Szalai, J. (1993). Predictive value of clinical features in diagnosing obstructive sleep apnea. *Sleep, 16*(2), 118-122.

Horne, J., & Östberg, O. (1976). A self-assessment questionnaire to determine morningness-eveningness in human circadian rhythms. *International Journal of Chronobiology, 4,* 97-110.

Hurwitz, T. D., Engdahl, B. E., Eberly, R., & Mahowald, M. W. (1997). Treatment of obstructive sleep apnea with continuous positive airway pressure is associated with improvement in symptoms of posttraumatic stress disorder in former WWII prisoners of war. *Sleep Research, 26,* 378.

Johns, M. (1991). A new method for measuring daytime sleepiness: The Epworth sleepiness scale. *Sleep, 14*(6), 540-545.

Kovacevic-Ristanovic, R., Cartwright, R. D., & Lloyd, S. (1991). Nonpharmacologic treatment of periodic leg movements in sleep. *Archives of Physical Medical Rehabilitation, 72*(6), 385-389.

Kryger, M. H., Walid, R., & Manfreda, L. (2002). Diagnoses received by narcolepsy patients in the year prior to diagnosis by a sleep specialist. *Sleep, 25*(1), 35-41.

Kushida, C. A., Rao, S., Guilliminault, C., Giraudo, S., Hsieh, J., Hyde, P., et al. (1999). Cervical positioning effects on snoring and apneas. *Sleep Research Online, 2*(1), 7-10.

Littner, M. R., Kushida, C., Anderson, W. M., Bailey, D., Berry, R. B., Hirshkowitz, M., et al. (2004). Practice parameters for the dopaminergic treatment of restless legs syndrome and periodic limb movement disorder. *Sleep, 27*(3), 557-559.

Man, G. (1996). Obstructive sleep apnea - diagnosis and treatment. *Medical Clinics of North America, 80*(4), 803-821.

Mahowald, M. W., & Schenck, C. H. (2005). REM sleep parasomnias. In M. H. Kryger, T. Roth, & W. C. Dement (Eds.), *Principles and Practice of Sleep Medicine* (pp. 897-916). Philadelphia: Elsevier Saunders.

McCall, W. V., Reboussin, B. A., & Cohen, W. (2000). Subjective measurement of insomnia and quality of life in depressed inpatients. *Journal of Sleep Research, 9,* 43-48.

Mendelson, W. B. (2005). Hypnotic medications: Mechanisms of action and pharmacologic effects. In M. H. Kryger, T. Roth, & W. C. Dement (Eds.). *Principles and Practice of Sleep Medicine* (pp. 444-451). Philadelphia: Elsevier Saunders.

Monti, J., & Monti, D. (2005). Sleep disturbance in schizophrenia. *International Review of Psychiatry, 17*(4), 247-253.

Montplaisir, J., Boucher, S., Poirier, G., Lavigne, G., Lapierre, O., & Lesperance, P. (1997). Clinical, polysomnographic, and genetic characteristics of restless legs syndrome: A study of 133 patients diagnosed with new standard criteria. *Movement Disorders, 12,* 61-65.

Morgenthaler, T., Kapen, S., Lee-Chiong, T., Alessi, C., Boehlecke, B., Brown, T., et al. (2006). Practice parameters for the medical therapy of obstructive sleep apnea. *Sleep, 29*(8), 1031-1035.

Morgenthaler, T., Kramer, M., Alessi, C., Friedman, L., Boehlecke, B., Brown, T., et al. (2006). Practice parameters for the psychological and behavioral treatment of insomnia: An update. An American Academy of Sleep Medicine Report. *Sleep, 29*(11), 1415-1419.

Morin, C. M. (2006). Cognitive-behavioral therapy of insomnia. *Sleep Medicine Clinics, 1,* 375-386.

Morin, C. M., Bootzin, R. R., Buysse, D. J., Edinger, J. D., Espie, C. A., & Lichstein, K. L. (2006). Psychological and behavioral treatment of insomnia: Update of the recent evidence (1998-2004). *Sleep, 29*(11), 1398-1414.

Morin C. M., & Espie, C. A. (2003). *Insomnia: A Clinical Guide to Assessment and Treatment.* New York: Kluwer Academic/Plenum Publishers.

Moscovitch, A., Partinen, M., & Guilleminault, C. (1993). The positive diagnosis of narcolepsy and narcolepsy's borderland. *Neurology, 43,* 55-60.

National Heart Lung and Blood Institute. (2006a). *Facts About Insomnia.* Retrieved July 31, 2008 from http://www.nhlbi.nih.gov/health/public/sleep/inso/inso_whatis.html

National Heart Lung and Blood Institute. (2006b). *Facts About Narcolepsy.* Retrieved July 31, 2008 from http://www.nhlbi.nih.gov/health/dci/Diseases/nar/nar_what.html

National Heart Lung and Blood Institute. (2008). *Facts About Sleep Apnea*. Retrieved July 31, 2008 from http://www.nhlbi.nih.gov/health/dci/Diseases/SleepApnea/SleepApnea_WhatIs.html

National Institute of Mental Health. (2001, February 21). The Numbers Count: Mental Disorders in America, Anxiety Disorders. Retrieved July 31, 2008 from http://www.nimh.nih.gov/publicat/numbers.cfm

National Institutes of Health, National Institute of Neurological Disorders and Stroke. (2007, June 22). NINDS Sleep Apnea Information Page. Retrieved July 31, 2008 from http://www.ninds.nih.gov/disorders/sleep_apnea/sleep_apnea.htm

National Sleep Foundation. (2002). *"Sleep in America" Poll*. Retrieved July 31, 2008 from http://www.sleepfoundation.org/site/c.huIXKjM0IxF/b.2417355/k.143E/2002_Sleep_in_America_Poll.htm

Netzer, N., Stoohs, R., Netzer, C., Clark, K., & Strohl, K. (1999). Using the Berlin Questionnaire to identify patients at risk for the sleep apnea syndrome. *Annals of Internal Medicine, 131,* 485-491.

Nordgard, S., Hein, G., Stene, B. K., Skjostad, K. W., & Maurer, J. T. (2007). One-year results: Palatal implants for the treatment of obstructive sleep apnea. *Otolaryngtology - Head and Neck Surgery, 136*(5), 818-822.

Ohayon, M. M. (2000). Prevalence of hallucinations and their pathological associations in the general population. *Psychiatry Research, 97*(2), 153-164.

Ohayon, M. M. (2003). The effects of breathing-related sleep disorders on mood disturbances in the general population. *Journal of Clinical Psychiatry, 64*(10), 1195-1200.

Ohayon, M. M., & Shapiro, C. M. (2000). Sleep disturbances and psychiatric disorders associated with posttraumatic stress disorder in the general population. *Comprehensive Psychiatry, 41,* 469-478.

Ozaki, S., Uchiyama, M., Shirakawa, S., & Okawa, M. (1996). Prolonged interval from body temperature nadir to sleep offset in patients with delayed sleep phase syndrome. *Sleep, 19,* 36-40.

Papp, L. A., Klein, D. F., & Gorman, J. M. (1993). Carbon dioxide hypersensitivity, hyperventilation, and panic disorder. *American Journal of Psychiatry, 150,* 1149-1157.

Puhan, M. A., Suarez, A., Lo Cascio, C., Zahn, A., Heitz, M., & Braendli, O. (2005). Didgeridoo playing as alternative treatment for obstructive sleep apnea syndrome: Randomized controlled trial. *British Medical Journal, 332*(7536), 266-270.

Romanow, J. H., & Catalano, P. J. (2006). Initial U.S. pilot study: Palatal implants for the treatment of snoring. *Otolaryngtology - Head and Neck Surgery, 134*(4), 551-557.

Sadeh, A., Hauri, P., Kripke, D., & Lavie, P. (1995). The role of actigraphy in the evaluation of sleep disorders. *Sleep, 18*(4), 288-302.

Sadock, B., & Sadock V. (2000). *Comprehensive Textbook of Psychiatry* (7th ed.). Philadelphia, PA: Lippincott, Williams & Wilkins.

Schenck, C. H., & Mahowald, M. W. (1990). Polysomnographic, neurologic, psychiatric, and clinical outcome report on 70 consecutive cases with REM sleep behavior disorder (RBD): Sustained clonazepam efficacy in 89.5% of 57 treated patients. *Cleveland Clinic Journal of Medicine, 57,* S9-S23.

Schenck, C. H., & Mahowald, M. W. (1996). REM sleep parasomnias. *Neurologic Clinics, 14*(4), 697-720.

Schramm, E., Hohagen, F., Grasshoff, U., Riemann, D., Hajak, G., Weess, H. G., et al. (1993). Test-retest reliability and validity of the Structured Interview for Sleep Disorders according to *DSM-III-R. American Journal of Psychiatry, 150*(6), 867-872.

Schroder, M., & O'Hara, R. (2005). Depression and Obstructive Sleep Apnea (OSA). *Annals of General Psychiatry, 4,* 13-30.

Seligman, L. (1998). *Selecting Effective Treatments: A Comprehensive, Systematic Guide to Treating Mental Disorders.* San Fransisco: Jossey-Bass.

Sharafkhaneh, A., Giray, N., Richardson, P., Young, T., & Hirshkowitz, M. (2005). Association of psychiatric disorders and sleep apnea in a large cohort. *Sleep, 28,* 1405-1411.

Sher, A. E., Schechtman, K. B., & Piccirillo, J. F. (1996). The efficacy of surgical modifications of the upper airway in adults with obstructive sleep apnea syndrome. *Sleep, 19*(2), 156-177.

Spoormaker, V. I., & van den Bout, J. (2005). Depression and anxiety complaints: Relations with sleep disturbances. *European Psychiatry, 20,* 243-245.

Stiasny, K., Oertel, W., & Trenkwalder, C. (2002). Clinical symptomatology and treatment of restless legs syndrome and periodic limb movement disorder. *Sleep Medicine Reviews, 6,* 253–265.

Szuba, M. P., Dinges, J. D., & Kloss, D. F. (2003). *Insomnia: Principles and Management.* Cambridge, UK: Cambridge University Press.

Tan, T. L., Kales, J. D., Kales, A., Soldatos, C. R., & Bixler, E. O. (1984). Biopsychobehavioral correlates of insomnia, IV: Diagnosis based on *DSM-III. American Journal of Psychiatry, 141,* 357-362.

Tasali, E., & Van Cauter, E. (2002). Sleep disordered breathing and the current epidemic of obesity: Consequence or a contributing factor. *American Journal of Respiratory and Critical Care Medicine, 165,* 562-563.

Vandeputte, M., & de Weerd, A. (2003). Sleep disorders and depressive feelings: A global survey with the Beck depression scale. *Sleep Medicine, 4*(4), 343-345.

Veasey, S. C., Guilleminault, C., Strohl, K. P., Sanders, M. H., Ballard, R. D., & Magalang, U. J. (2006). Medical therapy for obstructive sleep apnea: A review by the medical therapy for obstructive sleep apnea task force of the standards of the practice committee of the American Academy of Sleep Medicine. *Sleep, 29*(8), 1036-1044.

Vgontzas, A., & Kales, A. (1999). Sleep and its disorders. *Annual Review of Medicine, 50,* 387-400.

Walker-Engstrom, M. L., Ringqvist, I., Vestling, O., Wilhelmsson, B., & Tegelberg, A. (2003). A prospective randomized study comparing two different degrees of mandibular advancement with a dental appliance in treatment of severe obstructive sleep apnea. *Sleep and Breathing, 7*(3), 119-130.

Walker-Engstrom, M. L., Tegelberg, A., Wilhelmsson, B., & Ringqvist, I. (2002). 4-year follow-up of treatment with dental appliance or uvulopalatopharyngoplasty in patients with obstructive sleep apnea. *Chest, 121*(3), 1511-1518.

Weaver, T. (2001). Outcome measurement in sleep medicine practice and research. Part 1: Assessment of symptoms, subjective and objective daytime sleepiness, health-related quality of life and functional status. *Sleep Medicine Reviews, 5*(2), 103-128.

Youakim, J. M., Doghramji, K., & Schutte, S. L. (1998). Posttraumatic stress disorder and obstructive sleep apnea syndrome. *Psychosomatics, 39*(2), 168-171.

Young, T., Peppard, P., Palta, M., Hla, K. M., Finn, L., Morgan, B., et al. (1997). Population-based study of sleep-disordered breathing as a risk factor for hypertension. *Archives of Internal Medicine, 157*(15), 1746-1752.

Young, T., Peppard, P. E., & Taheri, S. (2005). Excess weight and sleep-disordered breathing. *Journal of Applied Physiology, 99*, 1592-1599.

Zuberi, N., Rekab, K., & Nguyen, H. (2004). Sleep apnea avoidance pillow effects on obstructive sleep apnea syndrome and snoring. *Sleep & Breathing, 8*, 201-207.

Biofeedback and Psychotherapy: Technology in the Clinical Setting

Jennifer Minkin, Maurice F. Prout, and Frank Masterpasqua

THE EMERGING DIRECTION IN PSYCHOTHERAPY: TIME TO GET TECHNICAL

Technology is an area that has been making tremendous strides worldwide – especially within the last decade – and its advancements are predicted to expand at an ever-increasing pace. Within this age of technology, the development of technological applications has also begun to make its way into the world of psychotherapy. Current indicators of this trend include the emergence of self-help Internet sites, computer-administered psychotherapy, virtual reality psychotherapy, interactive voice messaging systems, adjunctive palmtop computer psychotherapy, online support groups, and biofeedback. To date, researchers suggest that technology can offer several advantages to both the clinician and the patient in the clinical setting, such as providing more objective and precise information, as well as improved assessment and treatment outcomes; it is also suggested that increased patient motivation and compliance to treatment are likely to ensue as well (Newman, 2004).

These recent insights mark only the beginning of an era of psychotherapy and technology merging together, as many predict its integration is a direction rich with vast potential. However, as with any newer field of study, further research is still needed to gain insight into the full range of its therapeutic advantages. Despite the limited literature available thus far, researchers suggest that this integration of technology and psychotherapy is a highly promising avenue for the future of psychology and is expected to continue to grow substantially over the next decade or so (Newman, 2004).

BIOFEEDBACK: AN EMERGING FIELD IN THE AGE OF TECHNOLOGY

As mentioned above, biofeedback has been part of this evolving technological movement. Still considered a newly emerging field, the application of biofeedback within the professional health care arena surfaced only a little over 3 decades ago. Within this relatively short span of time, much focus of research has been directed toward investigating the efficacy of biofeedback therapy in itself as a means of treatment (Little, 2006). Many practitioners have also placed significant focus on incorporating a variety of therapeutic interventions in conjunction with biofeedback therapy (Schwartz, 1999), using biofeedback therapy as a complementary intervention along with the ongoing application of other treatment approaches. For the purposes of this contribution, attention will be directed toward using biofeedback instrumentation as a tool to *enhance* the effectiveness of traditional psychological assessment methods and interventions.

The psychophysiological information provided by biofeedback can be a beneficial adjunct to psychotherapeutic approaches on multiple levels. Within the clinical setting, "physiological responses can be detected and used to explore underlying physiological pathologies of psychological disorders as well as effective strategies for monitoring treatment progress and outcome" (Larkin, 2006, p. 165). In other words, the detection of covert psychological and physiological functioning displayed in objective, concrete measures can help clinicians generate more precise and comprehensive diagnoses, gain deeper insight into contributing factors of symptoms, choose more appropriate interventions that are better tailored to meet the specific needs of each individual clinical presentation, and better monitor the rate and degree of patient progression over the course of treatment.

For the patient, the ongoing feedback can enhance self-awareness and insight into factors affecting psychophysiological functioning, as well as facilitate the learning of behavioral skills in a more effective and efficient manner. In addition, the immediate concrete feedback of even subtle changes achieved during the treatment can serve to instill a greater sense of motivation, confidence, hope, self-efficacy, and sense of empowerment within the patient – which may subsequently lead to greater compliance to treatment and an overall more pleasurable therapeutic experience (Newman, 2004).

Overall, integrating biofeedback methods into existing assessment and intervention methods can be used as a means to reveal additional valuable information that may otherwise be inaccessible, which ultimately can help improve diagnostic and therapeutic outcomes of existing psychotherapeutic approaches. Further discussion of the advantages that biofeedback can bring to psychotherapy will be explored in more detail below following a brief overview of biofeedback and how it works in conjunction with psychology and physiology.

WHAT THE TECHNOLOGY REVEALS: AN OVERVIEW OF PSYCHO-PHYSIOLOGY AND BIOFEEDBACK

Psychophysiology refers to the study of the relationship and connections between the mind and bodily processes (Wickramasekera, 1976). Elmer Green (as cited in Schwartz & Andrasik, 2003), considered by many researchers to have been a key figure within the evolution of the field of biofeedback, explains that the psychophysiological principle is based on the notion that every change in the physiological state is accompanied by a change in the cognitive-emotional state. This change can be conscious or unconscious. Similarly, every change in the cognitive-emotional state – whether conscious or unconscious – is accompanied by a change in the physiological state. In other words, the core concept within the psychophysiological principle is based on the notion that the mind and body are connected and that changes in bodily functioning can cause or reflect changes in mental processes and behavior and vice versa. Thus, not only can the body reveal information about ongoing psychological elements (including psychological processes that may be difficult to access or out of conscious awareness), but changes in physiological processes can subsequently alter other cognitive and emotional processes (e.g., raising finger temperature can induce relaxation of the autonomic nervous system, simultaneously resulting in more relaxed cognitions and behaviors). Similarly, changes in mental processes can ultimately manifest changes in physiological functioning as well.

Rooted in the concept of psychophysiology, applied psychophysiology refers to the scientific study of the interrelationships of physiologic and psychological processes for diagnostic and therapeutic goals for individuals. In a general sense, it refers to a discipline that uses scientific knowledge – primarily psychophysiology – to facilitate change in physiological functioning. Schwartz (1999) explains that the term "applied psychophysiology" incorporates multiple facets, including assessment, diagnosis, education, treatment, and performance training. He states, "Applied psychophysiology includes a group of interventions and evaluation methods with the exclusive or primary intentions of understanding and effecting changes that help humans move toward and maintain healthier physiological functioning" (p. 5).

Rooted in the mind-body relationship and applied psychophysiology, the term "biofeedback" was coined around 40 years ago; since then, the term has been defined in various ways. Basmajian (as cited in I. Saito & Y. Saito, 2004) defined biofeedback as a technique to convey internal physiological processes to individuals to facilitate their manipulation of involuntary and imperceptible processes via auditory or visual signal equipment. E. E. Green, A. M. Green, and Norris (as cited in I. Saito & Y. Saito, 2004) defined biofeedback from a psychosomatic stance, stating that biofeedback is a method to assist patients in learning psychosomatic self-regulation. Schwartz and Beatty (as cited in I. Saito & Y. Saito, 2004) defined biofeedback as the use of electrical and electromechanical equipment as a means of providing information about physiological functioning; they explained that the ongoing information about psychophysiological processes and/or behaviors as they occur moment-to-moment displayed via biofeedback equipment are used to help regulate subsequent physical and psychological functioning (I. Saito & Y. Saito, 2004; Schwartz, 1999). Tortora and Anagnostakos (1990) offer yet another description of biofeedback: "In simplest terms, biofeedback is a process in which people get constant signals, or feedback, about various visceral biological functions. . . . By using special monitoring devices, they can control these visceral functions consciously to a limited degree" (p. 459).

In general, one of the most significant contributions of biofeedback research is its finding that the autonomic nervous system is in fact not entirely automatic, as studies have shown that visceral responses can be consciously regulated to some degree (Tortora & Anagnostakos, 1990). Thus, a key aspect of biofeedback that makes it such an invaluable technique is that it provides access to many psychophysiological processes once believed to be inaccessible and involuntary in nature. With the detection of such covert processes via highly technological measuring equipment, biofeedback enables more conscious control and regulation of these processes, thereby providing the individual the ability to achieve greater control over his or her overall health and well-being (AAPB, 2008).

BIOFEEDBACK:
HOW DOES IT WORK?

Biofeedback is considered a safe, noninvasive training technique geared toward helping individuals regulate mental and bodily processes by using signals from their own body to enhance both physical and psychological functioning. Based on the concept of the interrelationship of mental and physical processes, self-regulation of psychophysiological responses is achieved via ongoing feedback of such processes as they are recorded and displayed by measuring equipment. This self-regulation is a dynamic process; the individual gains the ability to regulate normally covert or unfelt internal processes by learning how to manipulate the signals displayed on the equipment from the attached sensors (Basmajian, 1989). Such displays enable individuals to observe subtle, internal psychophysiological responses usually difficult to detect, which can serve to help individuals acquire greater awareness - and subsequently greater voluntary control - over those responses.

Researchers posit that this increase of control of physiological functioning is a result of instrumental learning as the continuous feedback of changes acts as reinforcement for continued changes in either the same or opposite direction; in other words, autonomic behavior can be instrumentally conditioned within a stimulus-reinforcement paradigm (Hugdahl, 2001). The basis for these concepts evolved through the works of several key pioneers. Described in a publication by Kimble in 1961 (as cited in Hugdahl, 2001), it was suggested based on traditional learning theory that the conditioning of autonomic responses could be accomplished only via classical conditioning. In addition, Skinner's publication in 1953 asserted that instrumental, operant conditioning could be applied only to voluntary behavior (as cited in Hugdahl, 2001). However, contrary to these earlier studies, evidence of operant conditioning of autonomic responses was discovered as a result of Miller's work in 1964, in which he demonstrated the operant conditioning of blood pressure in rats. His discovery first opened the door for further research investigating the notion that humans could indeed regulate autonomic processes once believed to be involuntary in nature (Hugdahl, 2001).

Specifically, the mechanism of change within biofeedback is based on learning principles. The technological feedback provided by the sensors is represented by auditory cues and/or visual imagery. As the feedback cues enable both the clinician and patient to observe and monitor shifts in the patient's internal physiological processes as they occur, a greater awareness of these subtle internal processes is achieved, which can then facilitate improved ability to regulate those responses. Highly specific responses can be achieved that may otherwise not be possible without the technological feedback provided by the equipment; for example, an individual can learn how to relax individual muscles or raise finger temperature through the ongoing feedback cues (Little, 2006). This information is used by both the clinician and the patient to help gauge and direct the course and progress of treatment.

Biofeedback can be applied using a variety of measuring instruments, each used to feed back information about the body to help make changes in the body. Along with the technological advancements that have been made, more complicated electronic equipment has been developed that can detect internal bodily processes with far greater sensitivity and precision than a person can typically detect alone. This type of biofeedback instrumentation is composed of monitors that are secured to various parts of the body to detect and feed back vital internal bodily processes via a range of auditory and visual signals. The physiological processes that are most commonly measured with technological equipment include muscular tension, skin temperature, and sweat gland activity. Electromyographic (EMG) biofeedback is used to measure striate muscle tension, thermal biofeedback to measure peripheral skin temperature, and electrodermal activity (EDA) or galvanic skin response (GSR) to measure the electrical conductance on the skin. Other physiological activities also commonly measured in the clinical setting include cardiac measures (e.g., heart rate, blood volume pulse), respiration and breathing variables, and electrical brain activity (Little, 2006; Schwartz, 1999).

The ultimate goal of biofeedback is the self-detection of positive internal changes and generalization of self-regulatory skills within one's natural environment without the use of measuring instruments (Meichenbaum, 1976). In essence, the aim is for the individual to acquire a greater awareness of and connection with his or her own psychophysiology, as well as an improved ability to regulate and manage dynamic psychological and physical states as they arise in daily life experiences.

BIOFEEDBACK-ASSISTED PSYCHOTHERAPY: ASSESSMENT AND THERAPEUTIC BENEFITS

Biofeedback and psychophysiological monitoring can provide a range of benefits within clinical psychology, including its application to facilitate assessment, diagnosis, and treatment. Hugdahl (2001) further highlights this notion, stating that when exploring the uses of psychophysiology in clinical practice, a distinction should be made between using psychophysiological measurements for assessing the effectiveness of diagnosis and treatment and using psychophysiological methods directly for treatment purposes.

BIOFEEDBACK: FOR ASSESSMENT PURPOSES

Comprehensive and accurate assessment, in the initial stages and throughout the therapeutic process, is a vital element for both researchers and clinicians as it can play a key role in generating accurate diagnoses, choosing optimal treatment plans, monitoring the efficacy and progress of treatment, and determining treatment outcomes. The more precise the understanding of the nature and degree of symptoms experienced by the individual, the more accurate the diagnosis and appropriate treatment goals that can be established by the clinician. In a similar fashion, oversight of critical elements within a clinical presentation may lead to inaccurate or incomplete diagnoses, as well as the implementation of ineffective or even harmful therapeutic approaches.

In noting the importance of a thorough, comprehensive assessment, biofeedback instrumentation can be an invaluable aid for assessment and diagnostic purposes on multiple levels for both the clinician and the patient. "Assessment of psychophysiological reactions opens unique ways of understanding cognitive and emotional processes and provides insights that cannot be obtained by behavioral observation, interview, or questionnaire" (Wilhelm, Schneider, & Friedman, 2006, p. 201).

A core concept underlying the rationale for the additional benefit of using psychophysiological assessment for psychological disorders – especially anxiety disorders – is based on the three-systems model described in the work of Lang, Rachman, and Hodgson (as cited in Hugdahl, 2001). This model is based on Lang's theory, which posits that an emotional reaction has three components: a subjective experience, overt behavior, and physiological reactions. Due to the notion that every individual may be differentially sensitive to the three aspects of an anxiety response, it can be argued that clinical assessment should then involve measurements to address all three aspects. The three-systems approach for assessing anxiety disorders may reveal a more comprehensive picture of critical elements involved in each unique clinical presentation, thereby facilitating the ability to generate more accurate diagnoses and tailoring optimal treatment plans.

In general, the nature of the feedback – objective, concrete, and continuous psychophysiological measurements – can help provide further insight into the range of factors that may be contributing to the reported symptomology (Newman, 2004) as well as detect additional symptoms present that may otherwise go undetected – all in a manner that may more easily be conveyed by the clinician and more easily received by the patient. Furthermore, the scientific methodology involved in biofeedback technology can also add to the amount and precision of the information retrieved during the assessment process. Newman (2004) asserts that there is evidence that "technology can gather information of greater quantity and higher quality than clinician-administered assessments" (p. 142); this may include factors such as disclosure about sensitive areas (e.g., criminal history, sexual disorders, suicidality), as well as information that may be out of conscious awareness.

A specific structured approach of psychophysiological assessment is termed psychophysiological stress profiling (PSP). Within PSP, the clinician presents a series of stressors and recovery periods to the patient while he or she is attached to multiple biofeedback sensors in an effort to monitor various measures of physiological processes. The aim of the PSP is to identify specific stressors that induce stronger responses and/or psychophysiological systems or behaviors that are excessively reactive. The clinician is interested in determining not only the degree of reactivity to various forms of stressors, but also evaluating the patient's ability to recover after exposure to a stressor. In other words, the focus of the assessment is to determine how much the patient reacts to stressors and how quickly he or she adapts to and recovers from the impact of stressors and/or perceived threats. Patterns that are detected – including patterns of system activation and rate of recovery – can serve as helpful predictors of response to various interventions to alleviate degrees of reactions to stressors and enhance coping skills to better manage stress reactions. The rationale in using a PSP is based on the notion that the psychophysiological information conveyed through the assessment can help provide the clinician and patient with an additional understanding into the nature of the patient's unique ways of responding to stress.

Overall, the objective, psychophysiological information retrieved via biofeedback-assisted assessment can provide invaluable information that can be used to aid in the process of diagnosis, development and monitoring of treatment, and evaluation of treatment efficacy. More in-depth discussion into the nature of the information retrieved via biofeedback will be presented in this contribution to further illustrate how biofeedback can assist in providing a more holistic, comprehensive picture of the dynamic interrelationship among cognitions, physiology, and behavior.

Assessing the Effects of Cognitions on the Body

In traditional cognitive-behavioral therapy, much attention is geared toward identifying and monitoring cognitions in an effort to facilitate the development of healthier, more adaptive cognitive processes; strategies included in the cognitive-behavioral approach include cognitive restructuring, thought stopping, reframing, guided self-dialogue, and affirmations (Barlow, 2001). Specifically, cognitive behavioral interventions focus primarily on cognitions and overt behaviors; changes in psychophysiology may be assumed, but do not constitute the core element of treatment (Schwartz, 1999). Based on the notion that cognitions, physiology, and behavior are interrelated systems of functioning within the autonomic nervous system, using biofeedback to monitor physiological processes in relation to cognitions can help reveal information regarding the nature and impact of specific cognitions, as well as the impact of altering cognitive processes. Schwartz (1999) supports this idea, stating that practitioners who incorporate psychophysiologic interventions recognize the impact that regulation of psychophysiology can have on cognitions. Along the same lines, these practitioners also recognize the importance of changing cognitions in an attempt to change psychophysiological symptoms.

This concept was demonstrated in a study by Kremsdorf, Kochanowicz, and Costell (1981) in which they conducted two single-case design experiments to compare the effectiveness of biofeedback versus cognitive coping techniques for treating tension headaches. Although the findings suggested that emphasis on the modifying cognitive activity was the more efficient treatment for reducing tension headaches, the authors asserted that biofeedback may be valuable for investigating the physiological consequences of particular cognitive processes and in identifying specific cognitions with anxiety-provoking properties. Kremsdorf et al. (1981) state:

Biofeedback technology, in fact, may provide a singularly useful clinical tool with which to study the relationship between cognitive activity and resulting physiological arousal. An individual can receive direct and immediate feedback regarding his/her efforts to modify the cognitive activity that affects physiological responding. Also, the feedback of the body states offers an opportunity to identify particular cognitive processes that have anxiety-provoking properties. (p. 100)

Overall, the central goal in cognitive therapy is identifying thoughts that are maladaptive and replacing them with healthier ways of thinking. As illustrated above, biofeedback can help achieve both of those goals, as it can be a useful tool for assessing the quality and impact of specific cognitions; the psychophysiological information retrieved via ongoing monitoring can serve not only to assist the clinician and patient in detecting existing maladaptive cognitive processes, but also can help decipher healthier, more adaptive ways of thinking to benefit the patient's overall daily functioning and sense of well-being. Thus, biofeedback can serve as an invaluable tool in reflecting the nature and impact of cognitions, thereby helping to decipher the optimal direction in which changes can be made for the individual at hand.

More Than Words:
Physiology Can Reveal Psychology

Although cognitive therapy can be very effective for a range of problems and symptoms, some individuals experience internal conflicts and psychological issues that are beyond conscious awareness. In the latter case, working solely at the cognitive level may not suffice. Instead, attention directed toward physiological functioning may be more effective in accessing unconscious information. The rationale for working at a physiological level to address psychological processes is based on the psychophysiological principle referred to earlier, explaining that bodily functioning can reflect conscious or unconscious emotions; thus, for emotions that may be difficult to access, working with an individual's physiology as an alternate approach may be helpful.

Based on the notion that biofeedback equipment can measure and feed back covert physiological functioning that may be inaccessible otherwise, it seems plausible to suggest that biofeedback can be a valuable aid in accessing information stored in the body. In support of this concept, Little (2006) explains that biofeedback "helps bring into awareness unconscious thoughts and feelings that get expressed through the body, leading to potentially maladaptive ways of being and relating. As a therapeutic tool, biofeedback can provide a deeper level of self-understanding and control" (p. 1). Basmajian (1989) further explains that whether psychophysiological responses are exaggerated or reduced, biofeedback can serve as an adjunctive tool in providing an individual with information that can help facilitate the restoration or reinforcement of covert psychophysiological responses that may otherwise be difficult to access. In other words, access to deeper emotions found within the body can ultimately help shift or transform the nature and degree of the emotional experience within the individual.

In addition to helping reveal unconscious emotions, the nature of the measurements via biofeedback helps bring a degree of objectivity to this otherwise complex and vague area. Werbach (1977) makes reference to the objectivity biofeedback brings in conjunction with the surfacing of unconscious processes, stating, "in contrast to traditional psychotherapy, the information fed back is derived from the monitoring of physiologic events and provides an objective 'window' into the unconscious" (p. 376). He further posits: "When repressed thoughts or feelings, whether historic or transferential, have covertly altered physiologic activities, recognition of these cues through biofeedback may promote awareness of the repressed material" (Werbach, 1977, p. 378). As continuous feedback of physiological processes is made accessible to the clinician and patient, recognition of the internal cues that relate to changes in the moment may ensue that otherwise may be inaccessible through talk therapy alone.

In relation to this notion, Murphy (as cited in Werbach, 1977) mentions experimental literature exploring perceptual distortions of memory and thought which result as a coping mechanism to avoid awareness of stressful information. "He notes, for example, how a person may limit perceptual input by avoiding scanning of stressful images or by creating 'noise' through an increase in muscle tension, and suggest that biofeedback, by opening channels of information, may aid in overcoming self-deception" (p. 378). Thus, biofeedback can help break through the barriers of defenses – helping to make the unconscious conscious and allow for deeper emotional processing.

However, clinicians must be cognizant of the need to delve into repressed material in a careful, deliberate manner. "Adverse effects are possible . . . as they are with any other derepressive technique, when the process proceeds faster than the patient's ability to tolerate the resultant anxiety. Such effects would include psychotic reactions and depression" (Werbach, 1977, p. 380). Thus, although biofeedback can help reveal information that may have otherwise been inaccessible at the conscious level, exposing that delicate information must be done in a manner tolerable for the patient. Recognition and respect that defenses may have been developed as a coping mechanism is imperative, and the clinician must continuously use professional judgment to assess the amount of arousal the patient is able to tolerate in any given moment. In general, critical factors in implementing this approach include adequate clinical training, as well as a thorough assessment of the patient's ego strength, emotional support, and ample resources to cope with any challenging material that may surface during the process.

Initial Assessment:
For Diagnostic Purposes

Upon noting the range of objective information that can be retrieved via psychophysiological monitoring – including the nature and quality of cognitive processes, as well as unconscious psychological material – biofeedback provides access into additional physical and psychological functioning that may be unobservable to the naked eye. With this in mind, clinicians may find that incorporating biofeedback in the initial assessment and diagnostic process may be highly advantageous in yielding more precise and comprehensive diagnoses. This use of biofeedback for diagnostic purposes may be especially helpful for conditions or disorders that involve somatic symptoms, as well as clinical presentations in which suppression or repression of emotions or experiences may be out of conscious awareness (Barlow, 2001; Hugdahl, 2001).

Early exploration of this concept was conducted by Berman and Johnson (1985) in a research project geared toward the development of a psychophysiological assessment battery to be used for assessment and treatment of a variety of conditions:

> Through evaluating a variety of physiological systems under a variety of stress and nonstress tasks, an assessment battery could provide a standard framework for determining which physiological system was most appropriate to modify with biofeedback. The physiological systems recorded during the assessment could be modified to include the symptom-specific system for each individual. The first administration of the battery would serve as a validation of whether that system was indeed the maximally aroused system. (Berman & Johnson, 1985, p. 220)

More recently, Little (2006) mentions the use of a psychophysiological profile in the initial assessment to evaluate baseline responses and recovery time to moderate stressors administered by the clinician. A number of modalities can be used in this phase to help detect the individual's unique pattern of responding to stress and reveal specific areas in need of attention, which subsequently can be used to set treatment goals and develop a treatment plan specifically tailored to meet the needs of the individual at hand.

Ongoing Assessment: Monitoring Treatment Progress

Beyond initial assessment and diagnostic purposes, physiological measurements can also be used to help monitor how patients are responding to therapy. Clinicians can observe the immediate impact of specific elements of treatment in the moment and determine aspects of the intervention that are either helpful or counterproductive for the patient (Newman, 2004). In addition, ongoing, in-the-moment monitoring may not only assess the impact of intentional therapeutic strategies, but may also illuminate the effects of unintentional aspects within the therapy. Werbach (1977) explains that by monitoring physiology during treatment, the clinician "may also increase his awareness of his patient's responses to both interpersonal and intrapsychic stimuli" (p. 378).

In general, ongoing psychophysiological monitoring can help shed light onto the degree of progress made by the patient. From that information, the clinician can determine the effectiveness of the chosen treatment plan and decide whether any adjustment should be made regarding the nature of implemented techniques, as well as the patient's readiness for termination (Newman, 2004).

ASSESSING TREATMENT OUTCOMES AND EFFICACY

Beyond the benefits biofeedback can bring in initial and ongoing assessment processes, the psychophysiological information yielded from biofeedback equipment can be used to assess treatment outcomes and efficacy of specific interventions. An illustration of this is in a study conducted by Cote and Bouchard (2005), in which psychophysiological measures were used to assess the efficacy of virtual reality exposure (VRE). The rationale behind the study was based on the notion that most studies use self-report data to assess the efficacy of such treatments; in addition, physiological recordings have been most commonly used for therapeutic purposes, while the use of psychophysiological monitoring as a distinct outcome measure for the treatment of anxiety disorders is not as common in current publications. Thus, it was theorized that using additional objective measures of arousal and cognitive processes through psychophysiological monitoring would be a valuable source of data to further validate the usefulness of the treatment. Indeed, the psychophysiological data demonstrated positive change posttreatment – results that were concurrent with subjective self-report outcome measures. Cote and Bouchard (2005) conclude: "Hopefully, further controlled studies will include physiological and information processing measures when assessing the efficacy and cognitive mechanisms involved in VRE treatment" (p. 230). Overall, psychophysiological monitoring served as a useful objective measure in conjunction with self-report measures to demonstrate the significant therapeutic improvements that were gained from the treatment.

Biofeedback: For Therapeutic Purposes

Beyond assessment purposes, biofeedback can also be highly effective for therapeutic purposes. Such advantages include facilitating relaxation and physical functioning, the learning of coping skills, and the training of behavioral interventions. Additional benefits include the range of emotional impact it can instill within patients upon achieving success in these skills, as well as the overall more pleasurable therapeutic experience that can result. More in-depth discussion into the therapeutic benefits of biofeedback will be presented below.

Physiology Can Help Shift Psychology: A Bottom-Up Approach

Just as the body can reflect cognitive and emotional processes, learning how to consciously shift processes within the body can subsequently help shift the nature of psychological processes. One way to conceptualize this approach in comparison to traditional talk psychotherapy can be termed as a "bottom-up" approach, in which the use of physiological shifting is used as the mechanism of change. On the other hand, talk therapy can be conceptualized as a "top-down approach," in which the use of talk and verbal communication is used as the mechanism for change. Although working primarily with cognitive processes may be helpful on a variety of levels for many people, working with physiological processes can also be beneficial in the psychological healing process. In other words, steps taken toward achieving a relaxed body can ultimately help induce a relaxed mind and state of well-being.

The bottom-up approach is based on the notion that inducing more balanced, calm physiological processes can help induce calmer cognitive processes. Werbach (1977) explains: "Relaxation is a psychophysiologic event resulting in simultaneous intrapsychic and physiologic shifts. It appears to be an integrated hypothalamic response marked physiologically by generalized decreased sympathetic, and possibly increased parasympathetic, nervous system activity" (p. 379). As a more relaxed state ensues, not only can more relaxed cognitive activity occur, but also the individual can become more able to absorb and respond to therapeutic methods. "In a state of deep relaxation, the patient appears less prone to utilize habitual ego defenses and thus may be more receptive to therapeutic interventions. Repression decreases as relaxation deepens so that previously repressed material may become available" (Werbach, 1977, p. 379).

This method may be especially helpful for some individuals for whom confrontation of anxiety-provoking cues can actually exacerbate symptoms (e.g., as mentioned prior with the tendency for some PTSD patients to become retraumatized when exposed to stressors) (Hembree et al., 2003; Foa, Keane, & Friedman, 2000; Davidson & Conner, 1999). It can also be helpful for individuals who are "stuck" or have reached a standstill within the therapeutic progress; using an alternate route beyond traditional talk therapy may help access areas in need of attention that may be inaccessible or unresponsive through talk therapy alone. In support of this notion, I. Saito and Y. Saito (2004) assert that biofeedback is a useful approach in treating chronic symptoms and diseases when other interventions have been less effective. Using physiological feedback and monitoring during the therapeutic process can be a key element in accessing and treating areas that may have been difficult to reach via other approaches.

Enhanced Quality of Training and Additional Benefits

In behavioral therapy, various coping strategies are taught by the clinician for the individual to use for managing stress and anxiety and become more involved in constructive activity. Common coping skills include cognitive restructuring, cognitive rehearsal, self-reliance training, role playing, and diversion techniques (including physical activity, social contact, work, play, and visual imagery); relaxation methods are also used, including breath training, focusing techniques, and progressive muscle relaxation. Many factors can contribute to the success of such training efforts, including clinician expertise, patient characteristics, degree of pathology, amount of time and financial resources available, and general compliance with the treatment program (Barlow, 2001).

Beyond these factors – each of which may either enhance or impede success – biofeedback may be a useful tool to enhance training efforts of such coping behavioral techniques. This assertion is based on learning theories which posit that the constant feedback of successes can serve to reinforce additional success (Hugdahl, 2001). Continued feedback of even slight changes toward improved behavior modifications in the moment helps promote awareness of what "healthy" behaviors feel like, as well as provide a reward for the success. The increased awareness and immediate reward via biofeedback can reinforce continued improvement in behavior.

The slight detection of small changes may be especially helpful for individuals who may have difficulty in learning new behaviors. For example, for a person who cannot relax the trapezius muscles regardless of the clinician's suggestions and personal attempts, the biofeedback equipment's ability to detect covert muscle activity can help gain even a slight access to the muscle; with continued exposure and practice, access to conscious control of the muscle can develop and grow.

Multiple Modalities
Available for Diverse Needs

In multimodality biofeedback, several physiologic variables with one or more modalities for feedback are used. If one mode does not work, or the patient is having difficulty with modifying a symptom, state, or behavior, another mode can be used that may be more accessible to change. The key aspect within this concept is that the option of using multiple modalities enables the clinician to tailor the therapy to the patient's individual needs in the moment; if one approach is not effective, alternative methods can be applied until the clinician discovers the mode most appropriate and effective for the patient at the time. "The variable most closely related to the presenting symptom or the variable which appears to be best correlated to the patient's degree of 'activation' is usually selected. If the patient experiences difficulty in modifying this variable, another may then be selected for feedback or additional feedback channels may be introduced" (Werbach, 1977, p. 378). Not only can this yield more successful outcomes of the treatment itself, it can also prevent feelings of failure or despair within the patient as the right match is found for that particular individual and presenting problem.

Increased Self-Awareness

One of the critical elements in any type of change process within psychotherapy involves an initial awareness of the problem; identification and recognition of the problem is a significant aspect before real change can ensue. The ongoing psychophysiological monitoring can facilitate this process, as the patient gradually gains deeper insight into his or her perceptions and reactions to internal and external stimuli, including subtle reactions that may have otherwise been imperceptible to the patient. Werbach (1977) highlights this notion, commenting that biofeedback "may serve as an experiential adjunct to the psychotherapeutic process, perhaps by assisting them to develop their abilities to recognize and affect the internal events under scrutiny" (p. 376).

Increased Motivation,
Self-Efficacy, and Sense of Control

It should be noted that an especially valuable element of biofeedback involves the notion that it enables small changes in the healthier direction to be detected and rewarded as success, which subsequently facilitates further development and growth of these changes. This is especially helpful for clinical cases whereby subtle correct changes cannot be perceived or are perceived incorrectly by the individual. In conjunction with this concept, Basmajian (1989) highlights additional advantages that can be gained from biofeedback, including increased motivation, self-efficacy, confidence, and empowerment. He suggests:

> [B]y making the early signs of slight progress conspicuous, it can encourage and motivate the patients, relieve their sense of helplessness, and serve as a coping response to reduce symptoms of stress. Instead of having something done to patients, it teaches them to do something for themselves, increasing their confidence, or what has been called self-efficacy. This factor is particularly important when biofeedback is being used to treat symptoms that are elicited or aggravated by stress. (p. 9)

Even small indications of success can suffice to help develop greater self-efficacy, sense of control, and empowerment. I. Saito and Y. Saito (2004) explain that in addition to biofeedback therapy helping patients achieve a greater understanding of the correlation between the mind and body, it can also provide patients with a deeper understanding of their symptoms and motivation to partake in self-help treatments, thereby supporting more self control. Halley (1991) asserts that biobehavioral strategies such as biofeedback not only can facilitate improved functioning of the immune system, but are also well known for enhancing coping ability, assisting in increased feelings of control and building a greater sense of well-being. The strategies learned can provide tools to aid people in gaining a sense of control over elements that are within the scope of our individual influence, potentially fostering the achievement of a better quality of life and improved treatment outcome in the face of any illness or health state (Halley, 1991).

Newman (2004) also mentions the effect of technology on improving motivation within treatment, as well as additional benefits that may ensue as a result. He suggests that "technological applications may even motivate patients towards readiness for therapy or to comply with and apply assigned homework" (p. 141). Thus, the motivation that may result can help the patient not only commit to the therapeutic process, but also remain committed and invested in fully participating in the treatment.

I. Saito and Y. Saito (2004) also highlight the notion that the growth model (shaping) inherent in biofeedback, in which the treatment goals are broken down into smaller, graduated steps, can help make achievement easier to attain. Small successes are rewarded and reinforced, which can subsequently lead to more successes and overall performance enhancement.

Enhanced Overall Therapeutic Experience

Beyond its ability to enhance training of coping skills and behavioral interventions, biofeedback can positively impact additional psychological processes as well, such as greater self-awareness and insight, personal responsibility, self-efficacy, self-esteem, sense of control, and motivation. The overall therapeutic experience may also be more pleasurable as a result of continued feelings of success, which can subsequently lead to greater compliance and treatment outcomes.

Newman (2004) raises the question of potential effects that using technology may have on the therapeutic relationship and possible early termination, and explains that "research to date shows that contrary to many fears, technology need not compromise the therapeutic relationship, and in some instances technological interventions may even be preferred" (p. 142). For example, Ghosh, Marks, and Carr (as cited in Newman, 2004) reported that patients with panic disorder declined clinician-delivered therapy more so than computer-administered therapy. Additionally, in another publication by Ghosh and Marks (as cited in Newman, 2004), they reported higher compliance in a computer-administered condition than in individual therapy. Investigation into possible explanations for these individuals' preferences for technology would be an interesting avenue for further research.

PRACTICAL INFORMATION
FOR PROFESSIONALS

As mentioned above, biofeedback is currently used by health care professionals trained in a variety of areas, such as psychology, psychiatry, internists, nursing, physical and occupational therapy, social work, and counseling, and can be used as a complementary or alternate treatment for many diagnosed psychological, learning, and/or medical conditions. Such conditions include anxiety and stress, panic disorder, ADHD, sleep disorders, migraine and tension headaches, high blood pressure, muscle tension, incontinence, constipation, pain, gastrointestinal disorders, and more. Biofeedback training may also be used by coaches and educators to help people improve performance and functioning overall (AAPB, 2008). Overall, regardless of the specific condition or treatment population, biofeedback can serve as an invaluable tool for health care professionals who are invested in helping patients better identify and use their behavior, thoughts, and feelings in healthier, more adaptive ways.

Recommended Professional
Affiliations as Valuable Resources

Numerous avenues and resources are available for practitioners interested in pursuing further education and training in biofeedback and applied psychophysiology, including courses at universities (including distance and online didactic training), workshops, biofeedback organizations, mentoring programs, and journal publications. For professionals who are interested in learning more about biofeedback training, some of the most recognized professional associations to date that can serve as excellent resources include the following: The Association for Applied Psychophysiology and Biofeedback (AAPB), International Society for Neurofeedback & Research (ISNR), and the Biofeedback Certification Institute of America (BCIA). These organizations have been developed in an effort to advance the field of biofeedback, including providing information and resources for further education, research, and clinical practice. Additionally, the organizations listed above have developed websites and access to other publications that provide a wealth of information for both novice and experienced biofeedback clinicians. Such information includes an overview of biofeedback and how it works, disorders that can benefit from biofeedback training, educational resources and continuing education programs, cost of training, equipment information, data collection and management, insurance information, research and publications, guidelines for ethical practice, certification information, and other topics that are intended to help further educate and integrate biofeedback into mainstream medicine. For contact information, please refer to the resources listed at the end of this contribution (p. 76).

Certification for Biofeedback:
Why Get It and How?

As aforementioned, biofeedback can be used in both clinical and educational realms. In general, varying credentials are required (e.g., licenses, certifications) depending on the nature of health care services provided. However, the majority of states do not formally restrict who can provide biofeedback services. "Thus, a person with no clinical training of any kind nor any specialized training in biofeedback may claim to provide biofeedback services" (AAPB, 2007, Directory section).

In an effort to address the lack of formal established standards, as well as the varied nature and degree of training among the range of practitioners who integrate biofeedback and applied psychophysiology in their practice, the Biofeedback Certification Institute of America (BCIA) was established to grant certification to biofeedback practitioners and, in essence, to help set minimal standards for service providers (Schwartz & Andrasik, 2003). To date, the BCIA is the only institute recognized worldwide for biofeedback certification, and maintains firm policies and procedures set by an independent board of directors composed of distinguished biofeedback clinicians, researchers, and educators. Its mission is to protect the general public by establishing and maintaining standards of competence and clinical practice of biofeedback practitioners. Acquiring certification illustrates professionalism and adherence to strategically established standards as a health care provider (BCIA, 2007).

To receive BCIA biofeedback certification, health professionals are required to complete basic degree and educational requirements, learn to apply clinical biofeedback skills during mentorship, and pass a written examination. Furthermore, agreement to practice according to the Ethical Principles of BCIA and of their profession and in accordance with appropriate laws of their state is required. In addition, when treating a patient with a medical or psychological disorder, a BCIA certificant must have an appropriate license/credential for independent practice or agree to work under the supervision of another health care professional.

A more in-depth description of requirements is available on the BCIA website. It is important to note that certification does not guarantee competence, but does provide a credible index of fundamental knowledge and instrumentation proficiency. In addition, ongoing education and training is emphasized and required to maintain certification and help ensure competence among practitioners. BCIA can be contacted via telephone at 303-420-2902 or via the Internet* at http:www.bcia.org.

Certification Requirements:
A Note to Novice and Experienced Practitioners

Regarding education requirements, providers are encouraged to check the BCIA website for specific information. As a further note, in addition to the Entry Level General Biofeedback Certification, BCIA recently launched the option of Certification by Prior Experience. The latter option is available for "a select group of professionals who can demonstrate extensive training and experience and have been leaders through their various contributions to the field. We recognize that these professionals have training that goes beyond entry level and should not need to apply through our traditional certification process" (BCIA, 2007, Certification by Prior Experience section). Regardless of the type of certification received, once certification is granted to the provider, it is valid for 4 years thereafter. To maintain certification, 80 hours of continuing education are required, and the provider must attest that his or her license/credential has not been suspended, investigated, or revoked. "Recertification at four year intervals indicates providers have undergone continuous peer review of ethical practice and have continued to acquire knowledge of recent developments in the field" (BCIA, 2007, General Information about BCIA section).

BCIA's List of Universities Offering
Biofeedback Coursework

The BCIA website lists a number of universities nationwide that offer biofeedback coursework (including a distance learning and online option) and are regionally accredited academic institutions accepted by the U.S. Department of Education. It is advised that each institution be contacted directly for specific information regarding course content and availability. To see a complete list of didactic requirements for BCIA certification, refer to the blueprint of requirements listed on the website (http://www.bcia.org).

---

* Although all websites cited in this contribution were correct at the time of publication, they are subject to change at any time.

BIOFEEDBACK: WHAT HAS BEEN, WHAT IS NOW, AND WHAT IS TO COME

Although numerous studies and research have been established in the field of applied psychophysiology and biofeedback, its full potential has yet to be realized. Limited time and money, as well as the existence of approaches already proven effective, are just some factors that may be impeding the advancement of biofeedback thus far. For example, I. Saito & Y. Saito (2004) state, "There are many reports that have proved the effectiveness of BFT [biofeedback therapy] in treating anxiety. However, as a variety of excellent psychotropic drugs were already developed, BFT of anxiety tends to be used only in refractory cases" (p. 463). As with any new concept that extends beyond the scope of traditional practice, continued skepticism is expected regarding the areas of concern mentioned above, including the overall regard of biofeedback as a legitimate scientific practice and its value in the field. Furthermore, the notion of integrating biofeedback into psychotherapy is a specific area likely to raise many questions and concerns for professionals who have not been exposed to or trained in biofeedback, including the cost and benefit of taking on such an endeavor. Simply put: Is it worth it for clinicians to bring biofeedback into their existing practice, and, if so, how much will it really add to existing treatments?

Thus, although a wide range of biofeedback treatment protocols has already been established and empirically supported for a range of psychophysiological conditions, continued research efforts directed toward discovering the range of physical, cognitive, and behavioral changes that biofeedback can yield in treatment in still needed. It will be an exciting time in the field of psychology as further evidence is gained illustrating the value biofeedback can bring to helping individuals heal in mind, body, and heart.

CONTRIBUTORS

Jennifer Minkin, PsyD, is currently a Psychology Associate for Children's Hospital of Philadelphia. Prior to assuming this position, she helped establish the first Widener Biofeedback Clinic & Certification at Widener University, as well as participate in research aimed at developing biological methods to help assess cognitive performance in individuals. Her training is in clinical psychology, with special interests in psychophysiology and biofeedback, and also has been certified through the Biofeedback Certification Institute of America. Additionally, Dr. Minkin has earned a master's degree in special and elementary education. She may be contacted at CSH021, CHOP, 34th Street & Civic Center Blvd., Philadelphia, PA 19104-4399. E-mail: jiminkin@hotmail.com

Maurice F. Prout, PhD, ABPP, is currently professor at the Institute for Graduate Clinical Psychology at Widener University, Chester, Pennsylvania. He also directs the respecialization program housed within the Institute. His clinical interests include the treatment of anxiety and mood disorders as well as topics related to behavioral medicine. He is a Diplomate in Clinical Psychology and a Founding Fellow of the Academy of Cognitive Therapy. Dr. Prout can be reached at Widener University, Chester, PA 19013. E-mail: mfprout@widener.edu

Frank Masterpasqua, PhD, received his doctorate in psychology from Rutgers, The State University of New Jersey in 1980. He is professor at Widener University's Institute for Graduate Clinical Psychology where he teaches and supervises doctoral students in clinical psychology. He is licensed as a psychologist in Pennsylvania and is a member of the American Psychological Association. Dr. Masterpasqua teaches graduate courses in human development, positive psychology, statistical methods, and neurofeedback/EEG biofeedback. He has numerous publications including two published in *American Psychologist*, and a text - *The Psychological Meaning of Chaos*. He recently coauthored the first article on neurofeedback to be published in a journal published by the American Psychological Association. In 2005, he received Widener University's Lindback Award for excellence in teaching. Dr. Masterpasqua can be contacted at Widener University, Chester, PA 19013. E-mail: fmasterpasqua@widener.edu

RESOURCES

Association for Applied Psychophysiology & Biofeedback (AAPB). (2008). Retrieved September 18, 2008, from http://www.aapb.org

Barlow, D. H. (2001). *Clinical Handbook of Psychological Disorders: A Step-By-Step Treatment Manual* (3rd ed.). New York: Guilford.

Basmajian, J. V. (1989). *Biofeedback: Principles and Practice for Clinicians* (3rd ed.). Baltimore, MD: Williams & Wilkins.

Berman, P. S., & Johnson, H. J. (1985). A psychophysiological assessment battery. *Biofeedback and Self-Regulation, 10*(3), 203-221.

Biofeedback Certification Institute of America (BCIA). (2007). Retrieved May 30, 2007, from http://www.bcia.org/

Cote, S., & Bouchard, S. (2005). Documenting the efficacy of virtual reality exposure with psychophysiological and information processing measures. *Applied Psychophysiology and Biofeedback, 30*(3), 217-232.

Davidson, J. R. T., & Conner, K. M. (1999). Management of posttraumatic stress disorder: Diagnostic and therapeutic issues. *Journal of Clinical Psychiatry, 60*(18), 33-38.

Foa, E. B., Keane, T. M., & Friedman, M. J. (Eds.). (2000). *Effective Treatments for PTSD: Practice Guidelines From the International Society for Traumatic Stress Studies.* New York: Guilford.

Halley, F. M. (1991). Self-regulation of the immune system through biobehavioral strategies. *Biofeedback and Self-Regulation, 16*(1), 55-74.

Hembree, E. A., Foa, E. B., Dorfan, N. M., Street, G. P., Kowalski, J., & Tu, X. (2003). Do patients drop out prematurely from exposure therapy for PTSD? *Journal of Traumatic Stress, 16*(6), 555-562.

Hugdahl, K. (2001). *Psychophysiology: The Mind-Body Perspective.* Cambridge, MA: Harvard University Press.

International Society for Neurofeedback & Research (ISNR). (2008). Retrieved September 18, 2008 from http://www.isnr.org/

Kremsdorf, R., Kochanowicz, N., & Costell, S. (1981). Cognitive skills training versus EMG biofeedback in the treatment of tension headaches. *Biofeedback and Self-Regulation, 6,* 93-101.

Larkin, T. (2006). Psychophysiological assessment. In M. Hersen (Ed.), *Clinician's Handbook of Adult Behavioral Assessment* (pp. 165-185). San Diego, CA: Elsevier Academic Press.

Little, S. (2006). *Biofeedback.* Retrieved September 17, 2008 from http://www.healthandhealingny.org/complement/bio_how.asp

Meichenbaum, D. (1976). Cognitive factors in biofeedback therapy. *Biofeedback and Self-Regulation, 1*(2), 201-216.

Newman, M. G. (2004). Technology in psychotherapy: An introduction. *JCLP/In Session, 60*(2), 141-145.

Saito, I., & Saito, Y. (2004). Biofeedback training in clinical settings. *Biogenic Amines, 18*(3-6), 463-476.

Schwartz, M. S. (1999). What is applied psychophysiology? Toward a definition. *Applied Psychophysiology and Biofeedback, 24*(1), 3-10.

Schwartz, M. S., & Andrasik, F. (2003). *Biofeedback: A Practitioner's Guide* (3rd ed.). New York: Guilford.

Tortora, G. J., & Anagnostakos, N. (1990). *Principles of Anatomy & Physiology* (6th ed.). New York: Harper & Row.

Werbach, M. R. (1977). Biofeedback and psychotherapy. *American Journal of Psychotherapy, 31*(3), 376-382.

Wickramasekera, I. E. (1976). *Biofeedback, Behavior Therapy and Hypnosis: Potentiating the Verbal Control of Behavior for Clinicians.* Chicago: Nelson Hall.

Wilhelm, F. H., Schneider, S., & Friedman, B. H. (2006). Psychophysiological assessment. In M. Hersen, *Clinician's Handbook of Child Behavioral Assessment* (pp. 201-231). San Diego, CA: Elsevier Academic Press.

Anger Management Treatment

Carin M. Lefkowitz and Maurice F. Prout

As a nation, we are both captivated and disgusted by acts of anger and aggression. We see these acts as dangerous to society and have responded, in part, by instituting anger management training in various settings, including court-ordered classes, university campuses, and VA hospitals. Most attention is focused on chronically angry individuals who perform reprehensible violent acts: road rage violence, spousal abuse, and murder, for example. But difficulty with anger management is an all-too-common problem, and many individuals go through life experiencing significant occupational, physical, emotional, and social distress due to an inability to modulate and express anger appropriately. In fact, one third of community adults report that they experience anger almost every day (Kassinove & Tafrate, 2006). As an increasing number of individuals seek treatment (self-referred or court-mandated), there is a greater need for clinicians to understand chronic anger and develop the skills necessary to treat it.

Anger might be described as an automatic reaction, a feeling of antagonism, and a desire for justified revenge or vindication. At its best, anger can be energizing, empowering, relieving, and productive; at its worst, anger is destructive, unbridled, consuming, and uncontrollable (Novaco, 2000). Despite its adaptive benefits, anger is considered a negative emotion because individuals would generally prefer to not feel angry, and frequent or prolonged anger is correlated with several physical ailments (Dahlen & Deffenbacher, 2001; Lench, 2004). Indeed, effective treatment of chronic anger may lead to a decrease in future medical costs and mortality rates over the long run.

It is important to distinguish among the concepts of anger, hostility, and aggression, as they are often confused in the research literature, by clinicians, and by laypersons. Although these concepts overlap, clarification of each can aid understanding theories of anger management and implementation of interventions. Anger is the emotional state that can underlie both hostility and aggression. Hostility is the pervasive attitude that anticipates aggression in others and justifies aggressive responses in an individual. Aggression is any behavior intended to cause harm (Del Vecchio & O'Leary, 2004).

The focus of this contribution is the chronic anger that causes destruction (either self- or other-related), that is difficult to manage or control, and that causes distress to the actor and/or the people who surround him or her. Maladaptive anger is often identified by the elements of frequency, intensity, and duration. Chronically angry individuals feel anger more intensely and experience it in more situations and for longer amounts of time than those who experience "healthy" anger. It should be stressed that maladaptive anger is not always expressed; there is a significant subset of chronically angry individuals who are preoccupied with thoughts of past injustice and fantasies of revenge, but who do not openly express this anger (Kassinove & Tafrate, 2006). These individuals, whom we refer to as "anger suppressors," have an equal need for treatment, as they experience greater physiological arousal than "anger expressers" and are at an even higher risk for cardiovascular disease (Mayne & Ambrose, 1999). This contribution will focus on understanding and treating chronic anger in adults in an outpatient setting. A great deal of research has focused on treating maladaptive anger in children and adolescents, but this population falls outside the scope of this contribution.

THE PHYSIOLOGICAL, COGNITIVE, BEHAVIORAL, AND SOCIAL CORRELATES OF ANGER

The physiological reaction to anger is thought to have evolutionary roots as a survival response to threat and danger. When our ancestors experienced threat (such as a predator on the prowl), the physiological reaction known as the flight-or-fight response was automatically enacted. This reaction includes physiological activation of the cardiovascular, endocrine, limbic (especially the amygdala), and muscular systems. The activation helps the individual to focus attention to the threat and to temporarily increase pain/discomfort tolerance (Novaco, 2000). For example, the heightened arousal and attention might have helped our ancestors to track their predators and either escape or fight for survival. Observable physical reactions can include facial flushing, a tense and "puffed out" body stance, and a focused glare. These automatic reactions were likely adaptive in the past, as they served to intimidate the predator.

Unfortunately, what might have been adaptive and empowering for our ancestors can often prove detrimental in today's society. Anger can still be adaptive when it motivates individuals to confront a problem or threat, enables a quick and powerful response, and provides endurance to follow through on a solution. However, most modern challenges are predominantly psychological, not physical (Novaco, 2000). The same autonomic reactivity that leads us to focus attention on the threat might also prevent us from seeing the larger picture, and the natural inclination toward a quick and fierce reaction can hamper our abilities to problem solve or react in socially appropriate ways. Also, we know that the frequent and prolonged physiological experience of anger/hostility is associated with several coronary concerns (including heart disease, hypertension, and atherosclerosis [Lachar, 1993; Novaco, 2000]), and suppressed immune functioning (Del Vecchio & O'Leary, 2004), and that suppressed anger is associated with tension headaches (Hatch et al., 1991). Additionally, frequent and enduring muscle tension can cause significant pain and discomfort.

In addition to the predictable physiological reaction, anger is also associated with specific cognitive profiles. It is associated with several distortions that occur at the appraisal stage of stimulus interpretation. Berkowitz (1990) theorized that aversive stimuli automatically activate an emotional response, which then activates stereotyped cognitive, behavioral, and physiological reactions. Unfortunately, the combination of arousal and a tendency toward seeing the world in stereotyped ways often leads chronically angry individuals to distort stimuli in a way that begets more anger and distress. Some cognitive distortions commonly observed with anger are listed in Table 1 (p. 79; Kassinove & Tafrate, 2006).

Chronically angry individuals are especially sensitive to experiencing "slights" or insults from others, which can lead to selective attention to cues with a high provocation value (Novaco, 2000; Witte, Callahan, & Perez-Lopez, 2002). As chronic anger becomes ingrained, expectations about injustice and antagonism are formed, and these expectations focus individuals' attention on stimuli that meet these expectations, while ignoring disconfirming cues and evidence.

Table 1: Cognitive Distortions Commonly Made by Chronically Angry Individuals

---

- Overemphasizing importance: "It's awful" or "It's unacceptable."
- Misappraisals about the capacity to cope (secondary appraisal): "I can't deal with this."
- Justice-oriented demands: "He deserves better."
- Evaluations of others (fundamental attribution error): "She's a jerk!"
- Dichotomous thinking/focus on "shoulds": "There's a right way and a wrong way to do things."
- Overgeneralization: "Since she didn't respond, she must not want to work with me."
- Attributions of blame and misappraisals of preventability and/or intentionality: "It's all his fault. If he had thought more about it, it wouldn't have happened."
- Labeling: "He's a big idiot!"

Behaviorally, anger can be suppressed or expressed, and expression can take many forms. Most commonly, we expect anger to be expressed as physical or verbal aggression. Indeed, high levels of anger have been associated with various forms of aggression, including spousal abuse, child abuse, and road rage (Del Vecchio & O'Leary, 2004). However, Dahlen and Deffenbacher (2001) suggest that anger rarely leads to violent behavior. Novaco (2000) clarifies that aggression typically occurs when an individual experiences a very intense level of anger that increases physiological arousal while decreasing self-monitoring and inhibitory control. Anger is often expressed more subtly, through behaviors such as sabotage (occupational, social, etc.), withdrawing, using sarcasm, and manipulating others. Alternatively, some individuals may suppress angry feelings rather than express them (Kassinove & Tafrate, 2006). This approach can be based on the characteristics of the situation or characteristics of the individual, including cultural and gender characteristics.

It is not difficult to envision the many consequences that chronic anger can have on interpersonal relationships. Again, although "healthy" anger may enable individuals to end toxic relationships and ensure that they are treated fairly by others, chronic and maladaptive anger has a variety of negative effects on relationships. In general, chronically angry individuals have fewer and less-satisfying romantic, social, and occupational relationships. For example, chronically angry individuals report being single for longer periods of time, involved in fewer relationships per year, having more verbal conflict in relationships, and more physical conflict in current romantic relationships than did individuals who experienced "normal" or low levels of anger (Lench, 2004). Overall, chronic anger is associated with less social support (Dahlen & Deffenbacher, 2001). It is theorized that as angry individuals age, they may begin to alienate their friends until they only maintain a romantic relationship, which becomes the sole target of the individual's anger (Lench, 2004).

ASSESSMENT OF CHRONIC ANGER

Several self-report measures and structured clinical interviews have been devised to help clinicians assess pathological anger in their clients. Each tool provides a slightly different profile of anger. For example, tools may assess expression versus suppression of anger, or angry behaviors versus angry thoughts. A thorough review of each assessment tool falls outside the scope of this contribution, but a list of the most commonly used anger assessment tools is provided in Table 2 (p. 80). These tools can be used to assess treatment effectiveness by comparing scores both before and after treatment. Clinicians who work with individuals with chronic anger would be wise to understand these tools and determine which ones are most useful for their specific practice.

Table 2: Commonly Used Anger Assessment Tools

- Aggression Questionnaire (Buss & Warren, 2000)
- Anger Disorders Scale (DiGiuseppe & Tafrate, 2004)
- Anger Self-Report (Zelin, Adler, & Myerson, 1972)
- Cook-Medly Hostility Inventory (Cook & Medley, 1954)
- Minnesota Multiphasic Personality Inventory (MMPI-2; Butcher et al., 1989)
- Novaco Anger Inventory (Novaco, 1994)
- State-Trait Anger Expression Inventory (STAXI; Spielberger, 1991)

DIAGNOSES CORRELATED WITH ANGER MISMANAGEMENT

Many individuals are referred for treatment specifically because of their difficulties in managing anger. However, there are even more individuals receiving psychological treatment for disorders in which anger management is only one (albeit very significant) aspect of the presenting issues. A list of disorders from the *Diagnostic and Statistical Manual of Mental Disorders* (*DSM-IV*; American Psychiatric Association [APA], 1994) that are highly correlated with anger mismanagement is provided in Table 3 (below). This list is by no means exhaustive, as it focuses only on those disorders most commonly seen in clinical practice:

Table 3: *DSM-IV* Disorders Correlated With Anger Mismanagement

---

- Alcohol/Substance Abuse disorders
- Antisocial Personality Disorder
- Attention-Deficit/Hyperactivity Disorder (ADHD)
- Bipolar Disorder
- Borderline Personality Disorder
- Conduct Disorder
- Eating Disorders
- Intermittent Explosive Disorder
- Major Depressive Disorder
- Narcissistic Personality Disorder
- Oppositional Defiant Disorder
- Posttraumatic Stress Disorder
- Schizoaffective Disorder
- Schizophrenia
- Social Anxiety Disorder

Special attention in the research literature has been given to specific *DSM-IV* disorders in which maladaptive anger plays a significant role in the presentation and/or treatment of symptoms. For example, a subset of individuals with Social Anxiety Disorder experience intense anger at others when they feel negatively evaluated, or when they feel pressured into engaging in anxiety-provoking situations. Socially anxious individuals tend to experience more anger without provocation and a greater likelihood to express anger when criticized than do nonanxious individuals. However, due to their fear of being further criticized by others, these individuals are more likely to suppress anger, and those individuals who suppress their anger have higher levels of impairment and noncompliance with treatment (Erwin et al., 2003).

The relationship between Narcissistic Personality Disorder and maladaptive anger has also been investigated. Individuals high in narcissism were more likely to exhibit greater arousal of anger and to express anger verbally and physically. Men high in narcissism expressed anger in more physical ways than did women high in narcissism or men and women low in narcissism (McCann & Biaggio, 1989). Individuals who scored high on measures of entitlement and authority (which are both related to narcissistic personality disorder) tended to experience high levels of anger (Witte et al., 2002).

Much of the research investigating the relationship between Posttraumatic Stress Disorder (PTSD) and anger has focused on combat veterans. In one study of Vietnam veterans with PTSD, all participants reported serious arguments in the 6 months preceding initial assessment, 46% had threatened physical violence during these arguments, 36% destroyed property, 21% engaged in physical violence, 18% used a weapon to threaten another person, and 7% actually used a weapon to injure someone (Chemtob et al., 1997). A metaanalysis conducted by Orth and Wieland (2006) concluded that anger and hostility are significantly correlated with PTSD among adults. Individuals suffering with PTSD may be more likely to perceive situations as threatening, and their biologically predisposed survival (fight-or-flight) response may be heightened. Additionally, the tendency for rumination (related to the reexperiencing symptom cluster) may increase the likelihood of angry interpretations of stimuli. Finally, for survivors of trauma, anger may be a more acceptable emotional reaction to trauma-related stimuli; the other options of fear and depression may be more difficult to tolerate in some high-risk populations, such as veterans. Unfortunately, the tendency to react angrily to situations may beget violence, which can increase the likelihood that the survivor is exposed to more trauma in the future.

The relationship between anger and Eating Disorders has also received special attention. The research suggests that anger may be experienced and expressed in slightly different ways between individuals suffering from bulimia and anorexia. In one study, women with Eating Disorders who binged and vomited displayed higher levels of trait anger, while women who exercised excessively scored higher on measures of state anger. Women who displayed bulimic features scored higher on measures of anger suppression than did restricting anorexics and women without eating disorders (Waller et al., 2003).

Of course, many clinicians also work with clients referred for physical ailments. These clients often seek help in coping with the symptoms of the illness (e.g., pain management), coping with uncomfortable medical treatment (i.e., chemotherapy), or rehabilitation (following a traumatic brain injury). Many of these physical disorders are also associated with mismanaged anger. Some common physical ailments associated with anger are presented below in Table 4.

Table 4: Common Physical Disorders Associated With Chronic Anger

- Cancer
- Chronic Pain Syndrome
- Headaches
- Heart Disease
- Hypertension
- Stroke
- Traumatic Brain Injury
- Ulcers

Difficulties with anger management can precede these disorders or be intensified by these disorders. For example, hostility can both precede and exacerbate coronary diseases and ulcers. Trauma to the brain can damage emotional regulation centers, which can lead to a broad range of emotional dysfunction, including chronic anger; but anger and aggression can also make individuals vulnerable to sustaining brain injuries in the course of a physical confrontation. More generally, chronic anger can suppress the immune system, leaving individuals more susceptible to both acute and chronic diseases such as cancer, and can hamper the recovery process.

ETHICAL ISSUES

As when working with any client population, clinicians working with chronically angry individuals must be cognizant of the potential for ethical conflicts and concerns. Although clinicians are always advised to work from a preventative, rather than reactive, stance when it comes to ethics, this stance is particularly crucial when working with a chronically angry population. Difficulties with anger management can have a harmful (or even deadly) impact on individuals and those around them. Angry individuals themselves are vulnerable to a variety of physiological diseases as well as to injury as a result of aggression against others. Individuals who come in contact with chronically angry individuals (especially their family members) are also vulnerable to injury if violence and aggression follow from unmanaged anger. With so much at risk, clinicians must attempt to foresee potential problems to the best of their ability. Some relevant ethical considerations are discussed here.

It is important for clinicians and clients to understand that anger management therapy may be structured, but it rarely proceeds smoothly. There is a significant possibility that frustration will increase at the beginning stages of treatment due to the sometimes-challenging process of learning new behaviors and unlearning old behaviors that seem automatically evoked. Additionally, frustration and anxiety may increase again as individuals begin to face anger-provoking situations (in the course of cognitive behavioral therapy, discussed later) in real life. Clients need to be informed that emotional distress may temporarily increase at times in the course of therapy. Not only does this allow clients to give true informed consent, but this psychoeducation can also prevent fears of losing control and can motivate individuals to develop a "safety plan."

In addition to feelings of frustration and anxiety, violent behaviors and conflict might actually increase during the initial stages of anger management therapy, especially in couples-based therapy. Mayne and Ambrose (1999) suggest that this may be due to the prescribed increase in communication about conflict. Special considerations must therefore be made for this phenomenon when working with already-violent offenders. Appropriate steps might include informing family members and significant others of this possibility, requiring frequent monitoring of anger levels, offering twice-weekly (or more) sessions focused on relaxation training and other types of support in the early stages of therapy, early identification of situational triggers, and creation of a "safety plan" outlining when clients (or their significant others) might leave an escalating situation, where they will go, and how long they will stay there.

Clinicians treating clients with chronic anger may be more likely to be faced with a duty to warn. The ruling in *Tarasoff vs. Regents of the University of California* in 1976 requires mental health practitioners to warn an identified potential victim of possible harm. Although serious violent acts are relatively rare, the clinician must always be mindful of potentially dangerous situations and his responsibilities in such situations. The clinician has both a duty to the potential victim *and* to the client; it is particularly important that the chronically angry client fully understands the implications of the duty to warn before giving informed consent to treatment.

Simply because anger management treatment is successful, clinicians should never assure clients that treatment gains will be maintained permanently. While experiencing extreme distress, even clients who see the most improvements can temporarily revert to old, maladaptive ways of coping with stress due to primitive neural pathways guiding behavior (discussed later). While working with violent offenders (and their families), it is particularly important to share this caveat.

CONSIDERATIONS BASED ON CULTURE AND GENDER

Anger is often considered a universal emotion and is often recognized by the characteristic facial expressions associated with it (Thomas, 2006). But the experience and expression of anger, like many emotions, is influenced by society's prevailing cultural, religious, social, and gender-based guidelines. As with all clinical interventions, clinicians should include questions about culture and religion in intake sessions and should offer interventions that respect the client's culture and religious beliefs.

In general, within the United States, physical and verbal aggression are considered dysfunctional, while taking a "time-out" or engaging in open communication are considered more acceptable (Lench, 2004). Nonetheless, different standards are typically held for men and women. Men are typically praised for being assertive and direct, while women often feel pressured to suppress anger. Studies have shown that parents differentially reinforce anger expression and suppression in their male and female children, respectively (Thomas, 2006). Women are less likely to be physically or verbally aggressive than men, and may be labeled with adjectives such as "bitch" if they do express anger (McCann & Biaggio, 1989). However, women may be more likely to exhibit relational or social aggression when angry, such as excluding peers from social situations or spreading destructive gossip (Thomas, 2006). Because women's expression of anger does not follow our stereotyped notions of physical and verbal aggression, and because they may be less willing to voluntarily report feeling angry, the prevalence of anger in women may be overlooked.

Individuals from cultures outside the United States may have a very different experience and expression of anger. Even within the *DSM-IV*, several syndromes focus specifically on how individuals from different cultures experience anger (APA, 1994). Cultural standards determine what actions or situations elicit anger and how anger is permitted to be expressed (if at all). When working with individuals from cultures in which anger is suppressed or denied, it is important to remember that clients may not be willing to report their experience of anger accurately, even on what we consider to be objective self-report measurements. Therefore, when feasible, it may be useful to interview the individual's significant others or to focus on the expression of anger within therapy sessions (Thomas, 2006).

It is important to note that discussing anger with nonnative English speakers may be complicated and confusing; because anger is regarded so differently in other cultures, significant linguistic differences exist in descriptions of anger. Precise equivalents for English words related to anger might not exist in some other cultures. Therefore, there may be some benefit in encouraging bilingual clients to describe anger (and other emotions) in their native language; even if the therapist cannot fully understand the literal translation, the emotional content may be more easily and clearly conveyed within the session (Thomas, 2006).

Religious beliefs also play a significant role in how anger is experienced and expressed. The most well-known religions – Catholicism, Judaism, Hinduism, Buddhism, and Islam – dictate that followers should avoid feelings of anger. Anger (or wrath) is one of Christianity's seven deadly sins, while Hinduism warns that anger must be abandoned before one can join with the Brahman (Thomas, 2006). Additionally, religious guidelines may also impact how willing individuals are to learn new, assertive methods of managing anger. Religious guidelines should, therefore, always be considered when introducing anger management interventions.

NEUROPSYCHOLOGY AND ANGER

The psychopharmacological treatment of chronic anger is complicated by the fact that maladaptive anger is associated with many psychological and physical disorders. Nonetheless, the pattern of neurophysiologial activation during angry experiences guides pharmacological interventions. Autonomic arousal associated with anger is caused by an increase in adrenomedullary and adrenocortical hormonal activity. The andrenal medulla secretes catecholamines, epinephrine, and norepinephrine, while glucocorticoids activate the sympathetic nervous system's fight-or-flight response (Novaco, 2000). Within the central nervous system, the amygdala has been identified as being responsible for anger (and other emotions) processing. When anger centers in the amygdala become activated, signals are sent to the body to activate the fight-or-flight response. Researchers have found that emotional arousal often precedes cognitive interpretation of stimuli. This almost certainly has evolutionary roots; when our ancestors came in contact with predators, they needed to start running *before* they had the opportunity to ask, "What signs do I have that this animal is really going to hurt me?" and "What resources do I have?" Once anger is triggered and the fight-or-flight response is enacted, cognitive processes are activated which allow the individual to focus on specific cues of the stimuli. Again, information processing is not necessarily accurate at this time; the drive for survival is hardwired and dependent on the individual identifying the dangerous aspects of the situation, not the neutral or safe aspects (Mayne & Ambrose, 1999).

The more frequently anger is activated in the individual, the more ingrained the neural pathways from the brain to the body become. Each neural pathway represents a behavioral and/or cognitive response to an arousing stimulus. Cognitive behavioral therapy (CBT) serves to teach new coping responses and therefore develop new neural pathways. These observations imply that, for new coping skills to be learned and pathways to be built, anger must be activated within therapy sessions during skill acquisition. However, old pathways do not disappear – they only become less-preferred as new ways of responding are reinforced. Old pathways can be superseded, but this task requires patience and practice. Even then, because old pathways are so entrenched, the individual may temporarily revert to old ways of responding in the face of particularly intense arousal (Mayne & Ambrose, 1999).

PSYCHOPHARMACOLOGY

For individuals who display severe forms of aggression and require rapid stabilization, atypical antipsychotics might be most useful. The atypicals impact anger and aggression by regulating dopamine in the caudate nucleus. When very rapid control is necessary, these medications can be administered through intramuscular injections so that their effect will be observed within a day. When administered orally, they take effect within a week. Two aytpicals that have been found particularly effective in managing anger and aggression are olanzapine (Zyprexa) and risperidone (Risperdal) (Edwards, 2006).

Antidepressants such as fluoxetine (Prozac) and trazodone (Desyrel) have also been found to be effective in managing anger, although they require about 2 to 4 weeks to take effect. The antidepressants impact anger by increasing serotonin and norepinephrine levels, and are most appropriate for clients experiencing chronic anger comorbid with depression, anxiety disorders, or personality disorders (Edwards, 2006).

Finally, anxiolytics may be used to help clients manage anger. Anxiolytics increase brain levels of gamma-aminobutyric acid (GABA), which leads to a relaxation response. This class of drugs includes the commonly used benzodiazepines alprazolam (Xanax), clonazepam (Klonopin), and lorazepam (Ativan). These medications can quickly decrease the intensity of an angry response, but must be used cautiously and only in the short term due to a potential for abuse and rebound effect (Edwards, 2006).

Edwards (2006) posits that medication should never be prescribed to treat anger without understanding how it relates to the larger symptomatic picture and/or the individual's interpersonal dynamics. He does suggest that medications be strongly considered when anger is a prominent symptom of, or complicating factor in, underlying psychological or physical illness. Under these circumstances, it is most likely that the anger has a biological underpinning (as opposed to social or purely psychological) that can be treated with medication. Edwards also suggests that medication can be useful in decreasing dangerousness in chronically angry individuals who express anger through violence or extreme rage, and for individuals who are experiencing such severe occupational or social distress that it is impacting their functioning or response to treatment. For these individuals, psychotropic medication can slow reaction times, which will allow them to learn and apply new problem-solving and coping techniques.

COGNITIVE-BEHAVIORAL MODELS OF CHRONIC ANGER

Cognitive-behavioral interventions (most notably CBT) have been the most researched models in the chronic anger literature, so it is important to understand CBT theory as it relates to anger. Furthermore, Mayne and Ambrose (1999) have observed that more cathartic (as opposed to skill-building) therapies might actually perpetuate chronic anger. Cathartic expression or "venting" of anger can increase negative thinking and behavior. Mayne and Ambrose hypothesize that this phenomenon occurs due to the amplification of signals in the internal neural feedback loop.

Kassinove and Tafrate (2006) expanded the classic CBT information processing model of stimulus – appraisal – response to formulate a five-step anger episode model:

1. Trigger
2. Appraisal
3. Experience
4. Expression
5. Outcomes

The notion of trigger is identical to the "stimulus" concept in the CBT model. For the chronically angry individual, almost any stimulus can trigger anger, including current or remembered actions of another person and neutral stimuli.

Whether the stimuli will actually trigger anger depends largely on the individual's appraisal of the stimuli. As discussed previously, chronically angry individuals are likely to make cognitive misappraisals of situations. Cognitive distortions can take place at both the primary and secondary levels. At the primary level, chronically angry individuals are more likely to distort the meaning of the situation and to identify an intentional violation of rigid rules, undeserved attacks, and so on. Angry individuals focus on what "happened to them," while neglecting to consider their own responsibility in the given situation. They attribute their anger to the stable, personal, and controllable characteristics of the other person, neglecting to consider situational variables. At the secondary level, they make maladaptive assumptions about appropriate coping and may determine that aggressive responses are justified, for example (Novaco, 2000).

The experience of anger reflects a private event known only to the client, and consists of the intensity and duration of thoughts, images, and bodily sensations. Of course, any strong physiological and psychological arousal can impair information processing and lessen perceived control over behavior, which influences how anger is expressed. The arousal also leads to a decrease in objective self-monitoring, which can lead to impulsive or reckless responses that might not otherwise be enacted (Lench, 2004; Novaco, 2000). Although arousal activation eventually returns to baseline levels, recovery time can be prolonged if the individual engages in rumination or is exposed to additional arousing stimuli (Novaco, 2000).

The outcome of expressing anger of course depends on a variety of factors, including the actors, the situation, and the response. Expression of anger can be either reinforced or punished depending on the outcome or consequences of the behavior. Kassinove and Tafrate (2006) propose that, for the individual with chronic anger, certain responses become intermittently reinforced, making those responses resistant to extinction, creating a long-term habitual anger response. It is important to note that the reinforced response can be either an outright expression of anger (arguing, physical conflict, sarcasm, etc.) or suppression of anger. Due to avoidance conditioning, suppressing anger can be reinforced if it allows an individual to avoid conflict.

TREATMENT IMPLICATIONS

The focus in the anger management literature is on replacing negative coping skills with positive coping skills. Ineffective coping is associated with an increase in arousal and with a possible increase in aggression. This tends to aggravate the situation further, leading to more anger in the future. In contrast, effective coping strategies alleviate negative emotions by altering one's perception of self, others, and the environment (Lench, 2004). Effective coping enables individuals to affect the environment and express their anger in ways that encourage others to respond positively, which can increase feelings of self-efficacy and decrease emotional arousal. By decreasing arousal and increasing self-awareness and inhibition of behavior, aggressive responses may be decreased (Novaco, 2000).

Again, because CBT interventions have been the most studied and well-understood therapies for chronic anger, our discussion of available treatments is focused in this direction. In their metaanalysis of CBT interventions for anger management, Beck and Fernandez (1998) report that CBT interventions have a weighted mean effect size of .70, with individuals receiving CBT displaying 76% more improvement in anger management than control subjects. The results of a metaanalysis conducted by Del Vecchio and O'Leary (2004) suggest that not enough is yet known about the efficacy of other treatment models. Results of research focused on the efficacy of relaxation training, for example, varied tremendously from study to study. Additionally, the limited studies on non-CBT treatments used such varied techniques that even positive effects could not be ascribed to any specific intervention. Interestingly, however, there is little consensus in the literature as to which CBT interventions are most efficacious. Deffenbacher, Oetting, and DiGiuseppe (2002) used the Principles of Empirically Supported Interventions (PESI) to evaluate treatment options in the literature and identify those which could be considered empirically supported. Their review found empirical support for the treatment of chronic anger through the use of cognitive therapy and behavioral skill enhancement. However, they also found empirical support for relaxation training, as well as for relaxation training combined with cognitive and behavioral interventions. At the same time, a review by Mayne and Ambrose (1999) indicated that cognitive therapy alone had the smallest effect size (although still significant) on anger management. This is in contradiction to Del Vechhio and O'Leary's (2004) assertion that research most consistently supported the use of cognitive therapy.

The disagreement in the anger management literature suggests that although CBT interventions are highly effective for the treatment of chronic anger, no one intervention can be identified as superior to the others. Therefore, we suggest that, until one intervention or treatment package is found to be definitively superior to the others, a multicomponent approach incorporating several of these interventions is most clinically useful and likely to successfully treat chronic anger in our clients. Additionally, even as they assert that relaxation training alone might be the easiest approach to anger management, Mayne and Ambrose (1999) suggest that a multicomponent approach might be more satisfying to clients as gaining an understanding of how anger is enacted can add credibility to the treatment. Interventions that have received empirical support for anger management are presented below.

COGNITIVE THERAPY

Cognitive interventions are aimed at repairing the cognitive distortions that take place at the appraisal stage in the anger-episode model. As previously discussed, chronically angry individuals tend to view frustrating events as intolerable, unjustified, and intentionally caused by another person. They do not easily see their own responsibility for or contribution to the situation. Through a collaborative effort between clinician and client, more rational cognitions are developed to replace irrational and distorted cognitions associated with chronic anger. These cognitions are rehearsed in sessions, and homework assignments promote generalization by instructing clients to apply these skills to real-life situations.

The cognitive intervention with the most significant outcome (effect size = .81) on anger management is teaching problem-solving skills (Deffenbacher et al., 2002). Ineffective problem solving can take the form of misinterpreting the problem, choosing a solution prematurely without considering alternatives, and not foreseeing consequences. In contrast, effective problem solving is a multistep process requiring imagination, patience, and rational thought. Problem-solving training includes teaching how to identify a problem (including identification of the parties involved and situational factors), brainstorming solutions, assessing resources, anticipating consequences, choosing and enacting a solution, and assessing the success of the implementation. To garner the most benefit, problem-solving approaches should be combined with other skill building so that the individual can have a variety of positive coping skills to choose from.

Cognitive restructuring (CR) has also received statistical support (effect size = .51) in empirical studies of anger management (Deffenbacher et al., 2002). CR can be enacted in a number of ways, but all methods target distorted information processing and automatic thoughts. One example is the use of David Burns's (1999) "Ten forms of twisted thinking " (pp. 8-11) to help clients identify how cognitive distortions influence individuals to selectively attend to and misinterpret incoming information. Burns's examples of "twisted thinking" largely relate to the cognitive distortions associated with anger discussed previously. A brief review of Burns's distortions is provided in Table 5 (p. 88).

Another example of CR is the use of Socratic questioning (i.e., "What evidence do I have that this belief is true? What evidence do I have that this belief is false?") to challenge automatic thoughts. Once a cognitive distortion or irrational automatic thought is identified, client and therapist work together to replace it with a more rational perspective. For example, helping a client to consider mitigating circumstances in a situation (i.e., the other person just lost his job and is cranky) can defuse the client's focus on malevolence and promote a more neutral appraisal of an anger-provoking situation (Novaco, 2000).

Table 5: Ten Forms of Twisted Thinking (Burns, 1999)

1. All-or-nothing thinking: Viewing a situation in dichotomous or black-and-white terms
2. Overgeneralization: Viewing a single event as representative of total disaster; chronic and inappropriate use of the words "always" and "never"
3. Mental filter: Focusing on only one negative detail while ignoring the larger picture
4. Discounting the positive: Rejecting or minimizing positive experiences
5. Jumping to conclusions: Interpreting the situation negatively when there are few or no facts to support this view. Includes "mind-reading" and "fortune telling"
6. Magnification: Exaggerating the importance of problems and shortcomings
7. Emotional reasoning: Assuming that a situation is truly negative (i.e., hopeless) just because you feel that way (i.e., sad)
8. "Should statements": Setting high, rigid expectations for self and others that are rarely based in reality
9. Labeling: Attaching a negative label to yourself or others ("jerk," "loser," etc.), which are often useless and unrepresentative of real personal characteristics
10. Personalization and blame: Holding yourself or others personally responsible for behavior or an event that is not completely under anyone's control

---

One interesting example of CR is used in a group treatment program developed by the United States Substance Abuse and Mental Health Services Administration (SAMHSA) (Reilly et al., 2002). They use the A-B-C-D model (based on the work of Ellis [1979] and Ellis & Harper [1975]) to help participants understand how cognitions and interpretations influence behavior and consequences. In the model, "A" stands for "activating event," "B" represents beliefs about the activating event, "C" represents emotional consequences, and "D" reminds individuals to utilize Socratic questioning to assess whether their beliefs about the situation are accurate (dispute). An adaptation of their Participant Worksheet is provided on page 95.

The self-instruction component of CBT has also received statistical support (effect size = .69) in empirical studies of anger management. The process of self-instruction focuses on developing realistic and empowering self-dialogue. For example, within CBT anger management sessions, clients might verbally rehearse the skills that they have learned, including a step-by-step description of cognitive restructuring, relaxation training, and positive and encouraging self-statements (i.e., "I can learn to control my anger"). Once verbal rehearsal is mastered, these statements are rehearsed internally, at first on a regular basis, and later while being applied in real-life situations (Deffenbacher et al., 2002).

BEHAVIORAL THERAPY

Behavioral interventions aim to change learned associations and replace maladaptive coping responses (which may have previously been reinforced) with adaptive coping. Examples include relaxation training, social skills training, and self-monitoring.

Deffenbacher et al. (2002) found empirical support (effect size = .74) for the use of relaxation training for anger management. The resulting decrease in anger was maintained at 12- and 15-month follow-up. Although relaxation training was initially developed for use with anxious clients, it has been adapted for use with chronically angry individuals. As discussed previously, any type of emotional and physiological arousal can negatively impact information processing and rational thinking. Theoretically, then, decreasing levels of emotional and physiological arousal should allow clients to more effectively utilize rational coping skills. Relaxation training is therefore provided to clients experiencing chronic anger for two reasons: (a) to obtain an optimal level of arousal at which new skills can be learned and (b) to decrease arousal in the "real world" so that these skills can be applied. As clients feel more in control of their responses, their new feelings of self-efficacy can become reinforcing of new response patterns (Dahlen & Deffenbacher, 2001).

Relaxation training can include a variety of specific interventions, including breathing retraining, guided imagery, progressive muscle relaxation, and meditation, to name a few. Relaxation is often practiced with a hierarchical model of systematic desensitization. Situations that elicit anger are listed on a hierarchy in order of least arousing to most arousing. The situations are developed in collaboration with the client, so that each hierarchy represents the unique experience of each client. Initially, the client practices relaxation skills in the absence of arousing stimuli. The practice begins in the therapy session and continues daily outside of sessions. As clients master the relaxation techniques, they may begin to imagine themselves in the lowest situation on the hierarchy. Even imagining the situation will elicit some arousal, and clients practice decreasing their arousal using the relaxation techniques. With each successive mastery, application continues to other items on the hierarchy. At first the exposure is imaginal, but it later moves to real-life application in order to ensure generalization. Repetition of new responses to arousing situations results in extinction of previous responses and, possibly, habituation to anger arousal (Tafrate & Kassinove, 2006).

Social skills training is also widely used in the treatment of chronic anger. The interventions take place at the expression stage of the anger-episode model and focus on teaching clients appropriate ways to express anger to others. Chronically angry people may suppress anger (which does not allow resolution), or they may express anger in aggressive ways. Social skills training can include interventions such as assertiveness training, taking a time-out from arousing situations, and basic communication skills (including open-ended questions, perception checking, and receipt and provision of constructive feedback). Oftentimes, chronically angry individuals have never been taught to predict the impact of communication, nor received instruction (even appropriate role-modeling) in timing and phrasing of feedback. Like other cognitive and behavioral interventions, these skills are often practiced first during sessions in the form of role plays and imagined situations, then applied in real-life situations in a hierarchical fashion. Role plays provide an opportunity for clients to practice new skills without fear of embarrassment or failure. Initially, the therapist may play the role of the client in order to introduce new skills and provide the role modeling that may have been absent in the client's life. Next, the client might practice these skills in the role play, perhaps with verbal guidance from the therapist. With each repetition, the therapist's guidance decreases, but feedback is always provided at the end of the skit until the client is comfortable enough to apply these communication skills in real life. Ideally, both the therapist and client will offer suggestions on how to improve each role play. When applied in a group setting, group members practice these skills and get feedback from one another before applying them in the real world.

Another type of relevant behavioral intervention is self-monitoring. This technique is applied at the trigger stage of the anger-episode model and allows clients to become more skilled at identifying stimuli that commonly trigger angry reactions, as well as typical reactions to anger. This may include keeping a daily log of all situations that incite anger, the level or intensity of experienced anger (perhaps a 5- or 10-point Likert scale), the individual's cognitive and behavioral reactions, and the consequences of these actions. Clients are asked to identify behavioral, social, physiological, emotional, and cognitive cues or triggers (Reilly et al., 2002). For individuals low in self-awareness, simply learning this procedure may require time and practice. However, the results of the self-monitoring log can then be used to develop a hierarchy for later practice, to identify coping deficits, and to increase self-awareness of triggers. An adaptation of a self-monitoring log from SAMHSA's anger management protocol is provided on page 96.

MULTICOMPONENT TREATMENTS

One treatment package that combines cognitive and behavioral interventions is Meichenbaum's stress inoculation training (SIT; 1985). SIT is delivered in three stages. In the Cognitive Preparation stage, clients learn the ways in which cognitions (including distortions) influence anger. This step might include identification of cognitive distortions and automatic thoughts. In the second stage, Skill Acquisition and Rehearsal, clients learn and practice coping skills such as relaxation training, cognitive restructuring, and self-instructional training. In the third and final stage, Application, clients apply their new skills to successively more challenging situations. SIT and similar treatment packages have been found effective for treating chronic anger in a wide variety of populations (Dahlen & Deffenbacher, 2001).

Another multicomponent treatment was developed specifically for angry Vietnam War veterans suffering with PTSD and comorbid chronic anger (Chemtob et al., 1997). The 12-session treatment is CBT-based and includes the following interventions:

1. Self-monitoring of anger frequency, intensity, and situational triggers
2. Devising a hierarchy of anger-inducing situations (based on self-monitoring log)
3. Learning relaxation skills, including progressive muscle relaxation, guided imagery, and breathing retraining
4. Learning cognitive restructuring skills and self-instruction
5. Using role plays to teach communication skills
6. Practicing new skills while imagining arousing situations from hierarchy

Special attention was given to cognitive schemas related to combat experience, threat, survival and trauma, and how these schemas impacted current life.

Veterans who completed the treatment program reported significant effects on their experience of anger. They reported an increased capacity to control anger, which was maintained at 18-month follow-up. Although the treatment did not alter scores on measures of trait anger, it did decrease the intensity of participants' reactions to anger-provoking situations. Follow-up measures suggest that the treatment's main result was its enhancement of cognitive regulation of anger.

Schema-focused therapy (SFT) is a treatment package that has not yet been formally applied to anger management treatment. However, its theoretical underpinnings might hold promise for the future of anger management treatment. SFT is a unique combination of cognitive, behavioral, attachment, experiential, and object relations therapies. Originally developed to treat Axis II Personality Disorders, SFT identifies and aims to change maladaptive schemas that influence what stimuli individuals attend to, how they process information, and what coping mechanisms they utilize. SFT posits that maladaptive schemas develop in response to early childhood needs that were unmet, and that clients can benefit from learning adaptive methods of meeting core emotional needs (Young, Klosko, & Weishaar, 2003).

SFT may be particularly applicable to anger management in terms of its focus on the enduring and stereotyped patterns in which individuals interact with the world. Given the evolutionary roots of the drive for survival, and because anger schemas focus on detecting and responding to danger, these schemas often take priority over other schemas and guide information processing, making them an important target for intervention (Novaco, 2000). Preliminary research on the application of SFT to chronic anger has yielded interesting results. In a study of the Spanish version of the Schema Questionnaire – Short Form, anger was positively correlated with three specific schemas: Entitlement, Mistrust, and Insufficient Self-Control. At the same time, anger was negatively correlated with the schema of Self-Sacrifice (Calvete et al., 2005). If the results of this study can be replicated and specific schemas associated with chronic anger can be identified, SFT can be used to alter these schemas so that they become more flexible and adaptive.

The techniques generally used in SFT are briefly summarized in Table 6 below.

Table 6: Techniques Used in Schema-Focused Therapy

Cognitive
- Socratic questioning
- Identifying automatic thoughts
- Challenging cognitive distortions

Psychodynamic
- Empathic listening
- Exploration of transference
- Providing a corrective experience

Behavioral
- Extinguishing maladaptive behavior
- Learning adaptive responses
- Self-monitoring
- Imaginal and *in vivo* practice

Experiential
- "Empty chair technique"
- Imagery
- "Acting out" fear and anxiety

Given the fear of overstimulating neural pathways of anger that was discussed previously, some of the experiential techniques associated with SFT might seem contraindicated for use with anger management. Fortunately, some guidelines do exist for the use of SFT with angry individuals. While discussing treatment for individuals with borderline personality disorder, Kellogg and Young (2006) theorize that many of these individuals do not feel they have a right to express their emotions, particularly anger. Indeed, the diagnosis of borderline personality disorder largely focuses on vacillation between a dramatic expression of emotion (especially anger) and more withdrawn expressions of guilt and shame following emotional outbursts (APA, 1994). According to Kellogg and Young, when these clients feel unable to express their anger, they will suppress it and revert to "detached protector mode" (p. 451). The authors posit that it is important to validate clients' right to be angry and that cognitive restructuring and assertiveness training can be especially effective for this goal. When anger is expressed directly at the therapist within a session, Kellogg and Young recommend that the therapist use the following techniques to help the client express anger more appropriately:

1. *Ventilate:* Encourage the client to express anger and clarify its core in a respectful way. The therapist takes a neutral, fact-finding tone that allows the anger to be expressed fully.
2. *Empathize:* Therapist responds empathically to the client's pain AFTER the source of anger has been clarified fully (they suggest that displaying empathy during the ventilation phase can diffuse anger before it is fully expressed, reinforcing suppression). Therapist can acknowledge that the client's behavior has caused pain.
3. *Reality testing:* Therapist acknowledges those aspects of the situation about which the client was accurate, then point out those aspects of the anger that may have been caused or intensified by activation of a maladaptive schema.
4. *Rehearsal of appropriate assertiveness:* Once the anger has abated, the therapist helps the client rehearse more productive, appropriately assertive ways to express anger in the future.

Interestingly, this model incorporates many of the CBT interventions discussed previously. What SFT adds to other treatment models is its focus on the origins of maladaptive anger schemas and empathic understanding of unmet needs in childhood. This focus conveys a clear and nonjudgmental respect for the client's perspective, which can be a new and very different experience for the chronically angry individual. This integrative approach may indeed guide the future of anger management treatment.

Although several multicomponent treatments have been shown to be effective for chronically angry individuals, none has yet incorporated SFT. To rectify that deficit, we propose the following nine-session treatment program, which combines empirically supported CBT interventions with the most relevant components of SFT. We believe that the skills and interventions included in this model will be relevant for most individuals with chronic anger, but the specific focuses and topics discussed should, of course, be molded to each individual's specific presentation and needs. To that end, a thorough assessment that includes one of the anger assessment tools discussed previously should be conducted prior to the client's first session in order to identify the client's unique presentation and to determine whether a psychiatric referral is in order. As with all CBT models, the therapist-client relationship is considered collaborative; the therapist aims to elicit examples and possible applications from the client, who is considered the expert of his own life. If at any point in the course of treatment the client expresses anger at the therapist, the process of Ventilate, Empathize, Test Reality, and Rehearsal of Assertiveness set forth by Kellogg and Young (2006) should be followed by the therapist. Each weekly (except for last) session will last 1 hour. A brief description of each session's goals is provided below. For more detailed descriptions of each specific intervention, please refer to the previous section.

Session #1

- Give feedback from initial assessment and describe the treatment program.
- Explore physical, cognitive, and behavioral correlates of anger.
- Explore positive and negative consequences of anger.
- Introduce self-monitoring procedure and thorough description of the escalation phase of anger.
- For homework (HW): Week-long observation of anger levels, using self-monitoring log provided on page 96.

Session #2

- Review homework.
- Results of self-monitoring exercise may indicate a need for psychiatric referral if anger levels are consistently high and/or violence is experienced.
- Identify triggers for individual's anger. These may be social, cognitive, behavioral, or physiological.
- Identify physiological, cognitive, and behavioral cues that indicate increasing anger.
- Teach breathing retraining to dampen physiological arousal.
- HW: Continue to monitor anger levels and triggers, and practice breathing retraining daily.

Session #3

- Review homework.
- Begin discussion of A-B-C-D model, focusing specifically on the concept of activating events or trigger.
- Following review of anger triggers, identify which can be changed or avoided, and which must be dealt with for the individual client.
- Teach additional relaxation skills, such as progressive muscle relaxation (PMR) or guided imagery.

- For HW: Practice relaxation skills daily and make changes or avoid triggers, as appropriate.

Session #4

- Review homework.
- Continue discussion of A-B-C-D model.
- Pay special attention to beliefs and automatic thoughts that may suggest the presence of schemas related to entitlement, mistrust, and lack of self-control.
- Review common cognitive distortions and introduce Socratic Questioning (these interventions are considered "D" – disputing beliefs in the model).
- For HW: Practice relaxation skills; observe relationships between triggers and beliefs during the week; review list of cognitive distortions several times during the week.

Session #5

- Review HW.
- Continue review of A-B-C-D model, focusing specifically on disputing beliefs through the use of cognitive restructuring/Socratic questioning.
- Introduce concept of thought stopping.
- Introduce self-instruction in the form of developing positive coping statements to replace irrational, unproductive automatic thoughts.
- For HW: Practice thought stopping, cognitive restructuring, and self-instruction.

Session #6

- Review HW.
- Begin teaching problem-solving skills, applying the concepts of identifying the problem, brainstorming solutions, identifying resources, and enacting a solution to examples of stressful situations from real-life.
- Ensure that client is incorporating knowledge of cognitive distortions when identifying the problem, and that possible solutions include learned relaxation skills.
- For HW: Practice problem-solving skills in real-life situations.

Session #7

- Review HW.
- Introduce social skills training in the form of assertiveness training and general communication skills.
- Utilize role modeling and role-play to illustrate.
- Engage client in predicting how the other person in the confrontation might react to different presentations.
- For HW: Practice communication skills.

Session #8

- Review HW.
- Continue practicing social skills training, focusing on what did and did not work effectively for client during the week.
- Utilize role-playing exercises, with therapist providing feedback after each scenario.
- For HW: Continue practicing communication skills, and complete anger inventory for post-treatment comparisons.

Session #9 (Scheduled 2 Weeks After Session #8)

- Review HW.
- Review comparisons of scores on pretreatment and posttreatment assessments.
- Review course of therapy and ask client to assess his or her level of competence in each skill area.
- If client is clearly deficient in any skill, offer additional session focused on these specific skills.
- If client has met his or her goals, this serves as termination session.

SAMHSA's A-B-C-D Model
Participant Worksheet*

This worksheet will teach you about the A-B-C-D Model** as a form of cognitive restructuring.

The A-B-C-D Model

The A-B-C-D Model is consistent with the way some people conceptualize anger management treatment. In this model, *"A" stands for an activating event.* An activating event is any experience that inspires an emotional reaction. *"B" represents our beliefs* about the activating event. It is not the events themselves that produce feelings such as anger, but our interpretations and beliefs about the events. *"C" stands for the emotional consequences.* These are the feelings experienced as a result of interpretations and beliefs concerning the event. *"D" stands for dispute.* This part of the model involves identifying any irrational beliefs and replacing them with more realistic ways of looking at the activating event. The purpose of this exercise is to replace self-statements that lead to, or escalate, anger with ideas that allow you to have a more realistic and accurate interpretation of the event.

- What does each of the letters of the A-B-C-D Model stand for?

  _____

  _____

- List some of your irrational beliefs.

  _____

  _____

- What are some more realistic beliefs about the event?

  _____

  _____

---

* Adapted from *Anger Management for Substance Abuse and Mental Health Clients: Participant Workbook*, by P. M. Reilly et al., 2002. Rockville, MD: Substance Abuse and Mental Health Services Administration.

** Based on the work of Albert Ellis (1979), and Albert Ellis and R. A. Harper (1975).

SAMHSA's Self-Monitoring Log*

Check-In Procedure:
Monitoring Anger for the Week

In this session, you learned to monitor your anger and to identify anger-provoking events and situations. Each week we will review your homework and discuss the highest level of anger that you reached in the previous 7 days. You will also be asked to identify the event that triggered your anger, the cues that were associated with your anger, and the ways you managed your anger in response to the event. Please use the following format to check in at the beginning of each session:

```
1 ------- 2 ------- 3 ------- 4 ------- 5 ------- 6 ------- 7 ------- 8 ------- 9 ------- 10
Complete                                                               Very angry,
lack of anger                                                          loss of control
                            ANGER SCALE
```

1. What was the highest number you reached on the anger scale during the past week?

   _____

2. What was the event that triggered that anger?

   _____

   _____

3. What cues were associated with the anger-provoking event?

   Physical cues _____

   Behavioral cues _____

   Emotional cues _____

   Cognitive cues _____

4. What did you do to avoid reaching 10 on the anger meter?

   _____

   _____

For each day of the upcoming week, monitor and record the highest number you reach on the anger scale.

_____ M _____ T _____ W _____ Th _____ F _____ Sat _____ Sun

---

*Adapted from *Anger Management for Substance Abuse and Mental Health Clients: Participant Workbook*, by P. M. Reilly et al., 2002, Rockville, MD: Substance Abuse and Mental Health Services Administration.

Quick Reference Guide for
Electronic Anger Management Resources*

General Information
About Anger

The American Psychological Association offers a webpage with information and resources about anger:

http://www.apa.org/topics/topicanger.html

All About Counseling offers a nonjudgmental information page about anger, making it an appropriate resource for clients who are beginning to address problems managing anger:

http://www.allaboutcounseling.com/anger.htm

Treatment Resources

For free anger-management materials for clinicians, including a structured treatment program for groups, visit the U.S. Department of Health and Substance Abuse at:

http://www.samhsa.gov

For more information on Schema-Focused Therapy, including the Schema Inventory, visit:

http://www.schematherapy.com

Relaxation Techniques

Wikipedia.org and HelpGuide.org both offer organized links for information about specific relaxation techniques:

http://en.wikipedia.org/wiki/Relaxation_techniques
http://www.helpguide.org

---

*Although all websites cited in this contribution were correct at the time of publication, they are subject to change at any time.

CONTRIBUTORS

Carin M. Lefkowitz, PsyD, is a Staff Psychologist at the Villanova University Counseling Center, where she counsels and consults with students, families, and faculty. She is also an adjunct professor at Immaculata University and Widener University. Dr. Lefkowitz has written and presented in the areas of innovative and evidence-based treatments for psychological concerns. She may be contacted at Villanova University, 800 E. Lancaster Avenue, Villanova, PA 19085. E-mail: Carin.Lefkowitz@villanova.edu

Maurice F. Prout, PhD, ABPP, is currently professor at the Institute for Graduate Clinical Psychology at Widener University, Chester, Pennsylvania. He also directs the respecialization program housed within the Institute. His clinical interests include the treatment of anxiety and mood disorders as well as topics related to behavioral medicine. He is a Diplomate in Clinical Psychology and a Founding Fellow of the Academy of Cognitive Therapy. Dr. Prout can be reached at Widener University, Chester, PA 19013. E-mail: mfprout@widener.edu

RESOURCES

American Psychiatric Association. (1994). *Diagnostic and Statistical Manual of Mental Disorders* (4th ed.). Washington, DC: Author.

Beck, R., & Fernandez, E. (1998). Cognitive-behavioral therapy in the treatment of anger: A meta-analysis. *Cognitive Therapy and Research, 22*(1), 63-74.

Berkowitz, L. (1990). On the formation and regulation of anger and aggression: A cognitive–neoassociationistic analysis. *American Psychologist, 45*(4), 494-503.

Burns, D. (1999). *The Feeling Good Handbook* (rev. ed.). New York: Plume.

Buss, A. H., & Warren, W. L. (2000). *Aggression Questionnaire (AQ).* Los Angeles, CA: Western Psychological Services.

Butcher, J. N., Dahlstrom, W. G., Graham, J. R., Tellegen, A, & Kaemmer, B. (1989).*The Minnesota Multiphasic Personality Inventory-2 (MMPI-2): Manual for administration and scoring.* Minneapolis, MN: University of Minnesota Press.

Calvete, E., Estevez, A., Lopez de Arroyabe, E., & Ruiz, P. (2005). The Schema Questionnaire – Short Form: Structure and relationship with automatic thoughts and symptoms of affective disorders. *European Journal of Psychological Assessment, 21*(2), 90-99.

Chemtob, C., Hamada, R., Novaco, R., & Gross, D. (1997). Cognitive-behavioral treatment for severe anger in posttraumatic stress disorder. *Journal of Consulting and Clinical Psychology, 65*(1), 184-189.

Cook, W., & Medley, D. (1954). Proposed hostility and pharasaic-virtue scales for the MMPI. *Journal of Applied Psychology, 38,* 414-418.

Dahlen, E., & Deffenbacher, J. (2001). Anger management. In W. Lyddon & J. Jones (Eds.), *Empirically Supported Cognitive Therapies: Current and Future Applications* (pp. 163-181). New York: Springer.

Deffenbacher, J., Oetting, E., & DiGiuseppe, R. (2002). Principles of empirically supported interventions applied to anger management. *Counseling Psychologist, 30*(2), 262-280.

Del Vecchio, T., & O'Leary, K. (2004). Effectiveness of anger treatments for specific anger problems: A meta-analytic review. *Clinical Psychology Review, 24,* 15-34.

DiGiuseppe, R., & Tafrate, R. C. (2004). *Anger Disorders Scale (ADS).* North Tonawanda, NY: Multi-Health Systems.

Edwards, H. (2006). Psychopharmacological considerations in anger management. In E. Feindler (Ed.), *Anger-Related Disorders* (pp. 189-202). New York: Springer.

Ellis, A. (1979). Rational-emotive therapy. In R. Corsini (Ed.), *Current Psychotherapies* (pp. 185-229). Itasca, IL: Peacock Publishers.

Ellis, A., & Harper, R. A. (1975). *A New Guide to Rational Living.* N. Hollywood, CA: Wilshire Books.

Erwin, B., Heimberg, R., Schneier, F., & Liebowitz, M. (2003). Anger experience and expression in social anxiety disorder: Pretreatment profile and predictors of attrition and response to cognitive-behavioral treatment. *Behavior Therapy, 34,* 331-350.

Hatch, J., Schoenfeld, L., Boutros, N., Seleshi, E., Moore, P., & Cyr-Provost, M. (1991). Anger and hostility in tension-type headaches. *Headache: The Journal of Head and Face Pain, 31*(5), 302-304.

Kassinove, H., & Tafrate, R. C. (2006). Anger-related disorders: Basic issues, models, and diagnostic considerations. In E. Feindler (Ed.), *Anger-Related Disorders* (pp. 1-27). New York: Springer.

Kellogg, S., & Young, J. (2006). Schema therapy for borderline personality disorder. *Journal of Clinical Psychology, 62*(4), 445-458.

Lachar, B. (1993). Coronary-prone behavior: Type A behavior revisited. *Texas Heart Institute Journal, 20,* 143-151.

Lench, H. (2004). Anger management: Diagnostic differences and treatment implications. *Journal of Social and Clinical Psychology, 23*(4), 512-531.

Mayne, T., & Ambrose, T. (1999). Research review on anger in psychotherapy. *Journal of Clinical Psychology, 55*(3), 353-363.

McCann, J., & Biaggio, M. K. (1989). Narcissistic personality features and self-reported anger. *Psychological Reports, 64,* 55-58.

Meichenbaum, D. H. (1985). *Stress Inoculation Training.* New York: Pergamon Press.

Novaco, R.W. (1994). *Novaco Anger Scale and Provocation Inventory (NAS-PI).* Los Angeles, CA: Western Psychological Services.

Novaco, R. W. (2000). Anger. In A. Kazdin (Ed.), *Encyclopedia of Psychology* (pp. 170-174). Washington, DC: American Psychological Association.

Orth, U., & Wieland, E. (2006). Anger, hostility, and posttraumatic stress disorder in trauma-exposed adults: A meta-analysis. *Journal of Consulting and Clinical Psychology, 74*(4), 698-706.

Reilly, P. M., Shopshire, M. S., Durazzo, T. C., & Campbell, T. A. (2002). *Anger Management for Substance Abuse and Mental Health Clients: Participant Workbook.* Rockville, MD: Substance Abuse and Mental Health Services Administration.

Spielberger, C.D. (1991). *State-Trait Anger Expression Inventory: STAXI Professional Manual.* Lutz, FL: Psychological Assessment Resources.

Tafrate, R. C., & Kassinove, H. (2006). Anger management for adults: A menu-driven cognitive-behavioral approach to the treatment of anger disorders. *Anger-Related Disorders* (pp. 115-137). New York: Springer.

Tarasoff v. Regents of the University of California, 13 Cal.3d 177, 529 P.2d 533 (1974), *vacated,* 17 Cal.3d 425, 551 P.2d 334 (1976).

Thomas, S. (2006). Cultural and gender considerations in the assessment and treatment of anger-related disorders. In E. Feindler (Ed.), *Anger-Related Disorders* (pp. 71-95). New York: Springer.

Waller, G., Babbs, M., Milligan, R., Meyer, C., Ohanian, __., & Leung, N. (2003). Anger and core beliefs in the eating disorders. *International Journal of Eating Disorders, 34,* 118-124.

Witte, T., Callahan, K., & Perez-Lopez, M. (2002). Narcissism and anger: An exploration of underlying correlates. *Psychological Reports, 90,* 871-875.

Young, J., Klosko, J., & Weishaar, M. (2003). *Schema Therapy: A Practitioner's Guide.* New York: Guilford.

Zelin, M. L., Adler, G., & Myerson, P. (1972). Anger Self-Report: An objective questionnaire for the measurement of aggression. *Journal of Consulting and Clinical Psychology, 39*(2), 340.

Pro-Ana: Analysis and Implications for Treatment of Anorexia Nervosa

Mette Traae Brynolf

This contribution provides clinicians with useful and practical information relating to Anorexia Nervosa, the radical social movement of Pro-Anorexia (Pro-Ana), and how to work with the highly resistant client. Due to the limited information available regarding Pro-Ana, an extensive overview is provided to assist in the understanding of the added dimension this provides when working with clients diagnosed with Anorexia Nervosa. Further, the specific issue of resistance is examined in terms of natural response cycles and the Stages of Change Model, and examples of natural response cycles are provided. A counterintuitive stance with creative approaches to working with the highly resistant client is suggested and explained, and implications involving this stance are examined.

INTRODUCTION

Anorexia Nervosa is one of the most lethal and hard to treat psychiatric disorders (Crisp, 1997): its mortality rate is 20% (Crisp, 1997) and recidivism rates are over 50% (Harris et al., 2001). These facts clearly indicate that psychology as a profession is struggling with treating this disorder. Information regarding the Pro-Anorexia (Pro-Ana) movement and the impact it has on young people with this disorder becomes highly relevant for psychologists when looking at the high level of resistance to change and the profound aspect of denial of illness embedded in the disorder (Harris et al., 2001). One of the inherent characteristics of this disorder is high resistance to treatment (Crisp, 1997; Hall, 1985; Sargent, Liebman, & Silver, 1985). There is currently very limited psychological literature regarding the Pro-Ana movement and its relevance to psychological intervention. Thus, this author seeks to provide the clinician with information regarding this radical social movement and how it relates to psychological interventions in terms of resistance and compliance.

The main philosophy of the Pro-Ana movement is that Anorexia Nervosa is not an illness but a lifestyle choice (see, e.g., www.plagueangel.net/grotto).* Individuals involved in this movement are mostly people who meet criteria for the disorder. Extensive websites regarding Pro-Ana can be found on the Internet (e.g., www.plagueangel.net/grotto/; http://famine.brokensanity.org). This is a highly progressive social movement whose general stance is against seeing Anorexia Nervosa as a psychiatric disorder and thus against psychological

---

*All websites cited in this contribution are subject to change at any time.

treatment for Anorexia Nervosa. On many of the sites, resistance to treatment is encouraged and supported (e.g., www.plagueangel.net/grotto). There is an extensive literature base on different treatment approaches to Anorexia Nervosa (e.g., Crisp, 1997; Garner & Garfinkel, 1997; Werne, 1996), far too vast to be reviewed and discussed in this contribution. Rather, the focus will be on natural human response cycles in relation to the therapeutic relationship between client and clinician, specifically in terms of resistance, chaos, and control.

Resistance is examined through Threat Rigidity Theory (Staw, Sandelands, & Dutton, 1981), the aspects of chaos and control are examined through Chaos Theory (Briggs & Peat, 1999), and predictable response cycles are further examined through the Catalyst Model of Change (Fraser, 1998). Further, readiness for change and implications for treatment will be examined according to the Stages of Change model by Prochaska and DiClemente (Prochaska, 1999). These models are discussed in greater detail in terms of the impact of normal response cycles and the importance of assessing how ready the individual is for change before initiating an action-oriented treatment (e.g., cognitive behavioral treatment, interpersonal treatment, etc.). The relevance of these models is reviewed in terms of working with an individual diagnosed with Anorexia Nervosa, and especially clients involved with the radical social movement of Pro-Ana.

Finally, we suggest a creative counterintuitive stance the clinician can adopt when working with the highly resistant client, especially as it relates to Anorexia Nervosa and the radical social movement Pro-Ana. Certain principles relating to small changes that the clinician can introduce through this stance are provided. The importance of acceptance, empathy, and authenticity is examined and emphasized, and implications of this approach are examined in terms of importance for the therapeutic relationship.

ANOREXIA NERVOSA AND TREATMENT

Prevalence rates of Anorexia Nervosa are estimated to be from 0.5% to 1.0% of the general population (American Psychiatric Association, 2000; Wakeling, 1996). This is a fairly large number when considering that this does not cover people who do not meet the full criteria for the diagnosis and are likely given the diagnosis Eating Disorder Not Otherwise Specified (NOS). Some researchers claim that the diagnosis of Anorexia Nervosa is too narrow and that the disorder should rather be seen as a spectrum disorder. Garvin and Striegel-Moore (2001) propose that many people with symptoms of Anorexia Nervosa go undiagnosed due to not meeting the full criteria, and that this leads to the prevalence rates presented being lower than the actual number of people suffering from the effects of this disorder.

According to Steiger, Bruce, and Israel (2003), it is estimated that as many as 10% of school-age females in industrialized countries display what they refer to as "partial Anorexia Nervosa." These females could probably be considered to suffer from Anorexia Nervosa but may not meet full criteria according to today's diagnostic classification system. As stated by Powers and Santana (2002), the presentation of children with Anorexia Nervosa is diffuse and usually does not meet the criteria for diagnosis as adults would. According to Powers and Santana (2002), more adolescents are diagnosed with Eating Disorder NOS than adults, often due to the lack of amenorrhea in the adolescent. Thus it becomes hard to clearly define the diagnosis of Anorexia Nervosa for children (Powers & Santana, 2002). This is a problem when considering the rising number of young adolescents and children who are suffering from Anorexia Nervosa and who are possibly being affected by the Pro-Ana movement.

In the United States, results across five major studies indicate that there is no significant difference in the prevalence rates for Anorexia Nervosa among Whites, Hispanics, and Asian Americans. However, Zhang, Snowden, and Sue (1998) found that Asian Americans are much less likely to utilize mental health services and report problems relating to mental health, including Anorexia Nervosa. Thus, the results indicating the same prevalence rates for Whites and Asian Americans with regard to Anorexia Nervosa are alarming when the likelihood of underreporting by Asian Americans is taken into account.

Anorexia Nervosa is one of the most lethal and difficult to treat psychiatric disorders (Crisp, 1997; Neumärker, 2000). Anorexia Nervosa is regarded as the psychiatric disorder with the highest mortality rates. Several studies regarding mortality rates report different percentages, ranging from 10% to 25% (Crisp, 1997; Hersen & Bellack, 1999; Neumärker, 2000; Reijonen et al., 2003; Steinhausen, 2002). The number one cause of death is starvation, followed by suicide (Neumärker, 2000). The high mortality rates pose a serious challenge to the practicing clinician. With recidivism rates of around 50% that have not been reduced since 1978, there are clear indications that psychology as a profession is struggling with treating this disorder (Castro et al., 2004; Harris et al., 2001; Hersen & Bellack, 1999). This is despite extensive literature on different treatment forms of Anorexia Nervosa (Garner & Needleman, 1997; Harris et al., 2001). Based on this knowledge, the clinician is likely to feel urgency in intervening with the client suffering from Anorexia Nervosa to prevent harm or death by starvation or suicide. There is a dire need to intervene with an individual diagnosed with this disorder, yet the client often has an implacable resistance to change (Garner & Needleman, 1997).

In the literature, it is noted that people diagnosed with Anorexia Nervosa are perceived by clinicians as difficult to treat. One of the major factors contributing to this is the basic resistance to treatment and the profound denial of illness (Harris et al., 2001). Across the literature, the individual diagnosed with Anorexia Nervosa is characterized as behaving in a secretive, defiant, and resistant manner (e.g., Sargent et al., 1985). The resistance to give up control and to stop the starvation behaviors is to be expected when restriction and control is one of the very cornerstones of the illness. It takes a lot of control in order to maintain these stringent conditions in one's life, and thus it can be seen as inevitable that the individual will resist admitting illness and accepting treatment. This resistance and control is embraced and encouraged in the radical social movement of Pro-Ana.

THE PRO-ANOREXIA MOVEMENT AND RELEVANCE TO TREATMENT

History of Pro-Ana

There have been Pro-Ana websites on the Internet since 1994. The federal government made attempts to restrict these websites starting in 1996. These attempts were defeated after a campaign by the American Civil Liberties Union based on the "freedom of speech" argument (Barrett, n.d.). In the fall of 2001, there was an outcry in the media regarding Pro-Anorexia Internet websites (Dolan, 2003). The National Association of Anorexia Nervosa and Associated Disorders asked big Internet servers to remove Pro-Ana sites. The protest in 2001 led to some of the larger search engines, such as Yahoo, closing down websites containing Pro-Ana information. The reason for the protest was the provocative information contained on these sites, and the fear was that impressible teens would develop Anorexia Nervosa from reading this material. Holly Hoff of the National Eating Disorders Association stated in 2004 that "With the pressures to be thin in our culture, [these websites are] like placing a loaded gun in the hands of someone who is feeling suicidal" ("Girls who don't eat," 2005). The pressure from the public initially led to a decrease in easily accessible websites in 2001 but did not remove the websites from the Internet. Also, only websites in English were shut down, and thus all Pro-Ana websites in other languages (e.g., Spanish) on American search engines were still active.

Since the initial decrease in 2001, there has been a huge revival of these sites. In October of 2003 there was an estimate of over 400 Pro-Anorexia websites on the Internet (Dolan, 2003), and the number is continuously growing at an extremely fast pace. Pro-Ana websites are found all over the world and in most languages. A review of the websites today as compared to several years ago reveals that the overall movement is becoming more sophisticated and persuasive in its views. There has been a clear indication that the movement has developed from being rudimentary websites with personal suggestions to being a more organized network including web rings, paying membership sites, solidarity/membership bracelets, and elaborate rituals performed to seek help and guidance from "the goddess" of Anorexia Nervosa. When looking at the high number of visitors to these sites, it becomes relevant for practitioners to be aware of this movement and how this can affect treatment. This author's search on 10-07-2003 of the search term Pro-Ana on Yahoo.com (United States) yielded 530,000 results. The same search on 06-24-2005 yielded 5,700,000 results from the same search engine. These findings are consistent with the large number of visitors to some of the major Pro-Ana sites. For instance, this author was visitor number 1,971,162 for the year 2005 when visiting one major Pro-Ana site on 06-24-2005. One of the more recent Pro-Ana sites recently celebrated their "one millionth post" (www.proanamia.com/welcome.html). Due to the nature of these websites, and to the overall reaction to these websites in society, the web addresses are likely to change on a frequent basis. As such, although the information provided about these sites remains current, a site may or may not be currently available at the respective referenced web address.

In 2004, the first "essential guide" on Pro-Ana was published (Uca, 2004), and it has been widely distributed and is easily obtainable. It details what the Pro-Ana movement stands for and is essentially indistinguishable from a classic Pro-Ana website in book form. The book contains an explanation of the words used within the Pro-Ana movement, tips and tricks for starvation behaviors, "thinspiration," information on Pro-Ana as a religion, and member statements. On several Pro-Ana web forums, the members describe this as their Pro-Ana "handbook" that they carry with them wherever they go, utilizing it when needed for advice and inspiration. This is further an indication of the growth and sophistication of the Pro-Ana movement in recent years.

Overview and Relevance to Treatment

Pro-Ana is a progressive underground social movement that believes Anorexia Nervosa is a lifestyle choice of starvation behavior rather than a psychiatric disorder. People leading the underground movement tend to be people suffering from the disorder working hard to provide support and advice to others who may want to live with Anorexia Nervosa (e.g., http://famine.brokensanity.org; http://www.proanamia.com/welcome.html). These people usually do not see themselves as suffering from a disease, but rather as having chosen a lifestyle that is focused around Anorexia Nervosa. A common definition of Pro-Ana is that it stands for "proactive, volitional anorexia" (http://www.plagueangel.net/grotto). This is commonly referred to as "Ana praxis," referring to the practice of self-control and taking full control over their bodies by "practicing" Anorexia Nervosa, that is, starvation behavior (http://www.plagueangel.net/grotto).

Most claim that they are refusing to "teach" others these behaviors, but the vast majority of websites have multiple tips and advice relating to starvation behaviors (http://www.proanamia.com; http://community.livejournal.com/proanorexia). Most Pro-Ana websites have disclaimers that state that the content of the site may trigger certain starvation behaviors in people who are recovering, are already dieting, or who have a wish to be thin. These statements are often worded in such a way that, although providing a warning, they invite people who are "strong" and who have a strong will to be thin to examine the site further.

Control and will power are emphasized on all of these sites, and the practice of Anorexia Nervosa is seen as the way to be strong and have full control over oneself in a liberating manner (http://www.plagueangel.net/grotto). Certain websites have been operational for many years although they have changed location many times (e.g., http://www. plagueangel.net/ grotto; http://www.proanamia.com). These long-term websites are especially elaborate and provide extensive information relating to starvation behavior (e.g., http://famine. brokensanity.org; http://www.proanamia.com). Most Pro-Ana sites include similar information in addition to the disclaimer and introductory page. They usually include a tips and advice section related to starvation behaviors and how to hide the behaviors (e.g. http:// www.proanamia.com), and detailed explanations of the criteria for the different eating disorders (e.g., http://famine.brokensanity.org; http://www.mianaland.com/welcome.php), in addition to thinspiration, poetry and art, articles and quotations, and different chat-rooms or bulletin boards.

Many websites provide the reader with links to different articles that appear to support the notion that not eating or eating very little is healthy, such as studies indicating that eating less leads to a longer life (http://www.plagueangel.net/grotto), in addition to links to other sites, both diet and fasting sites, and other pro-eating disorder sites. Some sites include links to "recovery sites" as well. These links appear to be helping websites for people who have "gone too far" with their starvation. Some of these websites appear to be websites from professionals; however, upon closer examination they are often Pro-Ana (e.g., http://www. makaylashealingplace.dnswh.com). Most websites have recently joined large web communities where membership is required to access all the information on the sites (e.g., http:// community.livejournal.com/proanorexia); the person joins the specific chat sub-forum he or she is most compatible with in terms of age, gender, special interests, weight, trigger foods, and so on. The Pro-Ana movement is now also changing and spreading through other forms of media, such as YouTube, MySpace, and Facebook.

Some websites send out newsletters to their members, and all of the websites have some form of inspirational section, called "thinspiration." The "thinspiration" sections contain pictures of models and actresses who suffer from Anorexia Nervosa or pictures that have been digitally modified to make the individual in the picture appear extremely thin, most often with bones protruding and their faces looking emaciated; the modified images reflect people who appear to be much less than 85% of their ideal bodyweight. These pictures are intended to inspire the appropriate thinness (e.g., http://www.prettythin.com; http://www.prothinspo. com/). There are also images of severely obese people, something referred to as reverse thinspiration (e.g., http://www.prothinspo.com).

Since the start of Pro-Ana websites on the Internet, there has been a tendency to refer to "Ana" as a goddess (sometimes referred to as "Anamadim") and to refer to people who are "Pro-Ana" as "Ana's angels." Pro-Ana has also been described as a monotheistic religion, where the followers pray to the Goddess Ana and follow "sacred texts" (Uca, 2004). Since 2004, many sites have posted descriptions of elaborate rituals to perform in order to strengthen one's will to starve and rituals to "summon the Goddess." This can include rather elaborate relaxation exercises and self-suggestions in addition to a specific starvation plan that the individual will commit to for the next 4 weeks at a time (http://www.plagueangel.net/grotto). In 2002, "ana-bracelets" became highly popular. These are red bracelets sold over the Internet and worn to demonstrate solidarity for the Pro-Ana movement. In some chat-rooms on the Pro-Ana sites, young people write about wearing the bracelets to school and that it is a good way to recognize peers at school with whom they can talk freely about their wish to be thin and about the Pro-Ana movement.

Many of the Pro-Ana websites provide advice on how to keep starvation behavior from parents and anyone in a helping profession (http://www.proanamia.com/welcome.html). Some of these websites also contain information about how to appear compliant with Anorexia Nervosa treatment while hiding the disorder from the helping professions. There is an awareness that being diagnosed with Anorexia Nervosa will lead to greater pressure from parents and their surrounding support system about being "sick" and needing treatment. Thus, an individual who is involved with Pro-Ana and who is strongly against treatment does not want to meet full criteria for Anorexia Nervosa. The information provided regarding criteria will assist the individual in preparing for how to present to a helping professional in order not to meet full criteria for the disorder.

There is a very negative attitude toward any helping profession on most of these sites, often using quotation marks when writing about "doctors" and "professionals" and portraying an authority which is out to harm people rather than help (e.g., http://famine.brokensanity.org; www.plagueangel.net/grotto). Several websites have vast collections of statements made by professionals regarding Pro-Ana, and they are used in a manner to demonstrate that the helping profession's attitude is one of judgment and lack of empathy for people with Anorexia Nervosa. When reading these statements out of context and from the perspective of an individual with eating disorders, they can appear nonsupportive, and thus it is an effective tool to use in the fight toward seeing the helping profession as the "established authority."

To many young people, the webmasters who run Pro-Ana websites are people to be looked up to and whom they admire. Therefore, statements from helping professionals describing people running Pro-Ana websites in highly negative terms contributes to the negative impression of the helping professions not being supportive and empathic to people with Anorexia Nervosa. In the media, some clinicians have made remarks about Pro-Ana sites as being signs of desperation and the webmasters as building a rather destructive community for lonely and desperate people. On many of the more established sites, there are lists of quotations (from professionals) that people with eating disorders have been met with in their lives. The links to these statements are often labeled "idiot doctors" or similarly highly negative titles (http://famine.brokensanity.org; http://www.plagueangel.net/grotto). The following are examples of quotes regarding the helping professionals:

- "You're a smart girl, why don't you just stop?" (psychiatrist, again)
- "When I went to find a new psychiatrist, I stopped at this one office, and receptionist said, "No, we can't help you; Doctor ____ is only taking severe, chronic cases right now, she's very busy. You're fine, go home and make sure you eat 3 meals a day."
- "And then they dismiss you, flippant, and go back to their income of overprescribing psychotropic medication."
- "Well, she's drinking frappuccinos, so she must be doing better. They have a lot calories, you know." (psychiatrist.)
- "If she had an eating disorder she'd weigh a lot less." (my pediatrician, after mom told him I'd been diagnosed with anorexia.)
- "Or how about the time when I went to my new doctor, told him I'd suffered with various EDs, two miscarriages, and a history of hereditary depression, and he looked at me in the eyes, all austere and gentle, and said to me: "I want you to wake up, look at yourself in the mirror and say, 'I love you' to your reflection." (retrieved from http://famine.brokensanity.org, Answers/Idiot Doctors section).

These are a few examples of quotes found on Pro-Ana websites regarding previous negative experiences with helping professionals. Regardless if these statements are taken out of context and their authenticity cannot be validated, they are used on Pro-Ana websites as powerful testimonials about people from the helping professions.

Pro-Ana as a Radical Social Movement

According to Downing (2001), the use of the Internet to make radical societal changes in the form of resistance movements is powerful. Websites constructed and maintained by individuals rather than big organizations can be extremely powerful in eliciting change and participation in radical social movements (Downing, 2001). Through history, radical social movements have been a major cause for change in societies all over the world (Downing, 2001). Embedded in the term radical social movement is resistance toward authority and currently held beliefs (Downing, 2001). The Pro-Ana movement can be defined as a radical social movement, protesting and working against society's current view of Anorexia Nervosa as a psychiatric disorder. The power of this radical social movement is evident in the growth and spread of the movement, including the international awareness it has evoked. Further, in all radical social movements there exists a concept of secrecy and togetherness that strengthens the resistance (Downing, 2001). When looking at the Pro-Ana movement, secrecy and togetherness in the form of membership in chat rooms and wearing bracelets to identify other "members" is a very important aspect of the movement.

According to Martin, Hewstone, and Martin (2003), people holding a minority position on a given attitude are more likely to hold on to that opinion and less likely to change their attitude for a more majority-held position on a certain issue. Thus it can be concluded that people who adhere to the view of Pro-Ana (a minority position) are less likely to be persuaded to believe that Anorexia Nervosa is an illness (majority position), and thus it can be concluded they are likely to be more resistant to treatment than people who are not adhering to this radical social movement. This natural reaction of resistance in the face of perceived threat is addressed in depth in the following section, where the natural response cycles involved in threat, crisis, and chaos are closely examined.

NATURAL RESPONSE CYCLES

Regardless of theoretical orientation, the overall common goal for treatment of Anorexia Nervosa is for the individual to gain weight and become a psychologically healthy individual. One of the most important aspects regarding treatment becomes to keep the individual alive and to prevent the individual from dying of starvation (Bruch, 1985; Garner & Garfinkel, 1997; Garner & Magana, 2002, Harris et al., 2001). Most treatment approaches, including psychological approaches, make assumptions that the client is ready for change and ready to take action toward change (Connors, Donovan, & DiClemente, 2001). This becomes an essential problem when looking at the highly resistant client (Crisp, 1997). It becomes an even greater obstacle when considering the radical social movement of Pro-Ana, where secrecy is strongly encouraged, and resistance is continuously emphasized and supported (e.g., http://famine.brokensanity.org). Further, there is an overall suggestion within the Pro-Ana movement of false compliance. This false compliance is likely to greatly impact the therapeutic relationship, and it can lead the clinician and client to be locked into a countertherapeutic cycle based on natural responses to threat.

The natural response to threat can be described based on Threat Rigidity Theory as suggested by Staw et al. (1981), which broadly proposes that when people perceive a threat, they are more likely to act and respond in a well-learned or habitual manner. The theory suggests that the individual will react by ignoring peripheral information and will focus his or her attention more narrowly. Staw and Ross (1989) found that people tend to persist in their behavior in escalating situations even if they perceive it to be a losing course of action. Further, people will commonly react to threat by becoming less open to new ideas and less open to change (Griffin, Tesluk, & Jacobs, 1995). They will also narrow their choices to the most logical and conservative choices. Thus, anything seen as involving risk will be ruled out as a chosen response (Griffin et al., 1995). As an example, according to this theory, a clinician knowledgeable about the difficulty in treating Anorexia Nervosa is likely to perceive the client's resistance to initial treatment as a threat and will respond with well-learned compliance-based intervention models, often trying more of the same. The client will in turn respond in a habitual manner by increasing starvation behavior. Both persons will attend more narrowly, and persist in this manner, even when the resistance and the starvation behavior is escalating, and, according to the theory, both will be less open to new ideas and to changing their course of action. Finally, there is a risk that the clinician will not attend to barriers to therapy such as the client's involvement in the Pro-Ana movement in relation to resistance, due to narrowing his or her attention to the client's presentation and not attending to peripheral information. If the clinician does not ask the client for this information, the client is not likely to share his or her views. This highlights the importance of the informed clinician, who can address the issue of Pro-Ana with his or her clients and thus take some of the power out of the resistance to the helping profession.

This can further be explained through the Catalyst Model, which proposes that there is a predictable and cyclic reaction within systems to any crisis perceived within that system (Fraser, 1998). A system will perceive change as chaotic and threatening to the perceived state of typical, predictable patterns of their lives. There is an automatic focus on the crisis being a threat to the equilibrium of the system, and so the members of the system will behave in very predictable ways in order to help the individual in crisis and reestablish equilibrium (Fraser, 1998). The system is likely to utilize familiar solution patterns where the goal is to help the individual in crisis by pushing that individual to change back to a state of equilibrium which was maintained before the crisis (Fraser, 1998). Within this model, this is referred to as a "first order" attempt at change. However, if the members are not effective in solving the crisis, the natural progression is an escalation of the crisis at hand. In turn, when there is a perceived escalation, the system will react by trying even harder to resolve the crisis by doing even "more of the same," or utilizing the "first order" change again (Fraser, 1998).

This natural response is further explained by Chaos Theory, suggesting that each individual can be seen as a system that experiences both creativity and harmony, but also chaos (Briggs & Peat, 1999). Intrinsically, we are not likely to permit chaos in our lives, but rather to suppress chaos and thus suppress opportunities for change and creativity to take place. However, individuals usually find new openings and possibilities in chaos, and organization and control will simply lead to a struggle of power in which each person involved will become stronger in their held opinions and attitudes. Overly focusing on control leads to disease and maladjustment (Briggs & Peat, 1999). The theory further suggests that any destructive pattern, or system, is held in place by the outside world's collusion within the coupled feedback of the cycle (Briggs & Peat, 1999).

Anorexia Nervosa as a psychiatric disorder can appear chaotic. However, the opposite occurs. What really happens is that the individual's existence becomes rigid and closed, resistant to open and creative responses to the world. According to Perna (1997) and Briggs and Peat (1999), a certain amount of chaos is needed in order for change to be possible, and the chaotic phase of any system can be seen as creative. An individual with Anorexia Nervosa is terrified of letting go of control, and the rigidity and closed system he or she has created through communication with his or her surrounding environment is often influenced by the rigidity in interaction which leads to the downward spiral of "more of the same." Thus, even the smallest attempt at forcing through the resistance to treatment can lead to devastating effects in terms of amplifying the resistance and closing the system further. When the client is involved with the radical social movement of Pro-Ana, this resistance will be even higher.

It becomes evident that the expected and natural responses to threat will impact any therapeutic relationship, regardless of theoretical orientation or level of experience on the part of the clinician. According to the principles of the above-mentioned theories, if traditional compliance-based treatment is implemented as a "first order" attempt at decreasing the threat, the client is likely to respond with increased resistance. This cycle can result in a power struggle between client and clinician rather than a therapeutic relationship and potentially lead to an escalation of the crisis.

STAGES OF CHANGE MODEL AND READINESS TO CHANGE

To further complicate these predictable and natural cycles, most treatment approaches make a common assumption that the client is ready for change (Connors et al., 2001). Prochaska (1999) suggests that most psychological treatments are focused on taking action to change something about the individual seeking treatment. According to the Stages of Change Model by Prochaska and DiClemente (Prochaska, 1999), an individual is likely to progress through five stages before sustained change has occurred, and individuals can be at any of these stages at any given time. In the Precontemplation stage, the individual is not ready for change and may deny that there is a problem present, underestimating the benefits of change and overestimating the costs. This stage is followed by the Contemplation stage, where the individual is aware of the benefits of changing and equally aware of the costs. According to Prochaska (1999), this awareness is likely to cause great ambivalence for the client, which can immobilize the individual for great periods of time. In the following Preparation stage, the individual intends to take action in the immediate future and is ready for change. The following Action stage is where the client is likely to respond to action-oriented interventions, fully engaged in change behaviors. The focus of the final stage, Maintenance, is to maintain changes made and prevent relapse.

According to this model, as a rule of thumb, 40% of people will be in the Precontemplation stage, 40% in the Contemplation stage, and only 20% will be in the Preparation stage at all times. Thus, according to Prochaska (1999), action-oriented programs that only focus on immediate behavior change will not work for more than about 20% of all patients. When looking at treatment of Anorexia Nervosa through this model, the high recidivism rates are a natural reaction to action-oriented treatment being introduced at the wrong time, and when that treatment does not appropriately match the client's readiness to change. This becomes especially relevant regarding clients involved in the Pro-Ana movement. Further, information obtained from the Pro-Ana websites can aid to keep the person at the Precontemplation or Contemplation stages. If individuals with Anorexia Nervosa at this stage are forced to change through involuntary treatment, it can be hypothesized that they are likely to become even more resistant, and, because treatment is likely to fail, they are likely to become demoralized about their ability to change in the future.

CREATIVE OPTIONS AND THE COUNTERINTUITIVE STANCE

The Therapeutic Relationship and Acceptance

The most powerful way to influence the natural reactions examined in the previous sections is through the nature of interaction between clinician and client. The therapeutic relationship between clinician and client is viewed as a central component of treatment according to several theories and models (Hayes, 2004; Kohlenberg et al., 2004). According to recent studies, a greater emphasis on the therapist-client relationship is associated with better client outcomes (Kohlenberg et al., 2004). In terms of working with the highly resistant client, the therapeutic relationship has the potential of becoming the most profound place where change can be made. It is also the place where the client and therapist can benefit from interchanges that will lead to significant change in a fairly rapid manner (Hayes, 2004; Robins, Schmidt, & Linehan, 2004). Traditionally, the focus has been for the clinician to build rapport with the client by aligning *with* the client *against* the problem at hand. Thus, the emphasis is on the problem the client is experiencing or the dangerous consequences of the client's behaviors. Further, the focus is often to correct the client's deficits instead of focusing on the strengths inherent in the client's coping.

We suggest that the clinician take a different therapeutic stance in the relationship with clients involved with Pro-Ana in order to defuse the strong resistance to treatment and in order to avoid the predictable response cycles that are likely to influence the therapeutic relationship. The primary goal of the suggested counterintuitive therapeutic stance is to link with the client in a new and different manner to work with, not against, the client's resistance. In order to achieve this, the therapist has to focus on acceptance of the client, including a radical acceptance of the context the client presents with. Several treatment models look at acceptance as the cornerstone of a productive therapist-client relationship, such as Functional Analytic Psychotherapy (FAP) developed by Kohlenberg and Tsai (Kohlenberg et al., 2004), where the relationship is seen as a very important treatment component in itself. According to the concept of radical acceptance within Dialectical Behavior Therapy (Robins et al., 2004), it is crucial that the clinician is "getting it," meaning that he or she is opening up to the context the client brings. Thus, the goal of acceptance is to accept reality without any judgment and to see the client's distress as an understandable outcome based on the context, rather than a problem to be solved (Robins et al., 2004).

The importance of acceptance is also highlighted in Acceptance and Commitment Therapy (ACT), first introduced by Hayes, Strosahl, and Wilson (Hayes, 2004). Hayes (2004) emphasizes the need for a focus on accepting the client's context and function of psychological phenomena. This translates to a different conceptualization of problems, where an individual's reality is seen as a valid reflection of the interactions between the individual and his or her contexts. According to Hayes (2004), there needs to be a functional analysis conducted in order to assess what is successfully working for the client, and determination of whether an event will be targeted for change is based on how it works for the client in terms of function. This is similar to the proposed counterintuitive stance of acceptance when working with the highly resistant client, where the individual's level of readiness for overall change is assessed, and change is determined based on the client's contextual frames and what the client brings forth as not currently working. This new stance will then open the client to change and help the client "move" toward more readiness for change or a different stage of change.

A Counterintuitive Therapeutic Stance

This therapeutic stance on the part of the clinician can be adopted regardless of the clinician's theoretical orientation, and should be viewed as a transtheoretical stance that operates at a general level on the part of the clinician rather than a specific intervention. It is further counterintuitive in that the clinician will do something very different from, or the opposite of, what is expected by the client. In taking this stance, the clinician does not follow first-order interventions by taking immediate action to reduce distress or change what is perceived to be "wrong" or "maladaptive" by the surrounding system or by the clinician based on his or her clinical training. Thus, the stance represents the opposite of the natural reaction to crisis and threat on the part of the clinician as addressed in the previous sections. Moreover, it is meant to represent the opposite of a more traditional position taken by the clinician, where the aim is to link with the client through identifying the psychological problem that should be corrected and to help the client "fix" what is wrong through action-oriented interventions.

However, this counterintuitive stance must only be adopted if it feels authentic for the clinician to do so. The clinician must interact in an authentic and empathic manner, and the goal should be to build on the client's strengths and empower the client toward positive shifts in his or her perceptions. If a clinician does not feel comfortable with this stance, it should not be attempted due to the risk involved for the therapeutic relationship if this falseness comes through to the client who is already highly resistant to seek help.

The suggested stance should not be interpreted as a treatment model for Anorexia Nervosa, but rather a therapeutic stance that the clinician may adopt to help the client move toward a readiness to change, where action-oriented interventions, such as cognitive-behavioral treatment, can be successfully implemented. Further, it will prevent the clinician from becoming yet another individual that is part of the problem, according to the client. If this counterintuitive stance is carried out in a highly empathic and deliberate manner, it can be highly effective. The stance proposed here is counterintuitive in that it emphasizes aligning with the client involved with Pro-Ana in how he or she perceives the disorder, not necessarily in how the problem is defined as a psychiatric disorder. In order to do so, the clinician must be truly accepting and open to how the client views his or her world and how Anorexia Nervosa and Pro-Ana are viewed by the client. The clinician takes on more of a contextual and dialectical stance, where the client's perception is understood without judgment based on a subjective rather than an objective nature of reality.

Small Changes Leading to Large Shifts

The clinician's goal with this stance should be to make small changes both for the client and within the system surrounding the client. The goal is then that these small, significant changes become amplified through feedback cycles within the system (Briggs & Peat, 1999) until the individual is ready for change and at a stage where action-oriented intervention strategies can be successfully implemented. When looking at these small changes from the Stages of Change Model, the goal becomes to help the client "move" to the next stage.

According to the Catalyst Model, small shifts in the system's definition of the current situation, or any redirection of attention within the system, is likely to result in a significant difference within the system. Thus, such a small shift will lead to disproportionately large effects for the individuals in the system and for the overall system (Fraser, 1998). Chaos Theory proposes that even the smallest of changes, one way or another, will begin to amplify through feedback and lead to the unpredictable (Briggs & Peat, 1999).

Thus, simply doing *anything* different has the potential for making small and seemingly insignificant changes that have the potential to lead to significant major shifts (Briggs & Peat, 1999). Even the counterintuitive stance the clinician deliberately takes in the initial therapeutic encounter can be such a shift. The clinician may further incorporate several of the following creative options as part of the counterintuitive stance when interacting with the highly resistant client, especially those involved with Pro-Ana, in order to illicit these small changes.

Power-Down Positioning

One creative option is to take a power-down position when interacting with the client and the surrounding system. The clinician should be very attentive to the positioning he or she takes with the client, because this initial impression is likely to dictate the client's overall attitude toward the clinician. It is important for the clinician to adopt a deliberate position distinctly different from and most often the opposite of that of "helpful others" as discussed in previous sections. In doing this, the therapist has the potential to initiate a major shift in the client's perception already in the first interaction (Fraser, 1998). It is respectful to the client and to the view of the client as the authority figure and expert in relation to his or her own life.

In working with the client diagnosed with Anorexia Nervosa, it will be important for the clinician to be the first to address the Pro-Ana movement in a respectful and nonjudgmental manner with the client, in order to make the client aware that the clinician is informed and takes an accepting stance to the different view of Anorexia Nervosa. This can be a very powerful aspect of the beginning therapeutic relationship which can have an enormous impact on the client's resistance and the outcome of therapy. However, it is important to again point out that this positioning should only be adopted if the clinician is comfortable with it and it comes natural to the clinician. If not, the client is likely to pick up on this, and resistance is likely to increase.

Validation and Normalization

Another possibility of linking with the client and the surrounding system through the counterintuitive stance is to take a deliberate position of normalizing and validating (Fraser, 1998). An empathic validation of individual opinions and normalizing of reactions may lead to shifts within the system. Such validation can be very powerful and can lead to small shifts in the interaction between the people involved around the client. This may lead to a different pattern of interaction within the system which in turn will be amplified through feedback loops, as addressed through Chaos Theory (Briggs & Peat, 1999). If this further leads to a lessening in the rigidity of the system, it can lead to a decrease in overall resistance to change within the system, including within the client. Further, the clinician's validation can be understood as counterintuitive in that the clinician is accepting the client's reality without judgment and without pointing out the dysfunction, which is again the opposite of what the client expects. Through validation and normalization, the therapist instills hope and initiates an emotional and confiding relationship, which in turn will open the system to change.

From Deficits to Strengths

Another creative option with this counterintuitive stance is to link with the client and the system and to alter the direction of attention from deficits to strengths (Fraser, 1998). In the face of a crisis, people involved are most likely to view the deficits present and focus on the problems that are occurring. This is in accordance with Threat Rigidity Theory, which states that a natural reaction to threat is to narrow the focus in on the threat. Because a threat is described as an event that has potentially negative or harmful effects, there is an automatic focus on the negative and harmful (Staw et al., 1981). Thus, a clinician's focus on the positive relating to the client's coping, as opposed to the negative and harmful, is counterintuitive. According to Frank's Model of Common Factors, a hopeful clinician who is determined to help can have a profound positive impact on the client, and affect how the client views the possibility for change (J. D. Frank & J. B. Frank, 1991).

Go Slow with Change

Another aspect of the counterintuitive stance is that of encouraging clients to "go slow" (Fraser, 1998). The Catalyst Model suggests that the clinician should take the meta-position of "go slow messages" (Fraser, 1998), because the client has likely experienced a push for immediate change over a long time period and is likely to be very fearful of change. He or she may be maintaining the starvation behavior as a way of taking control in his or her life and as a way to resist change. Thus the "go slow" messages to the client, and to the system, become counterintuitive to the immediate changes the client is expecting and is fearful of. This message needs to be explained to the system involved, and can be explained based on repercussions for immediate changes within the system in the past. This meta-position on the part of the clinician is emphasizing the dialectical nature of the position of the client as intently wanting change, and yet terrified of change, and respects the importance of interplay between these two aspects (Robins et al., 2004). When the clinician suggests that the client "go slow," he or she sends a message that the opposing forces the client experiences are understood and respected by the clinician. Thus, this positioning can be utilized in the counterintuitive stance to link with the client and move the client to the next stage of change.

Addressing Previous Treatment Attempts

If the client has previously experienced "failed treatment," he or she is even more hyper-vigilant to the dangers associated with any change. Thus, the danger aspects of change need to be processed with the client before introducing any changes. The clinician can do this by predicting future patterns of escalation if the attempts at "first-order" change continue. By doing this in an empathic and accepting manner from a strength-based perspective and by explaining to clients that their reactions are natural responses to threat, it is likely to again validate and normalize their reactions. Again, this is likely to instill hope in the client and to send the message that the clinician is determined to help, which is one of the most important aspects of instilling hope for change (J. D. Frank & J. B. Frank, 1991; Snyder, Michael, & Cheavens, 1999). It will be important for the clinician to discuss both the expected escalation patterns related to the behaviors of the individual diagnosed with Anorexia Nervosa and the expected response patterns of the system as a whole.

In successfully doing this, the patterns of problematic solutions that are fueling the growing crisis and the rigid resistance on the part of the client with Anorexia Nervosa may be eliminated, because the client and system are informed about the predicted outcome if they continue utilizing "first-order" strategies. It may create a small shift in the solution strategies utilized by the system surrounding the client. This small change within the system may create a ripple effect in the patterns of communication and interaction within the system and can therefore potentially lead to major shifts within that system.

SUGGESTING NEW ACTIONS

Another creative option is for the clinician to introduce a small change to the system by suggesting that the system surrounding the client alter the solutions being employed (Fraser, 1998). This should only be done when the clinician has linked with the client and the surrounding system involved. New actions are likely to initiate new responses within the system, and these new patterns may open up the system and lead the client to being more open to change. If the system has become rigid in its solution-focused patterns and interactions, it is highly likely that the solutions employed to date are not productive, but rather destructive to the client and the support system involved. This suggested change should be counterintuitive compared to the "first-order" solutions already utilized by the system. This will likely create a counterintuitive reaction pattern within the system, and may lead to a ripple effect of changed interactions. By suggesting new solutions to the system in line with the client's strengths and current coping, there is a disruption in the escalating of the crisis. In this case, the clinician has opened up the system and made a small shift within the system, which then can be built upon and amplified, according to Chaos Theory (Briggs & Peat, 1999). This may again instill hope in the client, and can assist the client to move to the next Stage of Change.

Addressing Pro-Ana

When working with a client diagnosed with Anorexia Nervosa, it becomes crucial to address the Pro-Ana movement and the client's involvement with this movement at the onset of therapy. If the client is highly influenced by the philosophy and views of the Pro-Ana movement in relation to the helping profession, the client is not likely to be open and honest with the clinician. The client is likely to discuss aspects of his or her treatment with others involved in the Pro-Ana movement and is more likely to trust the views and opinions of his or her peers, who are looked up to, rather than those of a clinician who is feared and mistrusted. In the proposed stance, it is important to always have an open dialogue about Pro-Ana with any client diagnosed with Anorexia Nervosa in therapy, and for the clinician to bring this up with the client in an open and accepting manner. This is counterintuitive to what is expected by the client and is likely to facilitate the therapeutic relationship. According to Frank's Model of Common Factors (J. D. Frank & J. B. Frank, 1991), it is crucial that the client be able to rely on and trust the therapist's ability to help him or her in order for change to occur.

CONCLUSION

To summarize, there are several main points that emerge regarding the treatment of clients involved with Pro-Ana. First, there is an inherent need for control and resistance to treatment in Anorexia Nervosa, which is strengthened if the individual is involved with Pro-Ana. Secondly, there are natural and predictable response cycles to threat, crisis, and chaos that impact the clinician, the client, and the surrounding system. Third, these response patterns will impact most traditional treatment, regardless of theoretical orientation. Fourth, the client's readiness to change according to the Stages of Change Model has a major impact on treatment, and treatment that is not tailored to the client's stage of readiness is predicted to fail. Fifth, the suggested creative options will have great implications for the clinician who adopts the suggested counterintuitive stance and opens the dialogue regarding Pro-Ana with clients diagnosed with Anorexia Nervosa. By adopting this stance, the clinician is likely to counteract the normal response cycles of higher resistance and is likely to meet the client where he or she is in terms of readiness to change. Through positioning and introducing small changes to the client and the system surrounding the client, the clinician is likely to help the client move to a stage of readiness where action-oriented interventions can be successfully implemented. Regardless of the clinician's theoretical orientation, this stance and positioning can be a part of any intervention as it is transtheoretical. Further, it is suggested that the small changes introduced by the clinician have the potential to lead to major shifts within the client's context.

It can be concluded that a clinician taking this stance will also have a greater impact on the client. Through interacting with a clinician taking this stance, the client will experience acceptance and empathy, and the clinician is likely to be one of the few people outside Pro-Ana who do not focus on everything "wrong" with the client and who shows this understanding with empathy rather than judgment. The high suicide rate among people with Anorexia Nervosa indicates that many people suffering from this disorder feel demoralized and hopeless about being able to change their life. Thus, this form of interaction with a clinician who is hopeful and determined to help is likely to lead the client to become more hopeful.

CONTRIBUTOR

Mette Traae Brynolf, PsyD, is currently working as a staff therapist while completing her postdoctoral training at Michael T. Farrell, PhD, & Associates, a private practice in Cincinnati and Centerville, Ohio that specializes in providing psychological assessment and treatment for individuals with physical disabilities and chronic pain. Her training is in clinical psychology with special interest in multicultural issues, health psychology, eating disorders, and therapeutic resistance. She is also a clinical faculty member at Wright State University, School of Professional Psychology. Dr. Traae Brynolf may be contacted at 1159-E Lyons Road, Centerville, OH 45458. E-mail: mette.traae@wright.edu

RESOURCES

American Psychiatric Association. (2000). *Diagnostic and Statistical Manual of Mental Disorders* (4th ed. Text rev.). Washington, DC: Author.

Barrett, N. (n.d.). Wasting away on the web: Shocking internet websites are encouraging Anorexia as a "lifestyle." Retrieved October 7, 2003 from: http://www.btinternet.com/~virtuous/planetgrrlbabe/babearticles/wasting_away_on_the_web.htm

Briggs, J., & Peat, F. D. (1999). *Seven Life Lessons of Chaos – Timeless Wisdom from the Science of Change.* New York: Harper Collins.

Bruch, H. (1985). Four decades of eating disorders. In D. M. Garner & P. E. Garfinkel (Eds.), *Handbook of Psychotherapy for Anorexia Nervosa & Bulimia* (pp. 7-19). New York: Guilford.

Castro, J., Gila, A., Puig, J., Rodriguez, S., & Toro, J. (2004). Predictors of rehospitalization after total weight recovery in adolescents with anorexia nervosa. *International Journal of Eating Disorders, 36,* 22-30.

Connors G. J., Donovan, D. M., & DiClemente, C. C. (2001). *Substance Abuse Treatment and the Stages of Change.* New York: Guilford.

Crisp, A. H. (1997). Anorexia Nervosa as flight from growth: Assessment and treatment based on the model. In D.M. Garner & P. E. Garfinkel (Eds.), *Handbook of Treatment for Eating Disorders* (2nd ed., pp. 248-277). New York: Guilford.

Dolan, D. (2003, October 7). Learning to love Anorexia? "Pro-Ana" web sites flourish. *The New York Observer.* Retrieved 10-7-03 from: http://www.observer.com/node/47063

Downing, J. (2001). *Radical Media: Rebellious Communication and Social Movements.* Thousand Oaks, CA: Sage.

Frank, J. D., & Frank, J. B. (1991). *Persuasion and Healing: A Comparative Study of Psychotherapy* (3rd ed.). Baltimore, MD: Johns Hopkins University Press.

Fraser, J. S. (1998). A catalyst model: Guidelines for doing crisis intervention and brief therapy from a process view. *Crisis Intervention, 4*(2-3), 159-177.

Garner, D. M., & Garfinkel, P. E. (1997). (Eds.). *Handbook of Treatment for Eating Disorders* (2nd ed.). New York: Guilford.

Garner, D. M., & Magana, C. G. (2002). Anorexia Nervosa. In M. Hersen (Ed.), *Clinical Behavior Therapy: Adults and Children* (pp. 345-360). New York: John Wiley & Sons.

Garner, D. M., & Needleman, L. D. (1997). Sequencing and integration of treatments. In D. M. Garner & P. E. Garfinkel (Eds.), *Handbook of Treatment for Eating Disorders* (2nd ed., pp. 50-63). New York: Guilford.

Garvin, V., & Striegel-Moore, R. H. (2001). Health service research for eating disorders in the United States: A status report and a call to action. In R. H. Striegel-Moore & L. Smolak (Eds.), *Eating Disorders: Innovative Directions in Research and Practice* (pp. 153-172). Washington, DC: American Psychological Association.

Girls Who Don't Eat. (2005). Retrieved on June 24, 2005 from http://www.oprah.com/tows/pastshows/tows_past_20011004.jhtml

Griffin, M. A., Tesluk, P. E., & Jacobs, R. R. (1995). Bargaining cycles and work related attitudes: Evidence for threat-rigidity effects. *Academy of Management Journal, 38,* 1709-1725.

Hall, A. (1985). Group psychotherapy for anorexia nervosa. In D. M. Garner & P. E. Garfinkel (Eds.), *Handbook of Psychotherapy for Anorexia Nervosa & Bulimia* (pp. 213-240). New York: Guilford.

Harris, W. A., Wiseman, C. V., Wagner, S., & Halmi, K. A. (2001). The difficult-to-treat patient with eating disorder. In M. J. Dewan & R. W. Pies (Eds.), *The Difficult-to-Treat Psychiatric Patient* (pp. 243-271). Washington, DC: American Psychiatric Publishing.

Hayes, S. C. (2004). Acceptance and commitment therapy and the new behavioral therapies: Mindfulness, acceptance, and relationship. In S. C. Hayes, V. M. Follette, & M. M. Linehan (Eds.), *Mindfulness and Acceptance: Expanding the Cognitive-Behavioral Tradition* (pp. 1-29). New York: Guilford.

Hersen, M., & Bellack, A. S. (Eds.). (1999). *Handbook of Comparative Interventions for Adult Disorders* (2nd ed.). New York: John Wiley & Sons.

Kohlenberg, R. J., Kanter, J. W., Bolling, M., Wexner, R., Parker, C., & Tsai, M. (2004). Functional analytic psychotherapy, cognitive therapy, and acceptance. In S. C. Hayes, V. M. Follette, & M. M. Linehan (Eds.), *Mindfulness and Acceptance: Expanding the Cognitive-Behavioral Tradition* (pp. 96-119). New York: Guilford.

Martin, R., Hewstone, M., & Martin, P. Y. (2003). Resistance to persuasive messages as a function of majority and minority source status. *Journal of Experimental Social Psychology, 39*(6), 585-593.

Neumärker, K. J. (2000). Mortality rates and causes of death. *European Eating Disorders Review, 8,* 181-187.

Perna, P. A. (1997) Reflections on the therapeutic system as seen from the science of chaos and complexity: Implications for research and treatment. In F. Masterpasqua & P. A. Perna (Eds.), *The Psychological Meaning of Chaos: Translating Theory into Practice* (pp. 253-272). Washington, DC: American Psychological Association.

Powers, P. S., & Santana, C. A. (2002). Childhood and adolescent anorexia nervosa. *Child & Adolescent Psychiatric Clinics of North America, 11*(2), 219-235.

Prochaska, J. O. (1999). How do people change, and how can we change to help many more people? In M. A. Hubble, B. L. Duncan, & S. D. Miller (Eds.), *The Heart & Soul of Change: What Works in Therapy* (pp. 227-255). Washington, DC: American Psychological Association.

Reijonen, J. H., Pratt, H. D., Patel, D. R., & Greydanus, D. E. (2003). Eating disorders in the adolescent population: An overview. *Journal of Adolescent Research, 18*(3), 209-222.

Robins, C. J., Schmidt, III, H., & Linehan, M. M. (2004). Dialectical behavior therapy: Synthesizing radical acceptance with skillful means. In S. C. Hayes, V. M. Follette, & M. M. Linehan (Eds.), *Mindfulness and Acceptance: Expanding the Cognitive-Behavioral Tradition* (pp. 30-44). New York: Guilford.

Sargent, J., Liebman, R., & Silver, M. (1985). Family therapy for Anorexia Nervosa. In D. M. Garner & P. E. Garfinkel (Eds.), *Handbook of Psychotherapy for Anorexia Nervosa & Bulimia* (pp. 257-280). New York: Guilford.

Snyder, C. R., Michael, S. T., & Cheavens, J. S. (1999). Hope as a psychotherapeutic foundation of common factors, placebos, and expectancies. In M. A. Hubble, B. L. Duncan, & S. D. Miller (Eds.), *The Heart & Soul of Change: What Works in Therapy* (pp. 179-200). Washington, DC: American Psychological Association.

Staw, B. M., & Ross, J. (1989). Understanding behavior in escalation situations. *Science, New Series, 246*, 4927, 216-220.

Staw, B. M., Sandelands, L. E., & Dutton, J. E. (1981). Threat-rigidity effects in organization behavior: A multilevel analysis. *Administrative Science Quarterly, 26*, 501-524.

Steiger, H., Bruce, K. R., & Israel, M. (2003). Eating disorders. In G. Stricker & T. A. Widiger (Vol. Eds.), *Handbook of Psychology* (Vol. 8: Clinical Psychology, pp. 173-194). Hoboken, NJ: John Wiley & Sons.

Steinhausen, H. C. (2002). The outcome of anorexia nervosa in the 20th century. *American Journal of Psychiatry, 159*(8), 1284-1293.

Uca, E. (2004). *Ana's Girls: The Essential Guide to the Underground Eating Disorder Community Online.* Bloomington, IN: Author House.

Wakeling, A. (1996). Epidemiology of anorexia nervosa. *Psychiatry Research, 62*(1), 3-9.

Werne, J. (1996). Introduction. In J. Werne & I. D. Yalom (Eds.), *Treating Eating Disorders*. San Francisco: Jossey-Bass.

Zhang, A. Y., Snowden, L. R., & Sue, S. (1998). Differences between Asian and White Americans' help seeking and utilization patterns in the Los Angeles area. *Journal of Community Psychology, 26*(4), 317–326.

Websites Referenced in Text*

http://community.livejournal.com/proanorexia
http://famine.brokensanity.org
http://www.makaylashealingplace.dnswh.com
http://www.mianaland.com/welcome.php
http://www.plagueangel.net/grotto
http://www.prettythin.com
http://www.proanamia.com
http://www.prothinspo.com

*As noted at the beginning of this contribution, all websites cited are subject to change at any time.

Assessment and Treatment of Internet Addiction

Keith W. Beard

INTERNET ADDICTION: AN OVERVIEW

Although the Internet has many good qualities, mental health practitioners need to be aware of the problematic nature of Internet use for some clients. This contribution will cover the history of the Internet, the aspects of the Internet that make it appealing, the issues with defining problematic Internet use, how we may go about assessing if a person is engaging in problematic Internet use, some proposed criteria for diagnosis, and potential treatment options for problematic use.

BRIEF HISTORY

Parks and Floyd (1996) clarified how the Internet began in the late 1960s as a way to link a few universities and defense laboratories. This system was initially developed so the government could communicate with regions across the United States in order to maintain control after a nuclear war (Gackenbach & Ellerman, 1998). Between the 1960s and the 1990s, this new form of communication expanded and became more accessible to the general population. It was no longer confined to the government, universities, or technical users (Kiesler, Siegel, & McGuire, 1984).

The World Wide Web (WWW) is a part of the Internet. Gackenbach and Ellerman (1998) described how the WWW was created in 1989. It allowed local Internet systems to connect to other Internet systems so that information could be sent anywhere in the world. The WWW also allowed for the user to "click" on a term or word and this would automatically connect the user to other sites on the web. New words developed to describe the uses and users of the Internet. The term "Web" was used as a metaphor to illustrate how each site could be connected to another like a spider's web is interconnected.

Since its inception, Internet use has become widespread. According to Internet World Stats (2008), over 1.2 billion people are online. The use of the Internet has increased by 249% in the past 7 years. It is doubtful that these early developers of the Internet could have foreseen the significant impact their work would have on the world.

APPEAL OF THE INTERNET

There are countless reasons why people use the Internet. It is important for us to understand why people are drawn to the Internet, because this can help us understand why a person could be using the Internet in a problematic manner. Knowing this information may impact how best to treat the client.

According to Chou, Condron, and Belland (2005), there are five major needs that individuals try to fulfill online. The first relates to sexual behavior. Viewing online pornography as well as "cybersex" or "netsex" is often discussed in the media, and the Internet supplies almost an infinite amount of content for people to access. People engage in this behavior in order to fulfill biological needs as well as psychological and social needs. The second need that can be satisfied by Internet use is a desire for an altered state of consciousness. Individuals using the Internet may develop different online personas and seek to experience reality from different perspectives. The Internet may also provide a vehicle for relaxation, a place to escape from pressure, and a way to seek excitement. The third need addressed by the Internet relates to issues of achievement and mastery. Many people enjoy mastering software, games, and applications online. By engaging in these Internet applications, the person feels challenged, works to gain control, and is rewarded with success. This pattern is repeated as the person moves to the next level of difficulty in the software or game. The fourth need addressed by the Internet relates to a desire for communication and belonging. By routinely visiting particular chat rooms and sites, a sense of community and belongingness can develop. The final need addressed by the Internet is the development of relationships. Many individuals do not have sufficient social support. By going online, a person can make new friends, talk about problems, and get advice. According to King (1996) and Young (1997, 1998), Internet users take more emotional risks and express opinions that they are unable to express to others. This creates a need to continue these social interactions and receive the support that they are lacking in the real world. Unlike real world interactions, this support can quickly and easily end by no longer corresponding to the person. As a result, there is an illusion of companionship without the demands often placed on friendships.

Others believe that the Internet is attractive because it is accessible, affordable, and anonymous (Laaser & Gregoire, 2003; Leung, 2004). Of these, it is believed that anonymity is a primary factor in why people are attracted to the Internet (Beard, 2005, 2008; Beard & Wolf, 2001; Correll, 1995; Griffiths, 1997; Kiesler et al., 1984; Young, 1997, 1998). Unlike face-to-face communication, demographics have to be announced in order to be known (Correll, 1995). As mentioned previously, many Internet users take on different personas when online (Kandell, 1998; Suler, 1996; Young, 1997, 1998). The user may create different profiles with information about himself or herself. Young (1997, 1998) found that some users chose identities relating to an ideal self that represented the opposite of what the person was in real life, fulfilling unmet needs or representing an emotion or trait that may be repressed. The anonymity of the Internet can also create a feeling of safety and encourage more flirtation, overtures of friendship, and willingness to give positive and negative feedback (Harmon, 1998; N. B. McCormick & J. W. McCormick, 1992; Suler, 1996). It is not unusual in Internet culture to ask personal and intimate questions when users meet for the first time (Beard, 2008; Kandell, 1998; King, 1996; Suler, 1996; Young, 1997, 1998).

DEFINING PROBLEMATIC INTERNET USE

As the use of the Internet grows, so does the concern that this technology is being used in a maladaptive manner (Beard, 2008; Beard & Wolf, 2001; Ng & Wiemer-Hastings, 2005;

Song et al., 2004; C. K. Yang et al., 2005; Yellowlees & Marks, 2005). There have been instances of marital distress, failing in school, losing jobs, and accumulating debt as a result of the person's Internet use (Beard, 2002; Leung, 2004; Yellowlees & Marks, 2005). Using the Internet in a problematic manner has had dire consequences for some people.

The Question of Addiction

The term "Internet addiction" has been commonly used to describe problematic use. This term was quickly adopted by the media and general public in their attempt to identify those who are using the Internet in a maladaptive way (Beard & Wolf, 2001). Although the most popular term utilized is "Internet addiction," it is my position that this term does not accurately reflect the phenomenon of excessive Internet use. There are common behaviors and symptoms when comparing excessive Internet use and a chemical addiction. However, excessive Internet use does not involve the presence of a substance, which is a primary factor when diagnosing a chemical addiction. Moreover, Young (1998) compared problematic Internet use with pathological gambling. This suggests that problematic Internet use may be better classified as an impulse control disorder or behavioral addiction rather than trying to equate or classify it with the chemical addictions.

The debate over whether or not Internet addiction is even a "real" disorder continues (Beard & Wolf, 2001; Kaltiala-Heino, Lintonen, & Rimpela, 2004; C. K. Yang et al., 2005; Yellowlees & Marks, 2005). Additionally, it has not been determined if problematic use of the Internet warrants its own distinct diagnosis or if it is a symptom of some other disorder such as depression, anxiety, social phobia, impulse-control disorder, or obsessive-compulsive disorder (Kaltiala-Heino et al., 2004; C. K. Yang et al., 2005; Yellowlees & Marks, 2005).

The question is also raised as to whether it is the Internet that is addictive or the content or applications being used on the Internet that are addictive in nature (Beard, 2005; Chou et al., 2005; Kaltiala-Heino et al., 2004; Yellowlees & Marks, 2005). The two most common activities engaged in online are email exchanges and web surfing (Leung, 2004). However, applications that tend to encourage more interaction, such as instant messaging and gaming, tend to be more captivating and potentially result in problematic Internet use (Beard, 2005; Chak & Leung, 2004; Chou et al., 2005; Leung, 2004; Ng & Wiemer-Hastings, 2005; Niemz, Griffiths, & Banyard, 2005; Song et al., 2004; Yellowlees & Marks, 2005).

Development and Incidence of Problematic Use

Laaser and Gregoire (2003) suggest that four stages occur in the development of problematic Internet use. According to these authors, in stage one, the behavior becomes unmanageable. Even though there is intent to stop, there is an inability to do so. In the second stage, the authors propose an increase in neurotransmitter tolerance which results in a desensitization of the neuron receptor sites. The third stage is characterized as escalation, in which an increased amount of a neurotransmitter is needed in order to achieve the same level of excitation or stimulation. The final stage is described as medication of the mood, and is characterized by the person engaging in behavior and/or thoughts to help maintain their level of excitement or pleasure.

Several studies have investigated how much different groups (e.g., children, adolescents, young adults, and clergy) use the Internet in a maladaptive way (Beard, 2008; Kaltiala-Heino et al., 2004; Laaser & Gregoire, 2003; Leung, 2004; Simkova & Cincera, 2004; Yoo et al., 2004). Despite the lack of consensus for what constitutes problematic Internet use, it is estimated that somewhere between 6% and 30% of online users use the Internet in a maladaptive way (Kaltiala-Heino et al., 2004; Laaser & Gregoire, 2003; Yellowlees & Marks, 2005).

Limitations

It should be noted that several researchers are quick to point out that research on problematic Internet use is limited, and the research that has been completed has been problematic (Beard & Wolf, 2001; Kaltiala-Heino et al., 2004; Laaser & Gregoire, 2003; Leung, 2004; Niemz et al., 2005; Yellowlees & Marks, 2005). For example, there are different definitions for what constitutes problematic Internet use. Also, there are a variety of different ways that have been proposed to determine if someone meets the various proposed criteria. Additionally, the populations used to study this phenomenon are often biased and underrepresented, recruited from the Internet, or obtained from universities and colleges. That being said, the research on problematic Internet use has resulted in some promising data and is helping to push the research into new and exciting directions. With the popularity of the Internet and the possible problems that can result, there is little doubt that continued exploration into this topic will continue, and there are still many questions to be examined.

For the purposes of this contribution, problematic Internet use will be broadly defined as one's use of the Internet that creates psychological, social, school, and/or work difficulties in a person's life.

ASSESSMENTS

The following section will explore characteristics, traits, personality factors, and psychological disorders that have been associated with problematic Internet users. Additionally, assessment tools, such as test instruments and clinical interview questions, will be reviewed.

Characteristics

Certain characteristics of individuals who may be more susceptible to developing problematic Internet use have been found. Media attention has stereotyped those who are engaging in problematic Internet use as predominantly young, full-time students, computer-oriented, and male (Chak & Leung, 2004; Niemz et al., 2005; Scherer, 1997; Simkova & Cincera, 2004; Young, 1996, 1998). Niemz et al. (2005) report research in which students studying hard sciences (e.g., chemistry, computer science, engineering) were more likely to spend significantly more time online than those in other fields, with the most common major for students who fit the criteria for problematic Internet use being computer science. However, with the increased availability of the Internet to diverse populations, these demographic characteristics are likely to change; for example, there has been an increase in problematic Internet use in female, non-full-time students (Leung, 2004; C. K. Yang et al., 2005).

C. K. Yang et al. (2005) found that excessive users appear to have a distinctive personality profile when compared with nonusers, minimal, and moderate users. As a result, these researchers feel that there are certain clusters of symptoms that may predispose a person to be preoccupied with the Internet.

C. K. Yang et al. (2005) state that problematic Internet users tend to be absent-minded, have difficulty making decisions, are often absorbed in their thoughts, are intellectually curious, are scientific, and are unaware of particular people and the physical world around them. They are typically unconcerned with everyday matters. They tend to obtain a great deal of satisfaction from Internet activities instead of getting that satisfaction from more typical outlets such as social activities or friendships. Their individuality can lead to their rejection from group activities and continued pursuit of solitary activities. Although these people do not dislike others, they simply do not feel the need to obtain their agreement or support on matters.

Problematic Internet users tend to show less empathy toward others (Sattar & Ramaswamy, 2004; C. K. Yang et al., 2005). Engelberg and Sjoberg (2004) agreed with this finding and expanded on it, stating that frequent users of the Internet had lower emotional intelligence. As a result, they had more difficulty understanding how emotional perception can be useful in social contexts.

C. K. Yang et al. (2005) go on to say that excessive Internet users are unconventional, imaginative, willing to explore new ideas, and creative, but can be impractical and unrealistic about situations. When these people become overly imaginative, their beliefs and expectations can become fantastical. Consequently, they may fail to see the practical limitations of their ideas. This can result in their demonstrating expressive outbursts when things do not go their way. They are also more irritable, hostile, and aggressive. Laaser and Gregoire (2003) support this, suggesting that problematic Internet users may have repressed anger which can more easily be expressed online. In the "real world" the person may be more likely to engage in passive-aggressive behaviors and remarks.

Additionally, there is a sense of control with the Internet (Chak & Leung, 2004; Laaser & Gregoire, 2003; Leung, 2004). As previously mentioned, Internet users can talk to or ignore others with the click of a button. Chak and Leung (2004) found that the more people felt as though they had control over their own life, the less likely they were to be addicted to the Internet. The opposite was also found in their study. If participants had an external locus of control and felt that others or chance had control over their lives the more likely they were to be addicted to the Internet.

C. K. Yang et al. (2005) also describe how problematic Internet users can be self-sufficient, self-motivated, resourceful, and independent. Although these are often seen as positive personality traits to have, these users can get used to taking action on their own and can have some difficulties compromising with others. Consequently, pride and frequent engaging in intellectualization are often found in those who use the Internet in a problematic manner.

Being socially withdrawn, isolating, shy, introverted, lonely, nervous, and having attachment issues are all personality factors that have been examined with problematic Internet users (Chou et al., 2005; Engelberg & Sjoberg, 2004; Laaser & Gregoire, 2003; Leung, 2004; Sattar & Ramaswamy, 2004; S. C. Yang & Tung, 2004; C. K. Yang et al., 2005). Chak and Leung's (2004) findings suggest that those with poor social skills, such as being shy, are drawn to the Internet to get these social and emotional needs met. The development of relationships may occur that would otherwise be too terrifying to engage in if one were in the "real" world. So, it is often thought that these social aspects of the Internet are what are most addictive for a person (Ng & Wiemer-Hastings, 2005). These online relationships help them with their difficulty with intimacy (Laaser & Gregoire, 2003).

Users may have low self-esteem (Leung, 2004; Sattar & Ramaswamy, 2004). Niemz et al. (2005) support this notion, stating that self-esteem is a good predictor of Internet addiction as well as the amount of time that the user spends online per week. However, the relationship between self-esteem and Internet use is not clear. For example, low self-esteem may be a consequence rather than a cause of the Internet addiction.

Other researchers (Leung, 2004; S. C. Yang & Tung, 2004; C. K. Yang et al., 2005) go on to say that these people tend to have poor social relationships, few or no friends, high family conflict, poor coping skills, and increased social isolation. They tend to be unhappy with their physical appearance, have a decreased sense of well-being, and poor coping patterns. Cognitively, these people may engage in black-and-white thinking (Laaser & Gregoire, 2003). They also tend to blame others for their behaviors (Laaser & Gregoire, 2003).

C. K. Yang et al. (2005) claim that those who engage in problematic Internet use report and exhibit significantly more psychiatric symptoms than those who use the Internet less frequently. Several researchers have discussed how those who suffer from depression and anxiety may be more prone to develop Internet addiction (Chou et al., 2005; Laaser & Gregoire, 2003; S. C. Yang & Tung, 2004). In particular, S. C. Yang and Tung (2004) suggest that those with depression, anxiety, and low self-esteem are more likely to be drawn to the Internet and its addictive features. Additionally, people who are addicted to the Internet may also be more likely to be addicted to other substances or activities (Beard, 2005; Yoo et al., 2004). Other comorbid problems reported by problematic Internet users include phobias, sleep disturbances, obsessive-compulsive symptoms, and psychosomatic complaints (C. K. Yang et al., 2005). Furthermore, there is growing suspicion that those suffering from Attention-Deficit/Hyperactivity Disorder (ADHD) may also be susceptible to addictive behaviors like using the Internet in a maladaptive manner (Laaser & Gregoire, 2003; Yoo et al., 2004). Yoo et al. (2004) find that both the inattentive and the hyperactive-impulsive types had positive correlations with Internet addictive symptoms. The Internet may be attractive because of the constant stimulation and minimal delay for reward. Additionally, the Internet may help the person with ADHD compensate for poor social skills and get needed social interaction.

When examining the personality disorders, Laaser and Gregoire (2003) propose that a person with narcissistic personality disorder traits could be at risk for problematic Internet use. These people often grew up not feeling affirmed, listened to, or praised. There may also be a sense of entitlement. Interactions and behaviors on the Internet provide a substitute for these feelings. These unmet needs can be secured through their interaction and behaviors online. For example, by gaming online a user could gain recognition, attention, and potential idealization from others in an anonymous, faceless context that is under the person's control (Leung, 2004). This can be especially attractive to someone who is egocentric (C. K. Yang et al., 2005).

Furthermore, C. K. Yang et al. (2005) examined students and found that those who play virtual games excessively may have a more schizoid personality than other students. They explain that virtual games are often solitary activities, which feed into the person's inward-looking nature.

Assessment Tools

In terms of assessment instruments, several ways to determine if a person is using the Internet in a maladaptive way have been proposed. However, the value of these instruments or methods has been called into question (Mitchell, 2000). All of these instruments are checklists and considered self-report measures. Scherer's (1997) and Young's (1998) questionnaires were the first to be developed. Data collection occurred via telephone interview and online surveys. From there, Chou et al. (2005) report that the development of assessment instruments attempted to be more psychometrically sound by increasing the statistical analysis of the test items and moving from yes/no options for answering to a 4-point Likert scale. Interestingly, many of the more recent assessment instruments have been developed in Taiwan. A summary of these instruments can be found in Table 1 (p. 123).

Mental health providers need to keep an open mind and make sure to explore for potential maladaptive use of technology with our clients. People may not enter psychotherapy because of their problematic Internet use. Instead, these people may present with symptoms that helped to develop or maintain their problematic Internet behavior, such as depression, anxiety, relationship conflicts, trauma, or low self-esteem. As a result, a thorough initial intake interview is needed. Beard (2005) has generated a sampling of potential questions to ask someone during an initial evaluation for problematic Internet use. He proposes that problematic Internet use can be conceptualized based on the biopsychosocial model. Therefore, he believes that there are biological, psychological, and social aspects to the development and maintenance of problematic Internet use, and each of these should be assessed. The biological view recognizes that biological or neurochemical changes can happen in a person engaging in an addictive behavior. For example, there may be a combination of genes that make a person prone to developing addictive behaviors or an insufficient amount of a neurotransmitter, which is altered when the person is engaging in excessive Internet use. This may create an altered physiological state and help the body maintain homeostasis or create a sense of euphoria. The psychological view

TABLE 1: Assessment Instruments for Problematic Internet Use

Instrument	Questions	Reliability	Development
Diagnostic Questionnaire (DQ; Young, 1998)	8 Yes/no questions	None Reported	Based on a study with 396 dependents, 100 nondependents (online survey and telephone interview)
Clinical Symptoms of Internet Dependency (Scherer, 1997)	10 Yes/no questions	None Reported	Based on a study with 531 college students (online survey and telephone interview)
Pathological Internet Use scale (PIU; Morahan-Martin & Schumacker, 2000)	13 Yes/no questions	.88	Based on a study with 277 college students (paper-and-pencil survey)
Internet-Related Addictive Behavior Inventory (IRABI; Brenner, 1997)	32 Yes/no questions	.87	Based on a study with 563 online survey respondents
Chinese Internet Addiction Scale (CIAS; Chen & Chou, 1999)	28 questions on a 4-point Likert scale	.93	Based on a study with 1,336 students from National Taiwan University (paper-and-pencil survey)
Internet Addiction Scale for Taiwan High Schoolers (IAST; Lin & Tsai, 1999)	20 questions on a 4-point Likert scale	.85	Based on a study with 615 Taiwan high school students (paper-and-pencil survey)
Chinese IRABI Version II (C-IRABI-II; Chou & Hsiao, 2000)	40 questions on a 4-point Likert scale	.93	Based on a study with 910 Taiwan college students (paper-and-pencil survey)
Online Cognition Scale (OCS; Davis, Flett, & Besser, 2002)	36 questions on a 7-point Likert scale	.94	Based on a study with 211 college students (paper-and-pencil survey)

recognizes that principles such as classical and operant conditioning play a part in initiating and maintaining the behavior of those dealing with problematic Internet use. For example, physiological arousal and internal states, such as excitement, stimulation, pleasure, hope, and surprise, may be conditioned to occur to external cues such as turning on the computer or waiting for Internet information to be downloaded. Additionally, there could be reinforcing factors when online such as being able to gain and access information quickly. Likewise, engaging in online activities such as checking email may follow a variable ratio schedule of reinforcement. The Internet user gets a "payoff" of new email with the varying number of times the email is checked. The social view recognizes that there are familial, social, and cultural influences that prompt problematic Internet use. For example, the person may use the Internet to escape family conflict, increase social interaction, or feel pressured from peers to engage in various online activities. Additionally, family and peers may model problematic Internet use. For example, people may see those around them using the Internet to meet others, be entertained, and solve problems. Finally, because Beard views this problem as having at least some aspects of an addiction, questions related to relapse prevention are also included as part of his sample questions. His sample interview questions can be found on pages 131-132. You will note that the questions are clustered into categories revolving around potential biological, psychological, and social issues that might arise with someone who is engaging in problematic Internet use.

DIAGNOSIS

Most researchers who have developed criteria for problematic Internet use believe that although there may be chemical addiction aspects to the problematic Internet use, it is more of a behavioral addiction (Beard & Wolf, 2001; Kaltiala-Heino et al., 2004; Laaser & Gregoire, 2003; Ng & Wiemer-Hastings, 2005; Niemz et al., 2005; Song et al., 2004; Young, 1998). As a result, they have based the proposed diagnostic criteria on behavioral addiction standards and modeled their criteria on other behavioral addictions such as impulse control disorders. In particular, Beard and Wolf (2001) and Young (1998) have adapted criteria from the *Diagnostic and Statistical Manual of Mental Disorders* (*DSM-IV*; American Psychiatric Association [APA], 2000) for pathological gambling in an effort to develop consistent criteria for diagnosing problematic Internet use.

Young (1998) modified criteria for pathological gambling to fit Internet-related behaviors. Although there are 10 criteria for pathological gambling, Young modified only seven in the creation of her criteria. She felt that the remaining three criteria were not relevant to problematic Internet use (e.g., After losing money gambling, often returns another day to get even; Has committed illegal acts such as forgery, fraud, theft, or embezzlement to finance gambling; Relies on others to provide money to relieve a desperate financial situation caused by gambling [APA, 2000]). In addition to the seven modified criteria, Young (1998) added "Has stayed online longer than originally intended" to make her eight criteria. If a person had five out of the eight criteria, then the person exhibited problematic Internet use.

Although Beard and Wolf (2001) felt that Young's (1998) criteria were a positive step toward the development of criteria for problematic Internet use, they also felt that there were some problems with her standards. They believed that the first five criteria could account for numerous behaviors and would not necessarily constitute an "addictive" behavior. Therefore, they felt that all of the first five criteria had to be met. The remaining three criteria were separated out because they were seen as more problematic and influential in the person's daily functioning, ability to cope, and interactions/relationships with others. Therefore, they recommended that at least one of the remaining three criteria be met for a diagnosis of problematic Internet use.

Finally, Niemz et al. (2005) used Griffith's (1998) initial description of behaviors associated with problematic Internet use as a basis for their proposed criteria for problematic Internet use. Their list consists of seven areas that should be reviewed. If a person fit in three or more of these areas, then he or she was identified as Internet-dependent. A description of the different proposed criteria can be found in Table 2 (p. 125).

The issue of problematic Internet use is being taken seriously among medical and mental health professionals and there is a need to further examine the usefulness of some of the proposed criteria. In a report presented by the Council on Science and Public Health (CSAPH) to

TABLE 2: Proposed Diagnostic Criteria for Problematic Internet Use

Young's (1998) criteria	Beard & Wolf's (2001) criteria	Niemz et al. (2005) criteria
Five (or more) of the following:	All the following (1–5) must be present:	Symptoms consist of:
1. Is preoccupied with the Internet (think about previous online activity or anticipate next online session).	1. Is preoccupied with the Internet (think about previous online activity or anticipate next online session).	1. Increased preoccupation with online activities.
2. Needs to use the Internet with increased amounts of time in order to achieve satisfaction.	2. Needs to use the Internet with increased amounts of time in order to achieve satisfaction.	2. Tolerance (e.g., spending increased amounts of time in chat rooms).
3. Has made unsuccessful efforts to control, cut back, or stop Internet use.	3. Has made unsuccessful efforts to control, cut back, or stop Internet use.	3. Symptoms of withdrawal when not online (e.g., anxiety, depression).
4. Is restless, moody, depressed, or irritable when attempting to cut down or stop Internet use.	4. Is restless, moody, depressed, or irritable when attempting to cut down or stop Internet use.	4. Salience (whereby the Internet becomes the most important thing in the person's life).
5. Has stayed online longer than originally intended.	5. Has stayed online longer than originally intended.	5. Mood modification (where the Internet is used to change mood states).
6. Has jeopardized or risked the loss of a significant relationship, job, educational, or career opportunity because of the Internet.	At least one of the following:	6. Relapse (where the person returns to the addictive behavior, even after a period of abstinence).
7. Has lied to family members, therapist, or others to conceal the extent of involvement with the Internet.	1. Has jeopardized or risked the loss of a significant relationship, job, educational, or career opportunity because of the Internet.	If three or more are found then the person is considered Internet-dependent. The researchers go on to suggest that an addiction to the Internet can include any variety of application found from being online such as the process of typing, opportunities for communication, the lack of face-to-face contact, Internet content (e.g., pornography), or online social activities (e.g., chat rooms, multiuser domains, bulletin boards, and online games).
8. Uses the Internet as a way of escaping from problems or of relieving a dysphoric mood (e.g., feelings of helplessness, guilt, anxiety, depression).	2. Has lied to family members, therapist, or others to conceal the extent of involvement with the Internet.	
	3. Uses the Internet as a way of escaping from problems or of relieving a dysphoric mood (e.g., feelings of helplessness, guilt, anxiety, depression).	

the American Medical Association (AMA), it was recommended that the American Psychiatric Association review and consider the inclusion of a disorder involving excessive video game use and Internet overuse for the upcoming revision of the *Diagnostic and Statistical Manual of Mental Disorders* (AMA, 2007).

TREATMENT

As we continue to explore how to best assess and diagnose problematic Internet use, we also continue to investigate how best to treat difficulties that arise from Internet use. The likelihood of finding a therapist who specializes in treating problematic Internet use is small. It may be difficult to even find a therapist who will be open-minded to the notion of problematic Internet use and willing to fully examine the contribution of the Internet to the person's addictive behavior (King, 1996). As a result, treatment options are limited. At the onset, it should be noted that although some workable treatment approaches and techniques have been offered, Chou et al. (2005) concludes that few successful cases of treatment have been reported.

The following section will review different forms that treatment may take when working with a problematic Internet user. Then, a selection of intervention techniques that can be used with problematic Internet users will be highlighted. These interventions come from the general literature on intervening with addiction and specific intervention techniques recommended for treating problematic Internet use. Finally, issues related to relapse prevention will be examined.

Treatment Modality

Individual psychotherapy is the most common treatment modality that mental health providers will engage in when treating those with problematic Internet use. This treatment modality may be more comfortable for some clients because there is one-on-one attention and there could be an element of embarrassment or shame because of their Internet use and the consequences of that behavior.

Because problematic Internet use can impact many different parts of a person's life, there may need to be interventions in various aspects of the person's world. Therefore, a multidisciplinary approach may be effective. It is recommended that for successful treatment to occur, this team approach is needed, which could include psychiatrists, school counselors, social workers, faculty, parents, spouses, employers, and whomever else is consistently involved in the client's life (Young, 1998).

Family therapy is recommended by Young (1998). Psychotherapy may be necessary for those whose marriages and family relationships were disrupted and negatively impacted by problematic Internet usage. Additionally, the problematic Internet user will be returning to his or her family environment, which may have been contributing to the development of problematic Internet use to begin with.

Finding a support group could benefit the Internet user. Support can come from friends, family, or groups (Peele & Brodsky, 1991). Young (1998) explained that support groups can help the person gain insight into the origins of the addiction, feel validated, normalize the experience, decrease feelings of being alone, and instill hope that the person can get better. These factors may be important to the Internet user because this is a relatively new phenomenon. Local mental health or rehabilitation centers may have referrals. If no groups are available specifically for Internet addiction, then a support group for eating disorders or pathological gambling could be effective. These groups have similarities to Internet addiction because they are also nonchemical addictions and the assistance obtained can be generalized to the Internet user. Information about addiction can be obtained at these meetings. Even if the person only goes and listens to other's experiences, he or she will see similarities among others' situations. Internet support groups have developed on the Internet with members exchanging messages about the negative consequences their Internet addiction had created and coping strategies that were employed. Problems with online support groups include a lack of structure and consistency, as well as the fact that it encourages more Internet use.

Interventions and Treatment Models

Beard (2002) notes that from a biological standpoint, psychopharmacology can be used to treat problematic Internet use. Sattar and Ramaswamy (2004) agree, stating that for people who have problematic Internet and comorbid psychological symptoms, psychopharmacology can be used to aid them with this aspect of their addiction. For example, medication can help alleviate symptoms of anxiety or depression which could be a separate psychological problem or one that is contributing to the Internet use issues. Medication may also help to create homeostasis in the person or limit the sense of euphoria that comes from the Internet use.

As more research is done in this field, effective medications paired with psychotherapy may create better treatment outcomes, as is found in the treatment of other psychological disorders (Yellowlees & Marks, 2005). For example, medication, such as a selective serotonin reuptake inhibitor that has been an effective treatment for depression, is thought to provide additional benefits for patients with problematic Internet use (Sattar & Ramaswamy, 2004).

From a psychological standpoint, Beard (2002) proposes that classical conditioning intervention techniques may help break associations that have been with the Internet. For example, feeling lonely may be associated with logging on to the Internet in order to alleviate this feeling. The intervention would focus on breaking this association. This could be done by helping the user recognize how this emotional state is a cue for Internet use, helping the user recognize when the cue occurs, and helping the user find alternate ways to decrease his or her loneliness.

Young (1998) advised that pathological Internet users change their Internet use schedule. Changing the schedule may interrupt classically conditioned associations that have been made between certain times of the day and excessive Internet use. Another intervention she suggests is for the client to create "external stoppers." With this intervention, the person would use concrete things (e.g., time to work, to meet boss, etc.) that need to be done, to go to, or that prompt the user to help him or her log off.

Beard (2002) states that operant conditioning techniques can use rewards and punishments for Internet use. The strategy is to try and change the reinforcement or punishment that the user obtains from a behavior and/or helps the person receive reinforcement or punishment in a more appropriate manner. Additionally, operant conditioning interventions could be implemented to help a user who is engaging in certain Internet applications. One intervention that could be done is the development of a behavior modification plan.

Young (1996, 1998, 1999) has suggested using a combination of classical and operant conditioning techniques. One such intervention explores how to change the situation. This may include anything from altering the setting where the computer is kept or something as drastic as moving from a rural area to a more active city. By altering the environment, associations between the environment and Internet use can be extinguished. Likewise, having the computer in an isolated room could be negatively reinforcing by allowing the user to be left alone from a chaotic home environment. Once again, by changing the environment, a situation may be made in which the client is no longer reinforced for engaging in the same level of Internet use.

Cognitive behavioral therapy (CBT) is an appropriate intervention method for the treatment of Internet addiction (Beard, 2002; Yellowlees & Marks, 2005). The focus would be on identifying thoughts and triggers for excessive Internet use. There are numerous intervention strategies from this model that could be used (Beard, 2002; Chou et al., 2005).

Yellowlees and Marks (2005) propose that one intervention strategy would include cognitive restructuring connected to the Internet applications that are most used by the client. Additionally, there may be behavioral exercises that the client does as well as exposure therapy in which the client stays offline for increased amounts of time. Young (1998) offers numerous other CBT interventions that could be done. For example, she recommends that that client "practice the opposite." This would involve coming up with other activities to engage in instead of the Internet and constructing a new schedule that reduces Internet use or the time pattern for using the Internet. Another intervention she puts forward is "setting goals." It is important for the client to set clear and achievable goals which will enhance the client's sense of control. She also suggests using "reminder cards." These are tangible, portable reminders of what the Internet user wants to avoid (e.g., lost time with family) and the things that he or she wants to do (e.g., improved productivity at work). A "personal inventory" could be developed. With this, the user generates a list of every activity or practice that has been neglected or reduced since the problematic Internet use began.

M. H. Orzack and D. S. Orzack (1999) also suggest using Motivational Enhancement Therapy, which allows those who are having problems with their Internet use to work with their therapist in a collaborative manner on treatment plans and set attainable goals. The approach is largely client-centered, and treatment strategies train the client. Through planned and directed interventions, the client is motivated to use his or her own resources to create change. This treatment approach is less confrontational and more innovative than cognitive behavioral therapy. The researchers suggest that a combination of techniques from both approaches will yield the most benefits.

Additionally, a combination of CBT and psychodynamic techniques could be useful, if the person is engaging in online role playing. It might be important to explore what the person's role playing character is like, because it could be a projection of the client's inner desires. This may give the therapist a sense of what qualities the client may be missing or feel inhibited to express in the "real" world. The Internet may be used as a way to escape from reality and at least get some temporary relief from dealing with problems and inner conflicts (Sattar & Ramaswamy, 2004; C. K. Yang et al., 2005). If this is the case, while helping the person learn how to appropriately express these inner desires in the real world, it will be important to not limit the amount or type of Internet use until new coping skills have been taught, mastered, and can take the place of the Internet use.

From a social standpoint, Young (1998) feels that help is needed in order to expand the person's "social support." With this intervention, real-world friends and support can be organized and adapted to the user's particular needs and life situations. This will aid the person's dependence on online social support.

Education and training about the Internet and its effects could be an effective intervention strategy (Yellowlees & Marks, 2005). This type of intervention will be beneficial not only to the client but also to those who interact with the client and have witnessed the damaging effects of the person's problematic Internet use. Education may include understanding how and why the problem developed, what maintained the problem, and ways to intervene as well as to support the person who is dealing with this problem.

Additionally, interventions with family or peers may be needed, because they may be promoting, encouraging, enabling, and overlooking the problematic Internet use. Interventions may include learning ways to handle family crises and stabilizing the family (Stanton & Heath, 1997). Exploration into premorbid family problems is needed, because this may be a reason why the Internet user sought out the Internet (Young, 1998).

Another intervention is helping the client have more satisfying interactions with family members and peer relationships by improving communication skills (Beard, 2002). Goodman (1993) and Young (1998) stressed that both parties need to learn how to express what it is that they want the other to do. The language used needs to be structured in such a way that what is being said does not make the other person feel defensive, resulting in the communication becoming heated or terminated. Techniques may include learning how to construct "I statements," having the client paraphrase what has been said by the other person in order to convey understanding to the other person, and finding an agreed-upon and uninterrupted time to talk.

Finally, some argue that to best treat the Internet addict, the person must be aided in learning how to abstain from Internet use (Chou et al., 2005). Because the Internet is here to stay and becoming more and more of an integral part of our lives, this is probably not a realistic treatment option (Beard & Wolf, 2001). Instead, treatment should focus on moderation and controlled use, according to Young (1998).

Regardless of the treatment model used or specific interventions that are implemented, accountability is an important aspect to treatment (Laaser & Gregoire, 2003). Clients will need to be held responsible for their actions online and resulting consequences. Making clients answerable to their actions may be particularly important if they engage in defense mechanisms such as intellectualization or rationalization of their problem. Young (1998) remarks that the greatest difficulty in treating those with problematic Internet use is working through their denial of the problem.

Relapse Prevention

Recovering from any addiction carries the risk of relapse (Young, 1998). Relapse prevention involves both cognitive and behavioral components (Marlatt, 1985). Relapse prevention will be a necessary part of treating a problematic Internet user.

Many researchers (Fanning & O'Neill, 1996; Peele & Brodsky, 1991; Young, 1998) have recommended identifying high-risk situations where relapse may occur to help prevent the person from completing the relapse cycle. The client can then be taught ways to engage in alternate activities. It was also recommended that permission-giving thoughts to engage in the problematic behavior be identified. This may include a thought like, "An extra hour on the Internet won't hurt anything so it would be O.K. for me to stay on longer this time." Then, permission-denying thoughts can be generated to counteract them. This may include a thought like, "Staying online longer will make me want to stay online more. I know I will lose track of time and be late for work." Discussing relapse fantasies and past relapse experiences can also help in the identification of high-risk situations (Marlatt, 1985). Accepting urges and fantasies as natural, recognizing that they will pass, and reviewing the benefits of continuing the changes already made are cognitive strategies that help with cravings (Goodman, 1993).

Once high-risk situations have been identified, then coping skills need to be learned (Marlatt, 1985). Peele and Brodsky (1991) suggested that if clients begin to relapse, they try retreating to a quiet place and processing what they are doing. The person may also benefit from seeking support. Along with relaxation, imagery can be used to help the person cope with the urge to engage in the problematic behavior (Marlatt, 1985).

The next part of relapse prevention should involve educating the person on relapse prevention (Marlatt, 1985). For example, Fanning and O'Neill (1996) suggested reviewing the stages that people go through when dealing with any addiction (i.e., Precontemplation, Contemplation, Action, Maintenance) and how relapse occurs. A person can also be taught how to use a decision matrix in order to evaluate the benefits and consequences of engaging in the addictive behavior (Marlatt, 1985).

It has been proposed (Fanning & O'Neill, 1996; Marlatt, 1985) that the next part of relapse prevention involves helping the person develop a plan of action for situations in which the problematic behavior is initiated. A contract can be developed that the person will commit to if relapse begins. Reminder cards can also be made to help the person remember what needs to happen if relapse occurs. Practicing and using all of these techniques with various hypothetical situations can prepare the client for when a real situation occurs.

If a relapse situation occurs, it will be important for the user to review and analyze the elements of the situation in order to learn from it and avoid or be better prepared to handle similar situations in the future (Peele & Brodsky, 1991). Cognitive restructuring can assist the client in viewing the relapse as a mistake and attributing the behavior to the situation versus a personal weakness (Marlatt, 1985). Paradoxical intervention has also been used. A programmed relapse occurs when the client is required to engage in the addictive behavior under the supervision of a therapist in order to help the client experience a relapse and return to the target behavior with therapeutic assistance (Marlatt, 1985).

CONCLUSION

The debate over the existence of " Internet addiction" will undoubtedly continue for some time. Regardless of what term is used (e.g., Problematic Internet Use, Internet Addiction, Maladaptive Internet Use), it is clear that there are people developing a harmful dependence on the Internet. With the rapid increase of Internet use, mental health professionals are going to see more and more clients enter into treatment because of their problematic Internet use. As a result, our understanding of problematic Internet use needs to be expanded. There is a need for assessment instruments with demonstrated reliability and validity, which can be easily scored and administered. Moreover, diagnoses must be based on agreed-upon criteria, and treatment protocols must be developed and evaluated for their efficacy in assisting people dealing with this problem.

Sample Questions for an Interview With Someone Exhibiting Problematic Internet Use*

Presenting Problem

1. When did you begin to notice problems with your Internet use?
2. How long have you used the Internet?
3. What was going on in your life when you began using the Internet?
4. What was going on in your life when you began to have difficulties with your Internet use?
5. How much time do you spend on the Internet each day? Week? Month?
6. Do you ever feel preoccupied with the Internet (e.g., think about previous online activity or anticipate next online session)?
7. What is the longest amount of time you have spent using the Internet in one setting?
8. In what location does your Internet use occur?
9. What time of the day does the Internet use occur?
10. Who is around when you use the Internet?
11. What do you enjoy about the Internet?
12. What do you dislike about the Internet?
13. What Internet sites/applications (e.g., chat rooms, email, massively multiplayer online role-playing game [MMORP], multi-user domains [MUDs], instant messaging) do you use, and what effect do they have on you?
14. Have you ever stayed online longer than originally intended?
15. In what ways has your Internet use interfered with your daily activities?
16. Have you ever contemplated or tried cutting down on your Internet use but couldn't?
17. What helps or makes the situation better?
18. What hurts or makes the situation worse?
19. Have you ever lied to family members, therapist, or others to conceal the extent of your involvement with the Internet?
20. How did you feel when attempting to cut down or stop your Internet use?
21. Why did you decide to seek help now?

Biological Areas

1. Are you experiencing any health concerns? If so, please describe.
2. How have these health concerns been impacted by your Internet use?
3. What treatment have you received for these health concerns?
4. Does your Internet use interfere with your sleep?
5. How many hours a night do you typically sleep?
6. Does your Internet use interfere with eating regularly?
7. How many meals a day do you typically eat?
8. Have you recently gained or lost any weight?
9. What exercise patterns do you engage in?
10. What nonprescription medication do you take? How much? How often?
11. What prescription medication do you take? How much? How often?
12. What substances or behaviors do you or others feel you have been addicted to in the past?
13. What kind of alcohol do you currently use? How much? How often?
14. In the past, what kind of alcohol did you use? How much? How often?
15. What drugs do you currently use? How much? How often?
16. In the past, what drugs did you use? How much? How often?
17. Is there a history of addiction in your family? If so, who and what?

---

*From "Internet Addiction: A Review of Current Assessment Techniques and Potential Assessment Questions," by K. W. Beard, 2005, *CyberPsychology & Behavior, 8*(1), pp. 7-14. Copyright © 2005, Mary Ann Liebert, Inc. Publishers. Adapted with permission.

Psychological Areas

1. How do you feel before using the Internet?
2. What are your thoughts before using the Internet?
3. Have you ever used the Internet to help improve your mood or change your thoughts?
4. What is your environment like before using the Internet?
5. How do you feel while using the Internet?
6. What are your thoughts while using the Internet?
7. What is your environment like while using the Internet?
8. How do you feel after using the Internet?
9. What are your thoughts after using the Internet?
10. What is your environment like after using the Internet?
11. Have you ever felt anxious, depressed, or isolated when off-line?
12. How well do you think you cope with various events in your life?

Social Areas

1. How has your Internet use caused problems or concerns with your family?
2. What psychological/psychiatric illnesses have members of your family experienced?
3. What is your overall degree of satisfaction with your family?
4. How has your Internet use caused problems or concerns with your significant other?
5. What is your overall degree of satisfaction with your significant other?
6. How has your Internet use caused problems or concerns with your child/children?
7. What is your overall degree of satisfaction with your child/children?
8. How has using the Internet caused problems or concerns with your social activities and friendships?
9. What is your overall degree of satisfaction with your friendships?
10. How do others in your life use the Internet (e.g., email, Instant Message [IM])?
11. What is your overall degree of satisfaction with school/work?
12. How has using the Internet interfered with your performance at school or work?
13. Have you ever been in trouble with the authorities because of your Internet use?
14. What are your social/leisure/hobby activities?
15. How would you rate your social skills?
16. How would you rate your communication skills?

Relapse Prevention Areas

1. Do you believe that you have a problem with your level of Internet use?
2. What seems to trigger Internet use?
3. What do you see as the benefits and costs of continued Internet use?
4. What is your level of determination to change your current Internet patterns?
5. What plans have you implemented in the past to deal with your level of Internet use?
6. Have these plans worked?

CONTRIBUTOR

Keith W. Beard, PsyD, received his doctorate in Clinical Psychology from Wright State University in Dayton, Ohio. He is currently an associate professor in the Department of Psychology, the internship coordinator, and the Director of the Psychology Clinic at Marshall University in Huntington, West Virginia. In addition to teaching, he is a Licensed Psychologist and a Licensed Professional Counselor. He has a small private practice where he works with individuals and their families. He does consulting work and leads organizational workshops. His research interests include Internet addiction, psychological factors in mass media, men's issues, humor in teaching, and religion and psychology. Dr. Beard may be contacted at One John Marshall Drive, Huntington, WV 25755. E-mail: beard@marshall.edu

RESOURCES

Cited Resources

American Medical Association. (2007). *Emotional and Behavioral Effects of Video Games and Internet Overuse*. Retrieved Jan. 7, 2008 from http://www.ama-assn.org/ama/pub/category/17694.html#resolution

American Psychiatric Association. (2000). *Diagnostic and Statistical Manual of Mental Disorders* (4th ed. text rev.). Washington, DC: Author.

Beard, K. W. (2002). Internet addiction: Current status and implications for employees. *Journal of Employment Counseling, 39*, 2-11.

Beard, K. W. (2005). Internet addiction: A review of current assessment techniques and potential assessment questions. *CyberPsychology & Behavior, 8*(1), 7-14.

Beard, K. W. (2008). Internet addiction in children and adolescents. In C. Yarnall (Ed.), *Computer Science Research Trends* (pp. 169-180). Hauppauge, NY: Nova Science Publishers.

Beard, K. W., & Wolf, E. M. (2001). Modification in the proposed diagnostic criteria for Internet addiction. *CyberPsychology & Behavior, 4*(3), 377-383.

Brenner, V. (1997). Psychology of computer use: XLVII. Parameters of Internet use, abuse and addiction: The first 90 days of the Internet usage survey. *Psychological Reports, 80*, 879-882.

Chak, K., & Leung, L. (2004). Shyness and locus of control as predictors of Internet addiction and Internet use. *CyberPsychology & Behavior, 7*(5), 559-570.

Chen, S. H., & Chou, C. (1999, August). *Development of Chinese Internet Addiction Scale in Taiwan*. Poster presented at the 107th American Psychology annual convention, Boston, MA.

Chou, C., Condron, L., & Belland, J. C. (2005). A review of the research on Internet addiction. *Educational Psychology Review, 17*(4), 363-388.

Chou, C., & Hsiao, M. C. (2000). Internet addiction, usage, gratifications, and pleasure experience: The Taiwan college students' case. *Computers in Education, 35*(1), 65-80.

Correll, S. (1995). The ethnography of an electronic bar. *Journal of Contemporary Ethnography, 24*, 270-298.

Davis, R. A., Flett, G. L., & Besser, A. (2002). Validation of a new scale for measuring problematic Internet use: Implications for pre-employment screening. *CyberPsychology & Behavior, 5*(4), 331-345.

Engelberg, E., & Sjoberg, L. (2004). Internet use, social skills, and adjustment. *CyberPsychology & Behavior, 7*(1), 41-47.

Fanning, P., & O'Neill, J. T. (1996). *The Addiction Workbook: A Step-by-Step Guide to Quitting Alcohol and Drugs*. Oakland, CA: New Harbinger Publications.

Gackenbach, J., & Ellerman, E. (1998). Introductions to psychological aspects of Internet use. In J. Gackenbach (Ed.), *Psychology and the Internet* (pp. 1-26). San Diego, CA: Academic Press.

Goodman, A. (1993). Diagnosis and treatment of sexual addiction. *Journal of Sex & Marital Therapy, 19*, 225-246.

Griffiths, M. (1997). Psychology of computer use: XLIII. Some comments on "Addictive Use of the Internet" by Young. *Psychological Reports, 80*, 81-82.

Griffiths, M. (1998). Internet addiction: Does it really exist? In J. Gackenbach (Ed.), *Psychology and the Internet* (pp. 61-75). San Diego, CA: Academic Press.

Harmon, A. (1998). *Researchers Find Sad, Lonely, World in Cyberspace*. Retrieved Jan. 7, 2008 from http://www.nytimes.com/library/tech/98/08/biztech/articles/30depression.html

Internet World Stats. (2008). *World Internet users: November 2007*. Retrieved January 7, 2008 from http://www.internetworldstats.com/stats.htm

Kaltiala-Heino, R., Lintonen, T., & Rimpela, A. (2004). Internet addiction? Potentially problematic use of the Internet in a population of 12-18 year old adolescents. *Addiction Research and Theory, 12*(1), 89-96.

Kandell, J. J. (1998). Internet addiction on campus: The vulnerability of college students. *Cyberpsychology & Behavior, 1*, 11-17.

Kiesler, S., Siegel, J., & McGuire, T. W. (1984). Social psychological aspects of computer-mediated communication. *American Psychologist, 39*, 1123-1134

King, S. A. (1996). *Is the Internet Addictive, or are Addicts Using the Internet?* Retrieved Jan. 7, 2008 from http://webpages.charter.net/stormking/iad.html

Laaser, M. R., & Gregoire, L. J. (2003). Pastors and cybersex addiction. *Sexual Relationship Therapy, 18*(3), 395-404.

Leung, L. (2004). Net-generation attributes and seductive properties of the Internet as predictors of online activities and Internet addiction. *CyberPsychology & Behavior, 7*(3), 333-348.

Lin, S. S. J., & Tsai, C. C. (1999, August). *Internet Addiction Among High Schoolers in Taiwan.* Paper presented at the American Psychological Association annual meeting, Boston, MA.

Marlatt, G. A. (1985). Relapse prevention: Theoretical rationale and overview of the model. In G. A. Marlatt & J. Gordon, (Eds.), *Relapse Prevention* (pp. 250-280). New York: Guilford.

McCormick, N. B., & McCormick, J. W. (1992). Computer friends and foes: Content of undergraduates' electronic mail. *Computers in Human Behavior, 8*, 379-405.

Mitchell, P. (2000). Internet addiction: Genuine diagnosis or not? *Lancet, 355*, 632.

Morahan-Martin, J. M., & Schumacker, P. (2000). Incidence and correlates of pathological Internet use. *Computers in Human Behavior, 16*, 3-29.

Niemz, K., Griffiths, M., & Banyard, P. (2005). Prevalence of pathological Internet use among university students and correlations with self-esteem, the General Health Questionnaire (GHQ), and disinhibition. *CyberPsychology & Behavior, 8*(6), 562-570.

Ng, B. D., & Wiemer-Hastings, P. (2005). Addiction to the Internet and online gaming. *CyberPsychology & Behavior, 8*(2), 110-113.

Orzack, M. H., & Orzack, D. S. (1999). Treatment of computer addicts with complex comorbid psychiatric disorders. *CyberPsychology & Behavior, 2*, 465-473.

Parks, M. R., & Floyd, K. (1996). Making friends in cyberspace. *Journal of Communication, 46*, 80-97.

Peele, S., & Brodsky, A. (1991). *The Truth About Addiction and Recovery.* New York: Simon & Schuster.

Sattar, P., & Ramaswamy, S. (2004). Internet gaming addiction. *Canadian Journal of Psychiatry, 49*(12), 869-870.

Scherer, K. (1997). College life online: Healthy and unhealthy Internet use. *Journal of College Student Development, 38*, 655-665.

Simkova, B., & Cincera, J. (2004). Internet addiction disorder and chatting in the Czech Republic. *CyberPsychology & Behavior, 7*(5), 536-539.

Song, I., Larose, R., Eastin, M .S., & Lin, C. A. (2004). Internet gratification and Internet addiction: On the uses and abuses of new media. *CyberPsychology & Behavior, 7*(4), 384-394.

Stanton, M. D., & Heath, A. W. (1997). Family and marital therapy. In J. Lowinson, P., Ruiz, R. Millman, & J. Langrod (Eds.), *Substance Abuse: A Comprehensive Textbook* (3rd ed., pp. 448-454). Baltimore, MD: Williams & Wilkins.

Suler, J. (1996). *Why is This Thing Eating My Life? Computer and Cyberspace Addiction at the "Palace."* Retrieved Jan. 7, 2008 from http://users.rider.edu/~suler/psycyber/eatlife.html

Yang, C. K., Choe, B. M., Baity, M., Lee, J. H., & Cho, J. S. (2005). SCL-90-R and 16PF profiles of senior high school students with excessive Internet use. *Canadian Journal of Psychiatry, 50*(7), 407-414.

Yang, S. C., & Tung, C. J. (2004). Comparison of Internet addicts and non-addicts in Taiwanese high school. *Computers in Human Behavior, 23*, 79-96.

Yellowlees, P. M., & Marks, S. (2005). Problematic Internet use or Internet addiction? *Computers in Human Behavior, 23*, 1447-1453.

Yoo, H. J., Cho, S. C., Ha, J., Yune, S. K., Kim, S. J., Hwang, J., Chung, A., Sung, Y. H., & Lyoo, I. K., (2004). Attention deficit hyperactivity symptoms and Internet addiction. *Psychiatry and Clinical Neurosciences, 58*, 487-494.

Young, K. S. (1996). Psychology of computer use: XL. Addictive use of the Internet: A case that breaks the stereotype. *Psychological Reports, 79*, 899-902.

Young, K. S. (1997). *What Makes the Internet Addictive: Potential Explanations for Pathological Internet Use.* Retrieved Jan. 7, 2008 from http://www.netaddiction.com/articles/habitforming.pdf

Young, K. S. (1998). *Caught in the Net.* New York: John Wiley & Sons.

Young, K. S. (1999). Evaluation and treatment of Internet addiction. In L. VandeCreek & T. L. Jackson (Eds.), *Innovations in Clinical Practice* (Vol. 17, pp. 19-31). Sarasota, FL: Professional Resource Press.

Additional Resources

Center for Online Addiction. Website: http://www.netaddiction.com
Kimberly Young, PsyD

Computer Addiction Study Center at McLean Hospital, Harvard University. Website: http://www.computeraddiction.com/
Maressa Hecht Orzack, PhD

Center for Internet Behavior. Website: http://www.virtual-addiction.com/
Dave Greenfield, PhD

The Clinical Uses of Mindfulness

Robert B. Denton and Richard W. Sears

Much attention has been given in recent literature to the concept of mindfulness and mindfulness-based interventions, proving to be fruitful ground for both clinicians and researchers alike. But what is mindfulness? How can this be applied to clinical interventions? How should a clinician go about becoming competent to use this approach?

This contribution aims to familiarize clinicians with the most recent literature regarding mindfulness-based interventions and practice, and to identify ways to gain knowledge and competency in applying those concepts and intervention strategies in their own practice.

Mindfulness refers to an approach and a conceptual framework, not necessarily to a specific technique or an isolated theory. Basically, it means bringing a greater awareness of thoughts, feelings, and physical sensations into the therapeutic session and, ultimately, into daily life. For the practitioner, this means being more fully present and aware of what is going on in the therapy session. For the client, this means being more consciously aware of thoughts, feelings, and behaviors throughout the day. Use of mindfulness helps to discard old, unconscious, maladaptive patterns.

Use of mindfulness leads the client to a nonjudgmental understanding of the current situation, and therefore to greater acceptance. Acceptance of the current situation and one's feelings about the situation is a precondition for realistically being able to change them. Because this full acceptance can be difficult for clients, it has been termed "radical acceptance" (Linehan, 1993). Clients come to therapy because they are not happy with the way things are; however, in accordance with the concepts of mindfulness, they must accept the way things are before they can effect change.

The concepts of a mindfulness-based practice have shown utility in Western psychology for many categorized areas of mental affliction. These include things such as the reduction of anxiety (Astin, 1997; Gillani & Smith, 2001; Goldman, Dormitor, & Murray, 1979; Kabat-Zinn, 1990; Kabat-Zinn et al., 1992; Miller, Fletcher, & Kabat-Zinn, 1995; S. L. Shapiro, Schwartz, & Bonner, 1998; Tloczynski & Tantriella, 1998), preventing relapse in chronic depression (Segal, Williams, & Teasdale, 2002), increasing empathy (Lesh, 1970; Schuster, 1979; S. L. Shapiro et al., 1998), and increasing present-minded awareness or attention (Thompson, 2000; Valentine & Sweet, 1999; Walsh et al., 1978).

The application of mindfulness has been proposed as a way to help psychotherapists to be proficient in maintaining their own state of awareness and the awareness of their client in a therapeutic setting (Alexander, 1997; Bien, 2006; Chung, 1990; Epstein, 2003a, 2003b; Kabat-Zinn, 2003a). Collectively these authors state that mindfulness increases one's ability to be present and attuned to the here and now, an essential quality of a successful therapeutic encounter. According to Kabat-Zinn (1990), mindfulness has several qualities that influence one's attitude, which are nonjudging patience, *beginner's mind*, trust, nonstriving, acceptance, and letting go. These qualities help psychologists to engage in an effective therapeutic relationship with their clients.

"Beginner's mind" is a reference from the writings of Zen teacher Shunryu Suzuki (1970), who said, "In the beginner's mind there are many possibilities, but in the expert's there are few" (p. 21). Essentially, although our expertise allows us to use our experience to understand the situations faced by the client, we must also stay fresh to the unique presentation of the particular client with whom we are currently working. Inventing a new therapy for each client becomes a lesson in mindfulness as the clinician works to understand clients' particular frameworks from which they view and encounter the world.

HISTORY AND LITERATURE REVIEW

Mindfulness-based meditation originated from the teachings of Siddhartha Gautama, the historically referenced Buddha, and has been studied and practiced by generations for over 2,500 years (Hanh, 1990; Kabat-Zinn, 2003a). This practice is considered in some schools to be the backbone of the Buddhist teachings, and that which drives all other aspects of meditation practice (Hanh, 1990). Mindfulness has collectively been described as a state of being awake and fully present in the world during each passing moment (Alexander, 1997; Goleman, 1988; Kabat-Zinn, 1994). Atwood and Maltin (1991); Epstein (1984, 1990, 1995, 2003a, 2003b); Goleman (1988); Kabat-Zinn (1990, 1994, 2003a); Linehan and Kehrer (1992); Segal et al. (2002); Tart (1990); and Williams et al. (2007) each describe mindfulness as a practice that has significant implications for how individuals experience, understand, and make meaning of the world.

The first part of this contribution will describe the areas in which mindfulness practice has been theorized to be beneficial and where it has been empirically shown to be an effective tool in the practice of psychology and health. This synopsis aims to familiarize the beginning clinician with the literature base and support for the use of mindfulness to increase the clinician's skill set and as a clinical application for psychological intervention. The authors of this contribution have attempted to arrange the information into general themes so as to organize the current literature base.

Depression, Anxiety, and Stress Reduction

The concept of mindfulness practice to reduce stress and anxiety is as old as the teaching itself. Historically, the Buddha taught that there are "*four noble truths.*" These truths are that (a) suffering (or *dukkha*) is inherent in all existence; (b) suffering arises due to craving and attachment; (c) suffering can have an end; and (d) there is a *noble eight-fold path* which ultimately leads to *nirvana* (Keown, 2003). The first, second, and third of these are analogous with the concept Westerners may call psychological well-being and directly relate to the alleviation of anxiety, depression, and other areas of mental distress. The *Satipatthana Sutra,* the Treatise on the Four Establishments of Mindfulness, discusses (a) contemplation of the body, (b) contemplation of feelings, (c) contemplation of the mind, and (d) contemplation of mental objects (Soma & Pereira, 2004). The treatise provides teachings on how one can be liberated from the anger, anxiety, and fear in one's life by attending to the present moment and recognizing happiness, peace, and joy (Hanh, 1990).

In more recent years, Western practitioners of both psychological and medical science have recognized the potential for mindfulness-based practice in depression, anxiety, and stress reduction treatments (Astin, 1997; Austin, 1998, 2006; Kabat-Zinn, 1990; Kabat-Zinn et al., 1992; 2003b; Miller et al., 1995; Segal et al., 2002; S. L. Shapiro et al., 1998; Williams et al.,

2007). These authors as a group found that when individuals were instructed in mindfulness-based meditation, overall reports of anxiety and psychological distress decreased. Miller et al. (1995) also showed a more encouraging finding, that after 2 years of mindfulness-based intervention individuals maintained lower levels of anxiety. Kabat-Zinn's model for Mindfulness-Based Stress Reduction (MBSR) and Segal et al.'s (2002) Mindfulness Based Cognitive Therapy for Depression (MBCT) have both shown effectiveness in studies to warrant those approaches being recognized as an evidence-based treatment approach (Williams et al., 2007).

Mindfulness and radical acceptance are also integral components of Dialectical Behavior Therapy (DBT), one of the few evidence-based treatments for Borderline Personality Disorder (Linehan, 1993; Sneed, Balestri, & Belfi, 2003). Individuals with Borderline Personality Disorder often grew up in chaotic, traumatic environments and therefore have difficulties with emotional regulation. Through mindfulness and acceptance-based interventions, clients are taught to accept feelings as they are, not to push them away or grasp after them. In fact, it has been suggested that one of the key components that makes mindfulness effective in reducing anxiety is that it allows the client to experience the extinction of anxiety through interceptive exposure (Follette, Palm, & Rasmussen Hall, 2004). It has long been known that anticipatory anxiety and attempts to avoid anxiety tend to exacerbate symptoms.

Austin (1998, 2006), a neurobiologist, provides an in-depth look at the connection between meditation and its effects on brain function. He reviews current findings that suggest that there are biological changes that occur through the use of meditation that contribute to stress and anxiety reduction, increases in feelings of happiness, and sustaining attention.

Empathy Training

Lesh (1970) and Schuster (1979) began exploration of meditation practice as a means to increase one's ability and capacity for empathy. Rogers (1961) describes empathy as being the capacity for one to understand, be sensitive to, and feel what another person is feeling. In order to do this effectively, Stern (1985) identifies empathy as having "four distinct and probably sequential processes: (1) the resonance of feeling state; (2) the abstraction of empathic knowledge from the experience of emotional resonance; (3) the integration of abstracted empathic knowledge into an empathic response; and (4) a transient role identification" (p. 125). Of these, Stern identifies the second and third events as crucial elements for empathy. The attunement to affect (Step 1) is essential for the second two, but it alone is not sufficient for empathy. Stern identifies this extension of emotional resonance into an extrapolation of what it must be like to be that other person as the critical piece for an empathic response. Austin (1998) states "the root origins of this word, *empathy*, reflect the way we start with our own subjective state, and then project it out onto some other person or object" (p. 650). He feels that "empathy is limited to the observer's *perceptive*, imaginative side" (p. 650). In other words, it is the creative introspection that one has toward an outsider's feeling state. Mindfulness practice, by nature, helps to develop this personal introspective awareness and so offers a way for the individual to empathically experience another person. This is highlighted in the concept of what Epstein (2003a) identifies as nonjudging acceptance. As therapists, the ability to view our clients with a nonjudging attitude helps to create empathy for those individuals and their situation. Through this, they are more able to engage in a therapeutic process.

Norcross (2002) has worked to identify guidelines for the practice of empirically validated treatments and to identify and explicate common therapist factors that contribute to positive change. Of these, he identifies empathy as a key component in the relationship between therapist and client. Bohart et al. (2002), in their chapter on empathy, provide an argument toward the empirically validated relationship rather than the empirically validated treatment, citing literature that suggests that the relationship in therapy is a key component to change. They identify therapist empathy as being crucial for a positive psychotherapy outcome, and state that finding ways to increase the therapist's capacity for empathy is needed. In the Common

Factors literature, the therapeutic relationship, of which empathy is a primary factor, accounts for 30% of client change, while specific techniques account for only 15% (Hubble, Duncan, & Miller, 1999; Lambert, 1992).

One of the pioneers in using moment-to-moment awareness to enhance empathy in psychotherapy is Eugene Gendlin (1978; 1996), who called his approach "focusing." In addition to helping the therapist clearly empathize with the client, the client is taught to be more clearly aware of his or her own internal processes. Mindfulness practice is akin to Gendlin's purpose and an additional tool toward identifying those internal processes of both clinician and client. Schuster (1979) reviewed literature pertaining to empathy and mindfulness with the conclusion that "therapists experienced in mindfulness meditation should be able to inadvertently or deliberately move into direct moment-to-moment contact with their clients" (p. 76). Schuster also stated that "practice at mindfulness meditation can thus simultaneously enhance a therapist's professional skills and advance his or her evolution as a human being" (p. 76).

Lesh (1970) showed that applying Zen meditation training (which uses an approach similar to mindfulness) to master's level counselors led to greater empathy, particularly in those counselors who were initially low in the capacity for empathy. This increase in empathy was measured by those counselors' increased ability for affect sensitivity and openness to experience. Similarly, S. L. Shapiro et al. (1998) found that when medical and premedical students participated in an 8-week program based on Kabat-Zinn's Stress Reduction program (1982), there was an increase in those individual's overall levels of measured empathy.

More recently in this particular category, Block-Lerner et al. (2007) discuss the concepts of mindfulness-based training found within Kabat-Zinn's (1990) MBSR program, Segal and colleagues (2002) MBCT, Hayes, Strosahl, and Wilson's (1999) Acceptance and Commitment Therapy (ACT), and Linehan's (1993) DBT programs, and how these programs collectively impact the development of empathy in the individual. Although they assert that this may be a viable way to develop empathic connection in relationships, they also caution that these interventions need further research to support the claims that they as well as previous authors have made.

Present-Minded Attention

Yalom (2002) states that "accurate empathy is most important in the domain of the immediate present – that is, the here-and-now of the therapy hour" (p. 19). He refers to the here-and-now as the immediate events of the therapy hour as it is happening in the space created between the individuals present.

Thompson (2000) regards *zazen* (formal sitting meditation) as a practice in which "we sit with awareness, we observe, we become lost in thought, we awaken to the phenomenal present" (p. 538). He proposes that the "practice of zazen can help the clinician to become more aware of the fluidity of our presence as therapists and to capitalize on that awareness in our clinical practice" (p. 540).

Valentine & Sweet (1999) state that there is agreement in many previous studies (Brown, 1993; Goleman, 1977; Rao, 1989; Sethi, 1989) that meditation deals with the training of some type of attention, but that there are relatively few studies on the effect of meditation on attention. They state that previous studies such as Lesh (1970); Davidson, Goleman, and Schwartz (1976); Brown and Engler (1980); and D. H. Shapiro (1992) "revealed, firstly, that the practice of meditation leads to improvements in various aspects of attention, including increased sensitivity, concentration, openness to experience and decreased susceptibility to distraction and secondly, that such changes may increase as a function of duration of meditation practice" (p. 61). Other authors, such as Kabat-Zinn (1990, 1994, 2003a), Kabat-Zinn et al. (1992), Epstein (1995, 1998, 1999, 2003a, 2003b), and Chung (1990), also make claims that mindfulness is a method for increasing attention to the present moment.

Valentine and Sweet (1999) investigated this claim and conducted a study that compared the effect that both concentrative techniques and mindfulness-based meditation had on the training of attention. They found that both meditation practices lead to improved concentration and attention (as compared to a control group of nonmeditators) when individuals were subjected to a sustained attention task. Furthermore, they reported that long-term meditators showed a greater ability in attention compared to short-term meditators, suggesting that increased experience with meditation practice leads to greater improvements. In addition to this, there were also significant differences in performance between the concentration meditation group and the mindfulness meditation group, depending on whether the presented stimulus was expected or unexpected. Both groups performed equally well when a stimulus was expected, but the mindfulness group performed better on the attention task when there was an unexpected stimulus.

Given the nature of clinical practice, with its extended hours of mandated attention and the often unplanned spontaneous nature of the therapeutic hour, the therapist needs a way to cultivate the kind of attention described in the Valentine and Sweet (1999) study. Having shown its effectiveness, psychologists may regard mindfulness as a viable way to enhance their ability to be more present and attentive in the therapy hour.

Benefits to Clinical Practice

Alexander (1997) provides an in-depth look at the theoretical and practical aspects of cultivating mindfulness in the psychotherapist's clinical work. She provides a framework that attempts to incorporate theory and technique with direct experience and awareness of the clinician. She offers, in agreement with others, such as Epstein (2003a & 2003b), Chung (1990), and Twemlow (2001), statements suggesting that training in mindfulness can lead to a higher state of awareness and attunement to both the self and other such that it enhances the therapeutic process and client care. Although she does not describe how individuals should be trained, she offers suggestions on what she believes are important elements of such training. Her suggestions include involving the student in in-depth-oriented relational psychotherapy, formal practice in mindfulness-based meditation, an emphasis on instructors being mindfully engaged with their students, and to have a "seasoned" mindfulness meditation practitioner included in the school's faculty.

Twemlow (2001) provides another look into how the cultivation of mindfulness in the psychotherapist can help increase compassion, working in the here-and-now of the psychotherapy moment, and in strengthening therapeutic attention. He believes that Zen training for the therapist can help to fine-tune attention and thus strengthen the impact that the therapist has on the session.

Epstein (2003a) states that "mindfulness is a purposeful, nonanxious, reflective presence that can be applied to any aspect of practice" (p. 1). He believes that in the practice of medicine or psychology, mindfulness in the practitioner leads to a greater quality of client care. He defines what he calls four "habits of mindfulness" that can be taught to practitioners. These habits include "attentive observation" of oneself, "critical curiosity," "beginner's mind," and "presence" (Epstein, 2003a, p. 7). Attentive observation is defined as "observation of oneself to be aware of one's own filtering of perceptions" (p. 7). The habit of observing oneself allows examination of and adjustment to one's own perspectives and biases. Critical curiosity is defined as "tolerating awareness of one's own areas of incompetence, and inviting doubt" (p. 7). Beginner's mind is defined as "an ability to see a situation freshly, with a willingness to set aside categories that had previously been created" (p. 7). Presence is defined by "a connection between the knower and the known, undistracted attention on the task and the person, and compassion based on insight rather than sympathy" (p. 7). Epstein (2003a) believes that these qualities of mindfulness can not only help to cultivate more effective clinicians, but also to deepen their satisfaction with clinical practice.

Epstein (2003b) outlines what he terms an "8-fold teaching method" for teaching the four habits of mindfulness. These methods include "priming," "availability," "asking reflective questions," "active engagement," "modeling while thinking out loud," "practice," and "praxis."

Priming refers to the direct questions of what students observe in themselves before they engage in client interaction. Availability is having space set aside to practice mindfulness or to reflect on the moment. Asking reflective questions refers to the teacher's engagement with the student in asking questions that invite ambiguity or doubt. This is not to shake the student's confidence, but rather to allow him or her to create room for other possibilities. Active engagement involves the instructor's presence, physically and mentally, to participate in and to observe the student's actions. Modeling emphasizes the need for instructors to verbally go through their processes in front of students to actively show students how to formulate and reformulate hypotheses about treatment. Practice refers to the ongoing process of being mindful and to the neverending need to involve oneself in it. And finally, praxis is the learned ability to put one's knowledge into practice, or to apply the learned information in a clinical situation.

S. L. Shapiro et al. (2005) investigated the claims of previous authors by conducting an empirical study to determine the benefits of mindfulness-based practice for health care professionals. They determined through this study that an 8-week mindfulness-based stress reduction program based on Kabat-Zinn's MBSR (1982) was an effective prevention tool for burnout in health care professionals, as well as a means for improving client care.

GAINING COMPETENCY

Segal et al. (2002), Kabat-Zinn (2003a), and Williams et al. (2007) all emphasize the importance of individual practice for the practitioner. Segal et al. (2002) cite anecdotal data that Mindfulness-Based Cognitive Therapy for Depression was ineffective in affecting desired results when his team did not incorporate personal practice into their daily lives. However, once those clinicians began to practice and experience what mindfulness had to offer, the program began to work with clients as well.

To what may we attribute this change in effectiveness? The MBCT program was reported to be essentially the same, other than the personal practice of those involved in delivery. Mindfulness is, by nature, an exercise and ultimately an experience in awareness rather than an academically learned technique. By engaging in the very practice that is asked of clients, the clinician is learning to cultivate his or her own moment-to-moment awareness. The same pitfalls, blocks, advances, and insights that the clinician will experience allow him or her to more fully engage in coaching clients in practicing those skills. This may be likened to the psychoanalyst participating in his or her own analysis to gain insight into personal dynamics that facilitate his or her own ability to deliver an analysis to others. True, academic knowledge may assist in guiding one to the experience (hence this contribution), but it is important to participate in both and to not mistake the acquisition of read information for the experience itself. These authors, in agreement with previous authors (Segal et al., 2002; Kabat-Zinn, 2003a), suggest a personal practice for clinicians to gain competency in mindfulness-based practice.

When one talks about the need for "competency" in mindfulness, it is important for the clinician to distinguish this from the idea of "doing meditation right." A common mistake of beginning meditation students is to ascribe a value to how they are doing the meditation. One ascribes the description of a "good meditation session" because it was experienced as pleasant, or a "bad meditation session" because of discomfort or distraction. Goldstein (2003) writes that one should not place value on meditation based on the measure of pain or pleasure present in that time, but rather to let go of the value and accept things as what they are for the present moment with the understanding that that too will pass. In this spirit, the "competency" of practice is for the clinician to practice for the acquisition of recognizing the clinician's own experience of mindfulness. This facilitates understanding of the process that we ask our clients to engage in throughout treatment. Additionally, establishing this habit of mindfulness as a clinician, we offer ourselves the ability to track our reactions in thoughts, feelings, and actions that engage us in true experiential knowledge of the challenges and insights that may arise in the client we are instructing. In essence, there is no "right way" to becoming competent in the practice, which may seem contradictory to the outlined purpose of this contribution. The suggestions are, simply put, just the suggestions and guidance of learning principles, based on the experience of the cited theoreticians, practitioners, clinicians and authors of this contribution. Of course, when engaging in any new method of clinical intervention, it is best to seek supervision or consultation from an experienced clinician.

There are many ways in which a clinician may begin to gain knowledge and competency of practice, which include activities such as attending continuing education workshops offered in MBSR, MBCT, and DBT; reading more about the application of mindfulness-based practice in clinical settings in primary texts including those provided in this contribution's resource list; and to initiate practice on one's own. In general, there are significant advantages to completing workshops under the direction of a qualified teacher. This allows one to benefit from the experience of individuals who are familiar with mindfulness instruction and can help to avoid more of the common frustrations with beginning meditation practice. The difficulty for many individuals in attending workshops is often the cost in both time and money that often accompanies the trip. For this reason, engaging in personal practice and study with primary resources is often the most accessible way for clinicians to begin to familiarize themselves with the practice of mindfulness. As it is natural in the course of practice to become frustrated and to have questions along with insights and positive experiences, it is recommended that persons who practice have one or a group of others who also wish to explore the practice. In this way, each person in the group may support each other in their experiences and can discuss insights and applications in a supportive atmosphere. This contribution offers some suggestions for beginning practice in the form of suggested meditations that follow the conclusion (pp. 144-145), and recommends further reading for those who are interested in investigating the topic in more detail.

Although the purpose of this contribution is to familiarize the clinician with the literature base and rationale for the clinical application of mindfulness as well as the beginning stages of the clinician's becoming familiar with competency, the following case examples are provided to illustrate how principles of mindfulness may be introduced into individual treatment with clients, and the benefit of such interventions.

Clinical Case Example #1

Suzie Q* is a 57-year-old divorced white female who was seeking treatment in a community mental health center. Before beginning treatment with this therapist, she had worked with two other counselors over the duration of the previous year. Ms. Q reported symptoms associated with criteria for Posttraumatic Stress Disorder (PTSD) and of a Major Depressive Disorder. She reported having been witness to a family member's suicide and has since experienced her problems. She complained of sleep disturbances, hallmarked by repetitive nightmares, excessive thinking about the incident, heightened physiological arousal, feelings of responsibility and guilt, excessive crying, chronic and intense feelings of sadness, and a sense of hopelessness about the future which resulted in her believing that the only solution was suicide for herself. Ms. Q further reported having chronic health problems which included respiratory problems due to chronic smoking, which reportedly worsened in times of stress, and chronic pain in her back which necessitated the use of a cane.

---

*Names and characteristics in all case examples have been changed to protect privacy.

Ms. Q's previous therapists utilized a Cognitive Behavioral Therapy treatment approach and utilized symptom monitoring, relaxation training, thought stopping, and cognitive restructuring techniques. Ms. Q was vocal in stating that "nothing worked" and that if this current therapist "didn't help" that her case was "hopeless" and that suicide was the only alternative left.

Using the work that was previously done with Ms. Q, it was suggested that she continue to utilize her skills of symptom monitoring but to "tweak it" toward a different goal. Ms. Q was coached on the concepts of acceptance and nonjudgment, and was taught and led in a guided meditation on following her breath and following distractions in thought and awareness. She was given homework to utilize her skills of self-monitoring to simply be aware of thoughts that arise without judging them as "good or bad." Rather than attempting to push against, block, or stop those thoughts that she identified as negative, she was instructed to pay attention to them and to then gently redirect herself to her current activity and in being present with what she was doing. Ms. Q was instructed on the process of the "Body Scan" (Kabat-Zinn, 1990, pp. 92-93) and was given homework to participate in this at least two times per week. The body scan is a practice in which the participant systematically investigates each area of the body for physical sensations. This aims to help teach physiological awareness in the individual.

Over the course of 5 weeks, Ms. Q reported a decrease in the amount of time spent ruminating over the traumatic event, more time doing the things she enjoyed, an increase in her ability to concentrate, an increase in remembering positive memories of her loved one, a decrease in depressive feelings and suicidal ideation, and an increase in restful sleep. Ms. Q identified the most salient change element to be the acceptance of troubling thoughts and feelings and her ability to choose to engage in those thoughts or not in a nonjudging way. Although it was not a direct goal of Ms. Q's treatment plan, she further reported that the use of the body scan added a secondary benefit of being able to better identify the location of her pain and to relax into that pain, resulting in greater mobility and less experience of intense pain.

Clinical Case Example #2

John D. was a 43-year-old Caucasian male who came in to a community mental health center asking to see the on-call crisis therapist. His wife accompanied him into the session. He complained of severe anxiety. The client reported a history of panic attacks and was currently taking Alprazolam. A recent medical exam revealed no known physiological cause for the anxiety. The client reported that he drank two or three pots of coffee per day.

After taking a history of the presenting problem, the therapist noted out loud the client's breathing rate of approximately 40 breaths per minute (12-20 is considered normal). The client was asked to consciously slow his breathing rate and to breathe deeply from the diaphragm. This appeared to slightly reduce the client's anxiety level almost immediately.

The client was then asked if he felt comfortable participating in a breathing exercise. The client was asked to sit up straight in his chair and shade or close his eyes. He was asked to observe his breathing, noting the sensations produced by the inhalations and the exhalations. He was then asked to monitor the physical sensations and feelings in his body, and where these feelings were located. He was asked to simply watch these feelings rise and fall, trying not to control or alter the feelings. The client's wife also participated in the exercise.

The client was given psychoeducational information about the nature of panic, including the vicious cycle of anticipatory anxiety creating increased panic. He was instructed to learn to monitor the physical sensations of anxiety and to recognize that the sensations will pass. He was also told to monitor his caffeine intake and to follow up with his physician.

A 1-week follow-up revealed that the client's anxiety levels were significantly reduced. Though he still reported occasional panic attacks, the frequency and intensity of the attacks were reduced.

The previous case example illustrates that mindfulness need not be a specific technique that resembles formal meditation practice. The simple act of becoming more mindful of one's breathing, physical sensations, feelings, and thought content can significantly impact distressing symptoms.

CONCLUSION

It is the authors' hope that this contribution has provided an informative introduction to mindfulness-based practice and its clinical application. Although the authors attempted to provide a broad look at the background of this approach, this contribution should by no means be considered a complete information source for the topic but rather as a starting place for clinicians who are unfamiliar with the topic. The discussion regarding how to incorporate the lessons of mindfulness into a competency of the clinician is considered by the authors to be an area of future growth in the field. This, in conjunction with the brief case examples, is presented to inspire and interest readers into gaining further knowledge and training in the topic and thus sparking more individuals to benefit from the exciting and wonderful moments of mindful practice.

Instructions on Walking Meditation

Start by standing in a neutral body posture and focus your awareness on your breath. Allow your breath to rise and fall naturally. When you are aware of your breathing, begin to walk, taking only one step with each inhalation and exhalation. Allow your steps to be determined by your breath. If you have a longer breath, do not shorten it, but rather wait for the next step. As you are doing this exercise you may develop a series of statements to yourself, called a *mantra*. One example is as follows.

Breathing in, I take a step.
Breathing out, I take a step.
With each step I feel refreshed.
I am aware of myself in the moment.

Do this walking exercise for 10 to 20 minutes.

Instructions on Eating Meditation

Sit down at a meal or a snack and allow yourself a moment to be mindful of the activity in its entirety. First, be aware of the way your food looks. What are the colors? What are the visual textures and the arrangement of the food? Be aware of how your food smells. Does it smell fragrant? Is it pungent? Is it neutral in its smell? As you sit, prepare to take a bite of your food by being aware of the motion of your body bringing the food from its dish to your mouth. When the bite is in your mouth notice the flavor as it first hits your tongue. Notice the textures of the food. Chew your food with intention and with attention. Resist the urge to swallow the food until it is completely chewed. If you notice yourself focusing on the next bite of food, simply be aware of it and focus back to the current bite. Only after it is completely chewed and swallowed will you take the next. Do this for the remainder of your meal or snack and deeply ENJOY the nourishment it is giving your body.

Single Pointed Meditation – Concentration and Attention

For this exercise find a point of focus such as a light or candle in a dark room, a picture, or other object. Start by focusing on your breath. When you are centered in your breath, shift your focus to the object or light. Study that object. What shapes are there, what colors are manifesting? Watch the flame flicker; notice the wick in the center of the flame. If your attention wanders to noises or objects outside of the intended object simply acknowledge that your awareness was averted and shift it back to your intended focus.

Note: For a guided meditation, the facilitator may induce distracters by making loud clapping noises, ringing a bell, or making distracting motions. This allows for the student to develop sustained attention even in the most chaotic situation.

Meditation on
Person as a Healer

INSTRUCTION	PURPOSE
1. Breathing in, know that you Are breathing in. Breathing out, know that you Are breathing out.	Awareness of breath
2. Breathing in, know that you Are strong. Breathing out, know that you Can help others.	Strength/compassion
3. Breathing in, be mindful of The pain that is present in Others in the world. Breathing out, know that Pain can be alleviated through Compassion.	Awareness of suffering/ Awareness of compassion
4. Breathing in, be mindful of the Pain within our self. Breathing out, smile at our pain Knowing that it is transitory pain.	Awareness of the nature of pain

Guided Meditation for
Awareness of Thoughts

INSTRUCTION	PURPOSE
1. Breathing in, I know that I am breathing in. Breathing out, I know that I am breathing out.	Mindfulness of breath
2. Breathing in, I allow my Thoughts to come into awareness. Breathing out, I allow those Thoughts to occupy my attention.	Mindfulness of thought
3. Breathing in, I experience my thought Without judgment. Breathing out, I allow my current Thoughts to calm.	Nonjudging/letting go
4. Breathing in, I am aware of the Moment. Breathing out, I know that it is A wonderful moment.	Awareness of present

CONTRIBUTORS

Robert B. Denton, PsyD, is a Postdoctoral Fellow at the Wright State University School of Professional Psychology. He received his Doctorate in Clinical Psychology from Wright State University in Dayton, Ohio. Dr. Denton currently works at a Community Mental Health Center in Dayton, Ohio and has worked with both the children and adult populations. Dr. Denton has involved himself in the study of Eastern philosophy traditions for the past 9 years and has traveled to various monastic establishments, including those within the Tibetan Buddhist tradition and the Zen tradition of Thich Nhat Hanh and Soto Zen traditions, to gain further insights and teachings. Dr. Denton also trains in the martial art of Ninjutsu under the direction of Stephen K. Hayes. He has three beautiful children, who teach him more about life each day. Dr. Denton may be contacted at E-mail: robert.denton@wright.edu

Richard W. Sears, PsyD, MBA, is a core faculty member of the PsyD Program in Clinical Psychology at Union Institute & University. He received his Master of Business Administration degree and Doctorate in Clinical Psychology from Wright State University in Dayton, Ohio. Dr. Sears is a licensed psychologist in the state of Ohio, where he runs a private psychology practice. He is lead author of the book *Consultation Skills for Mental Health Professionals*. Dr. Sears is also a fourth degree black belt in Ninjutsu, and once served as a personal protection agent for the Dalai Lama of Tibet with his martial arts teacher, Stephen Hayes. He has studied the Eastern Wisdom traditions extensively. Dr. Sears may be contacted at 440 E. McMillan Street, Cincinnati, OH 45206. E-mail: richard.sears@tui.edu   Website: www.psych-insights.com

RESOURCES

Alexander, N. L. (1997). Balancing theory with presence: The importance of cultivating mindfulness in the psychotherapist. *Dissertation Abstracts International: Section B: The Sciences & Engineering, 58,* 6B (UMI No. 9735645).

Astin, J. A. (1997). Stress reduction through mindfulness meditation: Effects on psychological symptomatology, sense of control, and spiritual experiences. *Psychotherapy and Psychosomatics, 66,* 97-106.

Atwood, J. D., & Maltin, L. (1991). Putting eastern philosophies into western psychotherapies. *American Journal of Psychotherapy, XLV*(3), 368-382.

Austin, J. H. (1998). *Zen and the Brain.* Cambridge, MA: The MIT Press.

Austin, J. H. (2006). *Zen-Brain Reflections: Reviewing Recent Developments in Meditation and States of Consciousness.* Cambridge, MA: MIT Press.

Bien, T. (2006). *Mindful Therapy: A Guide for Therapists and Helping Professionals.* Boston: Wisdom Publications.

Block-Lerner, J., Adair, C., Plumb, J. C., Rhatigan, D., & Orsillo, S. (2007). The case for mindfulness-based approaches in the cultivation of empathy: Does nonjudgemental, present-moment awareness increase capacity for perspective-taking and empathic concern? *Journal of Marital & Family Therapy, 33*(4), 501-516.

Bohart, A. C., Elliott, R., Greenberg, L. S., & Watson, J. C., (2002). Empathy. In J. C. Norcross (Ed.), *Psychotherapy Relationships That Work: Therapist Contributions and Responsiveness to Clients* (pp. 89-108). New York: Oxford University Press.

Brown, D. (1993). The path of meditation: Affective development and psychological well-being. In S. L. Ablon, D. Brown, E. J. Khantzian, & J. E. Mack (Eds.), *Human Feelings: Explorations in Affect Development and Meaning.* Hillsdale, NJ: Analytic Press.

Brown, D. P., & Engler, J. (1980). The stages of mindfulness meditation: A validation study. *Journal of Transpersonal Psychology, 12,* 143-192.

Chung, C. (1990). Psychotherapist and expansion of awareness. *Psychotherapy and Psychosomatics, 53,* 28-32.

Davidson, R., Goleman, D., & Schwartz, G. (1976). Attentional and affective concomitants of meditation: A cross sectional study. *Journal of Abnormal Psychology, 85,* 235-238.

Epstein, R. M. (1984). On the neglect of evenly suspended attention. *Journal of Transpersonal Psychology, 16*(2), 193-205.

Epstein, R. M. (1990). Psychodynamics of meditation: Pitfalls on the spiritual path. *The Journal of Transpersonal Psychology, 22*(1), 17-34.

Epstein, R. M. (1995). *Thoughts Without Thinker.* New York: Basic Books.

Epstein, R. M. (1998). *Going to Pieces Without Falling Apart: A Buddhist Perspective on Wholeness: Lessons From Meditation and Psychotherapy.* New York: Broadway Books.

Epstein, R. M. (1999) Mindful practice. *Journal of the American Medical Association, 282,* 833-839.

Epstein, R. M. (2003a). Mindful practice in action (I): Technical competence, evidence-based medicine, and relationship centered care. *Families, Systems & Health, 21*(1), 1-9.

Epstein, R. M. (2003b). Mindful practice in action (II): Cultivating habits of mind. *Families, Systems & Health, 21*(1), 11-17.

Follette, V. M., Palm, K. M., & Rasmussen Hall, M. L. (2004). Acceptance, mindfulness, and trauma. In S. Hayes, V. Follette, & M. Linehan (Eds.), *Mindfulness and Acceptance.* New York: Guilford.

Fulton, P. R. (2005). Mindfulness as clinical training. In C. K. Germer, R. D. Siegel, & P. R. Fulton (Eds.), *Mindfulness and Psychotherapy* (pp. 55-72). New York: Guilford.

Gendlin, E. (1978). *Focusing*. New York: Bantam Books.

Gendlin, E. (1996). *Focus-Oriented Psychotherapy: A Manual of the Experiential Method*. New York: Guilford.

Gillani, N. B., & Smith, J. C. (2001). Zen meditation and abc relaxation theory: An exploration of relaxation states, beliefs, dispositions, and motivations. *Journal of Clinical Psychology, 57*(6), 839-846.

Goldman, B. L., Dormitor, P. J., & Murray, E. J. (1979). Effects of Zen meditation on anxiety reduction and perceptual functioning. *Journal of Consulting and Clinical Psychology, 47*, 551-556.

Goldstein, J. (2003). *Insight Meditation: The Practice of Freedom*. Boston: Shambhala Publications.

Goleman, D. (1977). *The Varieties of Meditative Experience*. New York: Irvington.

Goleman, D. (1988). *The Meditative Mind: Varieties of Meditative Experience*. New York: Putnam.

Hanh, T. N. (1990). *Transformation & Healing: Sutra on the Four Establishments of Mindfulness*. Berkley, CA: Parallax Press.

Hayes, S. C., Strosahl, K. D., & Wilson, K. G. (1999). *Acceptance and Commitment Therapy: An Experiential Approach to Behavior Change*. New York: Guilford.

Hubble, M. A., Duncan, B. L., & Miller, S. D. (1999). *The Heart and Soul of Change: What Works in Therapy*. Washington, DC: American Psychological Association.

Kabat-Zinn, J. (1982). An outclient program in behavioral medicine for chronic pain clients based on the practice of mindfulness meditation: Theoretical considerations and preliminary results. *General Hospital Psychiatry, 4*, 33-47.

Kabat-Zinn, J. (1990). *Full Catastrophe Living: Using the Wisdom of your Body and Mind to Face Stress, Pain, and Illness*. New York: Dell.

Kabat-Zinn, J. (1994). *Wherever You Go There You Are*. New York: Hyperion.

Kabat-Zinn, J. (2003a). Mindfulness-based interventions in context: Past, present, and future. *Clinical Psychology: Science and Practice, 10*(2), 144-156.

Kabat-Zinn, J. (2003b). Mindfulness-based stress reduction (MBSR). *Constructivism in the Human Sciences, 8*(2), 73-107.

Kabat-Zinn, J., Massion, A. O., Kristeller, J., Peterson, L. G., Fletcher, K. E., Pbert, L., Lenderking, W. R., & Santorelli, S. (1992). Effectiveness of a meditation based stress reduction program in the treatment of anxiety disorders. *American Journal of Psychiatry, 149*, 936-943.

Keown, D. (2003). *Dictionary of Buddhism*. New York: Oxford University Press.

Lambert, M. J. (1992). Implications of outcome research for psychotherapy integration. In J. C. Norcross & M. R. Goldstein (Eds.), *Handbook of Psychotherapy Integration* (pp. 94-129). New York: BasicBooks.

Lesh, T. V. (1970). Zen meditation and the development of empathy in counselors. *Journal of Humanistic Psychology, 10*, 39-74.

Linehan, M. M. (1993). *Cognitive-Behavioral Therapy for Borderline Personality Disorder*. New York: Guilford.

Linehan, M. M., & Kehrer, C. A. (1992). Borderline personality disorder. In D. Barlow (Ed.), *Clinical Handbook of Psychological Disorders* (pp. 396-441). New York: Plenum.

Miller, J. J., Fletcher, K., & Kabat-Zinn, J. (1995). Three-year follow-up and clinical implications of a mindfulness meditation-based stress reduction intervention in the treatment of anxiety disorders. *General Hospital Psychiatry, 17*, 192-200.

Norcross, J. C. (2002). *Psychotherapy Relationships That Work: Therapist Contributions and Responsiveness to Clients*. New York: Oxford University Press.

Rao, K. R. (1989). Meditation: Secular and sacred. A review and assessment of some recent research. *Journal of the Indian Academy of Applied Psychology. 15*, 51-74.

Rogers, C. R. (1961). *On Becoming a Person*. Boston: Houghton Mifflin.

Schuster, R. (1979). Empathy and mindfulness. *Journal of Humanistic Psychology, 19*(1), 71-77.

Segal, Z. V., Williams, J. M. G., & Teasdale, J. D. (2002). *Mindfulness-Based Cognitive Therapy for Depression: A New Approach to Preventing Relapse*. New York: Guilford.

Sethi, A. S. (1989). *Meditation as an Intervention in Stress Reactivity*. New York: AMS Press.

Shapiro, D. H. (1992). A preliminary study of long-term mediators: Goals, effects, religious orientation, cognitions. *Journal of Transpersonal Psychology, 24*, 23-39.

Shapiro, S. L., Astin, J. A., Bishop, S. R., & Cordova, M. (2005). Mindfulness-based stress reduction for health care professionals: Results from a randomized trial. *International Journal of Stress Management, 12*(2), 164-176.

Shapiro, S. L., Schwartz, G. E., & Bonner, G. (1998). Effects of mindfulness-based stress reduction on medical and premedical students. *Journal of Behavioral Medicine, 21*(6), 581-599.

Sneed, J. R., Balestri, M., & Belfi, B. J. (2003). The use of dialectical behavior therapy strategies in the psychiatric emergency room. *Psychotherapy: Theory, Research, Practice, Training, 40*(4), 265-277.

Soma, B., & Pereira, C. A. (2004). *The Way of Mindfulness: The Satipatthana Sutta 1949*. Whitefish, MT: Kessinger Publishing.

Stern, D. N. (1985). *The Interpersonal World of the Infant: A View From Psychoanalysis & Developmental Psychology*. New York: Basic Books.

Suzuki, S. (1970). *Zen Mind, Beginner's Mind*. New York: Weatherhill.

Tart, C. (1990). Extending mindfulness to everyday life. *Journal of Humanistic Psychology, 30*(1), 81-106.

Thompson, R. F. (2000). Zazen and psychotherapeutic presence. *American Journal of Psychotherapy, 54*(4), 531-547.

Tloczynski, J., & Tantriella, M. (1998). A comparison of the effects of Zen breath meditation or relaxation on college adjustment. *Psychologia: An International Journal of Psychology in the Orient, 41*(1), 32-43.

Twemlow, S. W. (2001). Training psychotherapists in attributes of "mind" from zen and psychoanalytic perspectives, part I: Core principles, emptiness, impermanence, and paradox. *American Journal of Psychotherapy, 55*(1), 1-39.

Valentine, E. R., & Sweet, P. L. G. (1999). Meditation and attention: A comparison of the effects of concentrative and mindfulness meditation on sustained attention. *Mental Health, Religion & Culture, 2*(1), 59-70.

Walsh, R. N., Goleman, D., Kornfield, J., Pensa, C., & Shapiro, D. (1978). Meditation: Aspects of research and practice. *The Journal of Transpersonal Psychology, 10*(2), 113-133.

Williams, M., Teasdale, J., Segal, Z., & Kabat-Zinn, J. (2007). *The Mindful Way Through Depression: Freeing Yourself From Chronic Unhappiness.* New York: Guilford.

Yalom, I. D. (2002). *The Gift of Therapy.* New York: HarperCollins.

Communications Training In Clinical Practice

Dennis E. O'Grady

Communication problems are at the heart of many challenges in life. The success or failure of your work and personal relationships depends upon how effectively positive communication skills are utilized as negative feelings and thoughts are shed. The *Talk to Me©* system (O'Grady, 2005) defines and teaches about two different styles of communicators – Empathizers and Instigators. Empathizers (E-types) and Instigators (I-types) think and speak differently when communicating with themselves and others. Because most people do not know about these differences, people assume that everyone else thinks and communicates as they do. Utilizing a format that likens communication to driving a car, *Talk to Me©* provides the understanding and insight needed to move beyond assumptions and begin communicating effectively in every dialogue in any situation.

WHY CAN'T WE ALL JUST GET ALONG?

It all boils down to communication skills. Everyone says so, everyone knows so. People listen to what they want to hear, and they hear it how they want to hear it. But the question is: How do you know the right strategy for getting talk partners to hear you – and work with you? After much research, we now know that when you're in conflict with a fellow communicator, chances are that person is your opposite communicator type – walking, talking, thinking, feeling, and problem solving entirely opposite from the way you do! Because we are often ignorant of communicator types, we end up blaming our fellow talk companion for the communication snafu and chaos AND lack of positive change results. Then our communicator car spins out of control, and we end up in the ditch, sputtering and needing a tow truck to rescue us.

Look Who's Talking!

The *Talk to Me©* system clearly demonstrates how *Empathizer* (E-types) and *Instigator-type* (I-types) communicators are opposites in their talk preferences. This is a radical departure from previously taught viewpoints that gender, gender role expectations, or personality style are solely in the driver's seat of communication. When you know your talk type and the talk type of your co-communicator, it is likely that you will figure out not only how to correct what's been going wrong, but also how to make small changes in the way you communicate, resulting in enhanced benefits for everyone. To date, my studies have involved over 470 of my clients who have achieved effective personal results by using the *Talk to Me©* system. The business version of the system has been implemented at such companies as Motoman, Inc.

(robotics), Dayton Freight Lines (shipping), and Morris South (machining industry), with impressive results, from top administration through the ranks of all employees.

Many of the communication clients with whom I work put it this way: "The light bulb came on for me after learning about my type and how my opposite type walks in different shoes. Now I have options that open new avenues of communication instead of closing them off."

CASE EXAMPLE #1: ARE GIVING COMPLIMENTS A SIGN OF WEAKNESS?

Do you most often dispense compliments freely or keep them to yourself? When you give compliments, what is your communication style? Do you feel that giving compliments is a sign of weakness, a form of manipulation, or both? Do you believe that people should just do what's right without expecting accolades? These are some of the thorny issues we brush against as we hike through the deep woods of interpersonal relationships. I love the e-mail I received from a male college student, who asked why compliments given to a female friend seemed to fall on deaf ears.

I Just Don't Understand Where the Issue Is

Here's what this young man wrote and how I helped explain that compliments are experienced very differently by *Empathizer* and by *Instigator* communicators. It's nothing personal . . . or peculiar!

Hi, Dr. O'Grady,

I sit here in the library, taking a break from studying for my first exam of the semester. The real reason that I thought to write to you is because of my female friend, Jill. It is a new milestone for me to have a really good friend, who happens to be a girl, and who is not my girlfriend. We talk so much that her roommate calls me her husband and refers to her as my wife! What perplexes me is that I have complimented her twice and neither time did I receive the response I had expected. I told her that I thought she was amazing, and that I really respected her. For me to say those things is extremely big, because I don't just go around giving out compliments. I give them when I really mean them, which is why I was kind of surprised and hurt by her response . . . or lack of response, actually. She didn't even acknowledge that I had just paid her a significant compliment. She just ignored it. When I kept pushing for a response, she said, "O.K. let's just forget about the whole thing. I think you're awesome, too."

I just don't understand where the issue is. I don't know if we just have different ways of accepting and responding to compliments, or what. Could it be that she is not recognizing that I am paying such a significant compliment or caring sentiment to her?

Please let me know what you think about the situation with Jill.

Thanks.

*Jack**

---

*Names in all examples have been changed to protect privacy.

The Instigator Viewpoint
On the Art of Compliments

Hi Jack,

I wanted to make sure I had time to digest your e-mail, so I waited until this morning to respond to you. I hope that is O.K. I am always glad to hear from you. I'll sound a little like your communications coach, which I am. Let me address your question, "Could it be that she is not recognizing that I am paying such a significant compliment or caring sentiment to her?"

Compliments are experienced very differently by Empathizer *(E-type) and* Instigator *(I-type) communicators. For comparison, remember that you and your mom are E-types, while your dad is an I-type. I should look like both E- and I-types since I've been working hard to adopt the strengths of my opposing communicator style. Jill sounds like an Instigator communicator, given her behavior. Her style isn't better or worse than yours; just different. Here are researched differences explained:*

I-types

1. *consider giving compliments unnecessary.*
2. *think needing compliments is a weakness.*
3. *try to put misunderstandings in the past by "forgetting about them."*
4. *don't like to feel vulnerable or to rely on others for help.*
5. *believe they can put a strong mind over difficult relationship matters.*
6. *are afraid that emotions will spin their communicator car out of control.*
7. *want to send all E-types to "Empathizer Island" when frustration mounts.*
8. *value Empathizers' ability to be true to their emotions.*
9. *love to solve problems.*
10. *are natural-born leaders.*

It's not a boy-girl thing, Jack. You are comfortable with nonmanipulative compliments. Your style is right on! I hope this helps clear up any confusing communication matters for you on this beautiful fall weekend, Jack! Thanks for talking with me. . . .

Communication Cliff Notes:
Compliments Are Experienced
Very Differently By Empathizer
And By Instigator Communicators

Empathizers freely give authentic praise, and they function best when their good works are recognized in words of genuine praise. *Instigators* believe that actions speak louder than words, and they function best when their genuine words are recognized in good works accomplished. So, it's not that women praise more than men, or that men praise to get their way; it's all about the communicator shoes in which you feel more comfortable. Can you tell the difference between the two communicators' types in the example above? Each type perceives the giving and receiving of positive feedback very differently.

WHAT TYPE ARE YOU?

Are You a Tuned-In Empathizer Communicator . . .

For now, let's typecast you on the fly.

1. Are your feelings easily hurt?
2. When you're in the driver's seat, is your mood affecting your output?
3. Do you back off or skim over important issues, so as not to create hard feelings?
4. Have you been told you are too "thin-skinned"?
5. Are you too good for your own good?
6. Do you feel you have trouble getting past the past?
7. Are you surprised when coworkers or family members can't "see the obvious"?

If you answered most of these questions "Yes," then chances are you are an E-type communicator. *Your viewpoint:* You have a bone to pick with I-types, who, from your vantage point, are too insensitive and coldly logical. This is a very important finding, because you can now begin to "adjust your driving style" to get better results with everyone in your communication circle – particularly those strong-willed I-types. You'll be able to tell the type of your cocommunicator – that person with whom you're talking at the time – with a few minutes of practice each day.

. . . Or a Get-Down-to-Business Instigator Communicator?

I'm frequently approached by trainees who say, "Well, I think I might be a mixture of both types, since I have traits of both types of communicators, Empathizer *and* Instigator. I don't like to be put into a box or labeled if there's a question about where I should be. Can't I be a combination of both types?" No, you can't. You can't walk on both sides of Talk Street at the same time. In fact, if you've been running this line of reasoning in your head, then chances are you're an Instigator communicator. But let's check to be sure . . .

1. Are your feelings difficult to hurt, because you believe, "It's nothing personal!"?
2. Are you able to put your mind over your mood?
3. Can you be impatient or get mad a little too easily?
4. Can you be pushy, or "over talk" and intimidating with your debating skills?
5. Have you been known to set the tone or mood in a family or work team?
6. When you're on a mission, can you be like a bull in a china shop?
7. Are you surprised when coworkers or family members don't read or use the map in front of their noses, to get from here to there?

If you answered most of these questions "Yes," then chances are you're an Instigator-type communicator who loves to fix problems and get things done. *Your viewpoint:* You have a bone to pick with E-types, who you think are too sensitive and emotional. Now, I'm not saying your heart is as cold as stone. I'm just saying you trust your head over your heart, and you put your faith in logic. This is a very important finding because you can begin now to "adjust your driving style" to get better results with each of your talk partners – particularly those brainstorming E-types.

The Communicator Prejudices on page 168 is a handy reference to see what your opposite talk type thinks and feels about your talk talk.

Test Your Typecasting Skills: Alpha Moms' Communication Style

Excellence in motherhood has again hit the newsstands! Have you heard of "Alpha Moms," the new breed of multitasking trendsetters who are kid-centric and who feel most relaxed while juggling lots of balls? Did you know that leading companies, such as Procter and Gamble, and big marketers alike are wagging their tails and drooling over them? Stay down now! "Alpha Moms" is the newest moniker created by Constance Van Flandern (Horovitz, 2007).

Alpha Moms – Instigators of Change?

Alpha Moms are instigators of change. But did you know that most Alpha Moms are also Instigator-type (I-type) communicators? Consider these comparisons:

1. *Multitasking experts.* An Alpha Mom is happiest multitasking. Instigator communicators like to save precious time to accomplish more, like talking on the phone while working on the computer.

   Downside: Alpha Mom I-types are less comfortable asking for help when they run into a problem that can't easily be solved.

2. *Progress-centric.* An Alpha Mom is kid-centric and hands-on, whether or not she works outside the home. Instigator communicators are progress-centered, love to solve problems, and embrace change as a way of life.

   Downside: Alpha Mom I-types can become very impatient and frustrated when their plans don't materialize fast enough.

3. *Tech-savvy happy.* An Alpha Mom enjoys finding out how new techno-gadgets work, because she is power-centered and loves to command the center of attention. Instigator communicators are perceived as strong personality types by family and associates.

   Downside: Alpha Mom I-types don't do well with boredom and can be neglectful of their romantic partners' needs.

4. *Enjoys debating and winning.* An Alpha Mom talks confidently and easily wins debates, taking pride in being the first to achieve a goal. Instigator communicators are world-class debaters and exceptionally strong-willed souls. They live by the rule: "If you aren't going to lead, then get out of my way!"

   Downside: Alpha Mom I-types are criticized for being too stubborn and covering up their insecurities while going after points to prove their self-worth, at the expense of a relationship.

5. *Influencers.* An Alpha Mom is an initiator and creator of social opinion, of what's popular or what is ditzy. Instigator communicators believe in making listeners quickly come around to their viewpoint.

   Downside: Alpha Mom I-types are criticized for listening with only half an ear and for not including the opinions of the quiet, meek, and shy contributors around the Communicator Table.

6. *Confident deciders.* An Alpha Mom makes up her mind and thrives on sharing her viewpoint of what way is the right way to reach a goal or solve a problem. Instigator communicators believe there is a right way and a wrong way to drive down the two-way Communicator Highway.

   Downside: Alpha Mom I-types can be negatively perceived as one-way communicators who are control freaks, too pushy, self-centered, strategic, blunt women who loudly talk over others.

Do You Prefer to be an Instigator of Change?

Horovitz's (2007) article, "Alpha Moms leap to top of trendsetters," provides a concise thumbnail sketch of Alpha Moms. An apt quote by Alpha Mom moniker-creater Van Flandern: "I'm at my Alpha Mommy-est when I have the most balls in the air: It's multitasking to the nth degree. It's like training for the Olympics. Most of all, it's fun."

My communication leadership research has determined that most natural-born leaders of both genders are Instigator-type communicators who love to lead and dominate in their chosen fields. Last, but certainly not least, my communication studies also found that an Alpha Mom Instigator communicator is more likely to be married to a "Beta Dad," who is an Empathizer-type communicator. Opposites do seem to attract, for better and worse.

Can You Change Your Communicator Type?

Although you cannot change your communicator type, you *can* adopt the strengths of your opposite type, avoid the negative traits of your own type, and choose more effective avenues of communication, based on your situation. (See The Communication Matrix on p. 166.) Before coming into this world, you and I are wired as either an Empathizer or Instigator communicator. Of course, if we follow the nature versus nurture theory, your family of origin will support or undercut your talk type. Thus, some E-types will sound like I-types because they hail from I-type families, and vice-versa. Although the only people who are truly a blend of both types are those who consciously use the *Talk to Me©* system, even those people will return to their preferred talking style when they are distressed.

In my clinical practice and teaching experiences, I've found that a majority of psychotherapists are E-types, and that a majority of supervisors are I-types. I-types are natural-born leaders, although E-types have the solutions to vexing organizational problems. Where do you fit on the spectrum of interpersonal sensitivity? In summary, Empathizer communicators are thinner-skinned, sensitive types who are critiqued for being too sensitive . . . taking things too personally . . . dwelling on the past . . . keeping things inside for too long . . . afraid of conflict . . . lovers of genuine compliments.

Conversely, Instigator communicators are thicker-skinned, insensitive types who are critiqued for being too insensitive . . . taking the position of "It's only business. It's nothing personal" . . . moving on quickly into the future . . . putting frustrations on others . . . rising to occasions of conflict . . . lovers of genuine accomplishments.

See how quickly you can identify your type?

What are the Percentages of Each Talk Type?

How many of each talk type are there running around? Statistically, about 40% of all people are Empathizer communicators, while 60% of all people are Instigator communicators. However, I usually advise that you think: by the flip of a coin, whoever you meet could be one type or the other. Being surprised is half the fun!

You won't reach any new destinations by way of the two-way Communicator Highway if you don't first know your communicator type. You have about an even chance of being either an Empathizer-type (E-type) or an Instigator-type (I-type) communicator. Historically, we all thought that gender or personality had everything to do with talk style. Now, with the advent of the *Talk to Me©* system, we know that this is not the case! For example, you can have two clients, each with passive-aggressive personality disorder, one of whom is a female Instigator client while the other is a male Empathizer client. Communication type is separate and distinct from every other variable with which you've been trained to interact. Life's going to get very interesting from here on out!

How Can I Easily and Reliably Determine the Types of my Clients, Colleagues, Supervisors, Friends, and Kids?

An easy way that you, your friends, and your clients can determine individual communicator types is to go to the link at www.drogrady.com which asks: *What's Your Type?* You will be taken to http://www.drogrady.com/type.php, where you will complete and submit a questionnaire. A free, private e-mail report will follow. (You are the only person who gets the results of this assessment.) There is, at most, a 7% error rate with this survey. In fact, you can complete the questionnaire as someone you know, guessing at the answers which you think would be given, and receive a report that will fairly accurately predict the communicator type of that person. However, if you'd rather know your type right now, instead of waiting to complete the survey, you can reasonably determine your type simply by looking at the lists of Empathizer and Instigator traits which follow later in this contribution.

If you are interested, you can download a free sample of the *Talk to Me©* system, from the *Talk to Me: Communication Moves to Get Along With Anyone* textbook, by going to http://www.drogrady.com/ttm_optin.php. In the first chapter, you can copy the New Insights Communication Inventory (NICI) and use the results as part of your initial client assessment session.

WITH WHOM ARE YOU TALKING, AN EMPATHIZER (E-TYPE) COMMUNICATOR OR AN INSTIGATOR (I-TYPE) COMMUNICATOR?

By the end of this contribution on results-driven communication training, you will know what your communicator type is and why adopting the strengths of your opposing communicator type is so crucial to effective communication, professional leadership development, and relationship communication in personal and parenting relationships. Glance at the following overview of opposing communicator traits to get a quick mindset for the two types of drivers on the Talk Highway.

Empathizer (E-Type) Communicators:

1. Experience the self as interpersonally sensitive.
2. Drive from their strength of empathy.
3. Have difficulty getting beyond the past, because failure and rejection pierce them to their core.
4. Feel negative when they are stressed then unexpectedly act out in negative behaviors.
5. Ding their opposite communicator type (I-types) for being too stubborn and hard-headed.
6. Listen inclusively with three ears, including what's said nonverbally.
7. Can become lost in the fog of feeling down, sad, and blue – their Achilles' heel.
8. Are empathy experts who are natural-born relationship rehabilitators.
9. Struggle with low self-esteem or the-glass-is-half-empty negativism.
10. Feel deeply about the impacts of a relationship in order to make life changes.
11. Are too thin-skinned; they take things too personally and their feelings get hurt too easily.
12. Regret thinking too much before speaking; bite their tongues too often.

13. Are prone to trying to please too much or telling you what you want to hear, and then holding grudges.
14. Negatively believe, "It's always your way or the highway!" when under severe relationship distress.
15. Secretly wish to be more assertive and speak more bluntly.
16. Are natural-born team players with strong intuitive skills to use in the game of life.

What about their opposite style drivers? Are we ever on the same page of the driver's education manual? Are the rules of the road the same or different?

Instigator (I-Type) Communicators:

1. Experience the self as interpersonally insensitive.
2. Drive from their strength of genuineness.
3. Forget the past and move on, because failure and rejection roll off the backs of I-types.
4. When stressed, think negatively and then unexpectedly talk out in negative words.
5. Ding their opposite communicator type (E-types) for being too soft and wishy-washy.
6. Listen selectively with one ear, with a goal to catch only the top headlines in the Daily Talk News.
7. Can become lost in the fog of impatience, irritation, and anger (their Achilles' heel).
8. Are strategic experts who are natural-born problem solvers.
9. Suffer from excessive self-esteem or the-glass-is-half-full thinking, which optimizes the negative.
10. Think deeply about impacts of a career, in order to make life changes.
11. Are too thick-skinned; they don't take things personally enough and their feelings don't get hurt easily enough.
12. Regret speaking too much before thinking and not biting their tongues often enough.
13. Are prone to displeasing too much or telling you what you don't want to hear, then withholding compliments.
14. When under severe relationship distress, negatively feel, "You're right. It IS my way or the highway!"
15. Secretly wish to be less aggressive and speak more diplomatically.
16. Are natural-born leaders with strong personalities, to use in the game of life.

Why Adopt the Strengths of Your Opposite Communicator Type?

Neither type is better or worse, just different. The objective of the *Talk to Me©* system is to enable you to understand your own and your opposite communicator type so well that you can adopt the strengths of your opposite communicator type at the Communicator Table. Being able to see the situation through your talk partner's eyes is what makes you a flexible and responsive communicator, one who is positive and who can look like *either* type in nonmanipulative ways when the situation warrants. You will be able to match the type of the client with whom you are working, to instantly build rapport, develop trust, set goals for change, and reinforce changes in ways preferred by either type.

Is this not exciting news? Is the couple with whom you're working not seeing the viewpoint of their opposite communicator types? Is the teenager in conflict with a parent, because mom or dad drive in a different lane on Talk Highway? Does your boss or supervisor not *get* what you're saying? Are the clients with whom you struggle the most your opposite communicator type? Undoubtedly so. When you are able to address communicator type differences, travel to new talk destinations will benefit all talk partners.

CASE EXAMPLE #2: CAN YOU TAKE A LITTLE CRITICISM WITHOUT GETTING ALL TICKED OFF?

Empathizer communicators (E-types) tend to take others' criticisms too personally while they offer criticisms too slowly. Instigator communicators (I-types) tend to offer criticisms too quickly while taking criticisms too impersonally. Do you issue criticisms too slowly or too quickly?

Giving and receiving feedback to encourage change is what good therapy and good communication is all about. Many people, though, have fat ears when it comes to an oversized ego. Can you take a little criticism without getting all ticked off? Can you help a client do likewise? That depends on whether your client is a thin-skinned and self-critical Empathizer or a thick-skinned and other-critical Instigator communicator. Would you like to get a feel for the difference, and will you NOW agree with me that many helpers or psychotherapists are Empathizer-type communicators?

What are Seven Disadvantages of *Not* Knowing Your and Your Cocommunicators' Types?

Empathizer communicators feel and talk differently than their Instigator counterparts. "You can't compare apples to oranges!" gets at the distinctions and preferences of each type. Not knowing if you're an apple or an orange, or if you are working with or against your communicator style, can create disadvantages:

1. You will feel hurt for too long (E-type) . . . or hurt the feelings of others without intending to do so (I-type).
2. You will feel down and dismissed (E-type) . . . or make others feel dismissed and unimportant (I-type).
3. You will be angry at yourself (E-type) . . . or be resented and disliked by others (I-type).
4. You will shy away from being a strong leader (E-type) . . . or not garner creative teamwork (I-type).
5. You will react to problems instead of resolving problems (E- and I-type communicators).
6. You will make less money (E-type) . . . or feel more stressed by the money you do make (I-type).
7. You will feel stuck and blame yourself for feeling bad (E-type) . . . or feel stuck and blame others for your feeling mad (I-type).

> **FIRST COMMANDMENT OF GOOD COMMUNICATION:**
>
> **LEARN YOUR TALK PARTNER'S COMMUNICATION TYPE.**

CASE EXAMPLE #3: THE MILLION-DOLLAR COMMUNICATION TOOL

Would you like to own a million-dollar solution to many of the key relationship communication problems your clients bring to your doorstep each and every day? O.K. then, here it is! If your client is an Empathizer-type (E-type) communicator, he or she doesn't ever want to hurt another person's feelings and so doesn't speak up forcefully. When the courage is mustered to finally speak up, the thought of being too intense or going to extremes makes for one very uncomfortable feeling.

If There's a Communication Gap or Disconnect

Many of my assertively coached, interpersonally sensitive, Empathizer communication clients put it like this:

> *I am perceived as being wishy-washy or needing direction so often it makes me frown. I-types perceive me as asking for help when I don't need it. I have trouble saying, "This is what I need now!" or "This is what I need for you to do for me." There's a disconnect. I'm not good at stating my opinion right up front, but if I were able, life would be a lot easier.*

Can you relate? Who would ever think that being sensitive could irritate communication matters?

To get through to the thicker-skinned Instigator-type (I-type) communicators in the world, the temptation for E-types is to listen to the I-types' opinions *before* stating their own opinions or conclusions. This is ineffective at best, and very confusing to the Instigator cocommunicator, at worst.

A Million-Dollar Communication Solution

So, that's why I say in *Talk to Me©* that Empathizers need to adopt the strengths of Instigators, and the Instigators should adopt the strengths of Empathizers. Here are some black-and-white statements (more easily heard by I-types) which my newly assertive E-types use to be more direct, clear, and upfront about their outstanding opinions, which will benefit everyone involved:

1. I'm not good at stating my opinion right up front, but I feel strongly that we should . . . .
2. This is my decision.
3. This is the way it is.
4. This isn't about you.
5. Don't be confused. I'm not asking for your help.
6. I don't need suggestions or solutions to the problem.
7. I've worked out the answers that will get us down the road on this one.
8. There's no room for debate.
9. I don't appreciate your raising your voice with me or talking over me. It shuts me down.
10. I'll ask for your help if and when I need it.
11. What would it be worth to you if my way is the right way to go?
12. My Achilles heel is that before I give my opinion, I want to hear others' opinions and include input that's relevant to the problem's solution.
13. This is what I need now. I need for this to be done.

Are you an E-type who goes along to get along? Enough, already, of the humble-to-a-fault act! Don't start backing down or justifying your decision. Your decision is final and not open for negotiation. I-types will pounce on your apparent indecision every time, and they will make it about *you*, instead of the issue. I-types know about *Conversational Coercion*.

Are You Wrong To Be So Direct?

Instigator communicators respect those who take a stand and won't back down. I-types love to debate, and they are expert debaters, so unnecessary debating with an I-type will make your E-type communication foggy. You need to be a clear and direct communicator who sends the implied message, "I mean business!" After all, if you can fix a problem, why act like you aren't sure of what you're doing?

With a Little Help From Yourself

With a little practice, you and your clients will spontaneously come up with responsive (vs. knee-jerk), nondefensive communication strategies that send the message, "I know what I'm doing. This is the era of the E-type leader, and you would be wise to follow me."

CASE EXAMPLE #4: LET GO OF *CONVERSATIONAL COERCION*

Conversational coercion is strategically manipulating the outcome of a conversation to gain the upper hand, in order to get your way. For example, I may say, "You're not listening!" when in truth, you're simply not agreeing with me. That example of conversational coercion is a twisted talk trick which shows that it's going to be "my way or the highway" for you. But at what expense? A good relationship?

Instigators Are the Best Debaters

Instigators, or I-types, will be the first to tell you that the very best ideas stem from a good, fierce debate. What they *won't* tell you is that their ideas aren't always right or the best idea on the block. Truth be told, we all want to get our way. It's just a plain old fact that Instigator communicators are masters at getting their pet ideas heard and acted upon. Are they good, or what? But there is a cost involved: Conversational coercion leaves feelings of frustration and misunderstanding, and it creates a disconnect with others. To put it dramatically, Empathizer communicators can feel conversationally mugged or raped and their confidence assaulted, after a round with the I-type using this tactic.

Techniques Used to Validate and Strengthen a Decision or Position

Coercive communication implies: "I'm doing the right thing here. . . . I'm fighting the fight for good, not evil. . . . It's a battle between right and wrong. . . . I'm taking responsibility, so just take my word on this." There are a multitude of pushy or coercive talk techniques:

- I'm a good person, and I'm not mean spirited, so . . .
- My intention is good, so you should . . .
- This is the right thing to do because . . .
- If it's a bad decision, it's because I made it with limited information. . . .

- If I had it to do all over again, I would make the same decision, based on what I knew. . . .
- Listen to me because I'm older . . . smarter . . . I care for you . . . I have more experience. . . .

"I'm in the right here because . . ." is a coercive talk technique that is a big lie told by small-thinking people. Negatalking coercive talkers hammer you with, "It's my way or the highway!" which is one-way communication of the worst kind. As a result, morale drops . . . coworkers or family members won't go the extra mile, or smile . . . your once-supportive team members leave . . . and your project is left with miles to go before completion. Poor communication can be likened to throwing opportunities and money right out your communicator car window! But that fact alone doesn't stop negatalkers who urge you to bite into the manure sandwich they try to stuff into your mouth.

Summed up, all coercive communicators intimidate their talk partners emotionally and send them packing on a guilt trip in this way: "Since I stand on moral ground, you should listen to me and do what I want you to do!"

Secrets of the Talk Trade

The above examples coerce cocommunicators into thinking that responsibility is exercised in a righteous or moral manner, when in fact, that may or may not be what's happening. A few secrets of the coercive talk trade from my Instigator (I-type) guy and gal pals:

1. I am a tough debater, but I realize I also limit talk options.
2. If you don't agree with me, I claim to be misunderstood.
3. Actually, I become frustrated that I'm not hearing from you what I want to be hearing.
4. Is this working for me? Not really. If the spirit of a conversation is to engage another person, then I shouldn't shepherd or steer them into a position that limits their options.
5. I shouldn't choose Empathizers' positions for them. But I do.
6. I can talk circles around my opponents. Conversational coercion really limits Empathizers' response options and flexibility.
7. This can precipitate a defensive posture with my E-type talk partner. Example: I limit the options so severely that my Empathizer talk partner has to fight his or her way out of a corner.
8. As an Instigator, I'm guilty of "Conversational Abuse," because I can focus the topic on a negative point and draw everybody into the fray.
9. Because I am an I-type, I have no doubt that a good defense (The Deflecting Defense) is a good first-strike offense.
10. As an I-type, I also believe that communication is a chess or poker game. You've got to play to win the point. It either forces agreement or makes the other player come up with a counterargument very quickly, or a siege will follow. Who cares more? Who will be the last one standing? Who will not surrender the point? Who will have the last word? I will!
11. As an I-type, I am doggedly determined, and my mental gyrations and exercises are incredibly exhausting to everyone involved. What I label as "damage control" is a real energy-drainer, and it often causes extreme relationship friction.
12. I can conversationally set the agenda and place individuals into positions they will have to defend. I say authoritatively, "Here's the issue . . . and here's what you think about it!"
13. Not only do I define the issue, but I also attempt to define how the people at the Communicator Table think about it.

14. True, conversational coercion has diminished utility when there is less of an emotional bond or connection, but I employ this approach professionally when someone isn't buying into my plan. I take pot shots when I can, but without trust present, my co-communicator doesn't listen to me.

15. I-types use verbal intimidation and re-directing. I can exert pressure and be verbally disquieting. I also create the urgency to hurry up and decide, because time is wasting.

16. Biggest drawback of being a tough-minded I-type? I can get my way, but it might be at the expense of finding a better way.

17. I restrain Empathizers with my I-type talk tactics. I jail rather than liberate. What is the enticement to enter into a conversation when you're told what to think, how to think it, when to think it, and you have an emotional connection turn out to be a burden rather than a blessing?

If You Seek to Create Communication Freedom

What should you do if you seek to deepen the bond, create communication freedom, be open and visible, and be free to come up with more effective ideas? You must recognize that throwing punches of conversational coercion simply does not work to accomplish positive intent.

I-Types – Try this Positive Self-Talk Tool:

I will practice changing my habit of dominating a conversation, which leads to disconnecting and quashing disagreement. I will practice traveling in a middle zone instead of always trying to monopolize the dialogue. I will stop limiting the options of my talk partners. Empathizers have a right to speak up, too. I will approach an emotional topic with a cool-headed openness for both input and possible outcomes.

Your Communication Rights

What are your communication rights and how do they help enforce a speed limit on drivers traveling along the Communicator Highway? We all know that respect is both given and earned. What do you and I want during intense times of respectful disagreeing?

1. *We want respect.*
2. *We want our opinions to be worth something.*
3. *We want our talk partners to actively listen to us.*
4. *We want positive effort put into communicating effectively with each other, because we want to.*
5. *We want our wisdom to be recognized, considered, and utilized when warranted.*
6. *We want to have genuine and trusting experiences with each other, during which we can be open and honest.*
7. *We want to be credited for progressing and becoming better communicators.*
8. *We want communication to be a two-way street instead of a one-way, dead-end alley.*
9. *We want what we have to say to have an impact.*
10. *We want to be able to speak assertively while being enlightened listeners.*
11. *We want to be able to process negative or positive feedback without taking it too personally or too impersonally.*

Respectful communication is built on a foundation of trust, fortified with an open exchange of ideas which could benefit everyone.

CASE EXAMPLE #5: WHY PARENT-TEEN TALK – OR CORRECTIVE FEEDBACK – IS A HARD NUT TO CRACK

Are you willing to tell teens something that will make them as mad as a hornet? Of course you are. You don't fear telling teens what they don't want to hear, because maybe they won't listen, or maybe they'll hate your guts, along with harboring a bad attitude toward you. I ran into the issue of giving corrective feedback with my new teenage driver recently. It's a hard nut to crack!

Teaching a Teen to Drive on the Two-Way Communicator Highway

The Driving Problem: I was stunned when I spotted my newly licensed teenage daughter driving down the highway with one hand on the steering wheel and the other hand holding a cell phone up to her ear. That wasn't the agreement! I was ready to let it rip to make my point.

Reactionary Knee-Jerk-Me-Jerk Feedback: I could have let loose and spewed from a nega-tive Instigator reaction (see The Communication Matrix on p. 166) like this: "Hey, Erin, what were you thinking? That's right! You *weren't* thinking!! Did you think you could get away with this? Fat chance. . . . Are you trying to get yourself killed? Young lady you've lost your driving privileges for a month!"

To Whom Are You Talking, By Type? Erin is a sensitive, Empathizer-type (E-type). If she were a thicker-skinned Instigator-type (I-type) communicator, I could have probably gotten away with dressing her down like that in private – but not in public. Why? Because I-types let the water of criticism run off their backs like the proverbial duck. However, Erin is an E-type communicator, and she might easily have written me off for a very long time – or for life! Why? E-types are very sensitive; like to be liked; fear disapproval or being harshly criticized; fear making mistakes or appearing foolish or stupid; tune in to the volume of the voice tone and amplify the negative words; take criticism to heart; replay criticisms in their mind so much they might have difficulty sleeping at night; criticize themselves for small mistakes; and, when defensive, throw up a wall or emotionally shut down in depression. Erin is a sensitive E-type communicator – a little criticism goes a long way!

Who Are You To Talk? What if the speaker – Dad, your boss, your mate or friend – is an I-type? Well, if my style were to be a straight shooter . . . a problem-solver . . . a mapmaker and responsible change-agent . . . a tell-it-like-it-is-type person when others are shying away from telling the truth – specifically, if I were an Instigator-type communicator – then I would be prone to switching talk lanes and saying something foolish that I would regret for a long time, such as, "You're going to turn out to be a dizzy female driver who ends up in an expensive accident like so many women, if you keep this up, young lady!" Not a good attitude for a young woman to adopt, I think. But wasn't the deal *no cell phones used while driving*, due to safety issues?

Talking to Anyone About Anything

Why does all this matter in the *Talk to Me©* system? *Knowing* that Erin is a sensitive, Empathizer-type communicator, and that I was *feeling* like an insensitive, Instigator-type communicator, I chose to deliver my corrective feedback thusly:

(Standing in the garage) *Erin, I am going to speak for 1 to 2 minutes and you are going to listen. This is about your driving. After I'm finished speaking, I will remain quiet while you talk to me for 1 to 2 minutes. There are to be no interruptions.*

I know I must have been seeing things. I passed you driving on Highway 48 and saw you with one hand on the steering wheel and one hand pressed up to your right ear. You were holding in your right hand what appeared to be your cell phone, and you appeared to be talking. It was about 3:30 P.M., and you would have been returning home from work. I just know this couldn't have actually taken place. . . .

The intent of the rule of "no cell phone use while driving" is to make sure you concentrate on your driving. You are a new driver, and a very good driver. However, statistics show that you have a good chance of getting into an accident when you're not paying attention. Only having one hand on the steering wheel is not paying attention. I know you are a careful and responsible driver, and I know this must have been a mistake, one that you won't repeat.

In terms of punishment, I am in my full rights as a parent to suspend your driving privileges for a week or longer. I am not going to do that. I figure you must have been excited to share your job news or whatever. But this won't happen again, I just know it. I consider this conversation sufficient to get the result that we all want – that of you being a safe driver. Perhaps later I will allow cell phone use, but for now, pull over and park whenever you need to take or make a call.

In fact, I don't care if the President . . . Pope . . . or your Papa calls, don't answer it! Now I've used my time, and it's time for you to talk.

Talking . . . Listening . . . Talking

Erin apologized for talking on her cell phone. She confirmed that she was talking on the phone to her mother, who had called. Erin worried that perhaps it was an emergency. She didn't feel dressed down by me, and I no longer felt upset and disappointed. My intent was to stress safety and clarify the rules, one more time. The rest was up to her. I have great faith in my daughter. If I had suffered from a case of "mistaken identity," that Erin was a tough-minded Instigator communicator instead of the sensitive E-type, I would have talked real tough – perhaps even yelled at her – and I would have lost the battle and perhaps the entire identity and psychological individuation war.

The lesson to be learned? Know the communication type of your talk partner. Otherwise, you're going to make people mad who don't need to be – and you're going to fail to make people uncomfortable, when they ought to be.

ARE YOU AN OPTIMISTIC DRIVER ON THE TWO-WAY COMMUNICATOR HIGHWAY?

Positive communicators are optimistic drivers on a *two*-way Communicator Highway. Their way is only one among many by which to travel. In contrast, *negative* communicators are closed-minded drivers on a *one*-way Communicator Highway. Their way is the *only* way to travel (and they're happy to tell you so).

Don't worry if all traits in any of the lists don't fit you exactly, because one size car doesn't fit all communicators. Just get a feel for the talk *pattern* for each type, then identify your talk partner's type to triple the power of your talk tools! Knowing your talk partner's and your own communicator types makes two-way, positive communication travel on the Communicator Highway more sane, predictable, and enjoyable. And, once you learn to use new talk road maps and new driving strategies, you'll find that life is a lot easier everywhere – and your communication trips will net greater, more positive results than you could have imagined.

Cliff Notes: Empathizer vs. Instigator
Communicators – Controlling Negative Emotional States

Bad communication makes people feel distressed. When life partners (or employees, bosses, kids, friends . . . any talk partners) feel bad, you don't get their best – of anything. Everyone loses something, and no one wins much. Are you an optimistic driver on the two-way Communicator Highway? Negative emotional states (feeling blue, anxious, angry, guilty) act like fog that makes traveling at normal speeds on the two-way Communicator Highway impossible. *The problem*: To get rid of negative emotions, we often hand them off by sticking them in the mind of a cocommunicator.

Keys to the Ignition of
Good Communication, Empathizer Style

Here, then, are a few key summary points about how Empathizer-type communicators drive and operate quite differently on the two-way Communicator Highway . . . in the lanes of *Emotions and Talks*.

Empathizer-type communicators:

- Are *intimidated* by the I-types' debating skills.
- *Desire* approval and recognition.
- By nature, are *shy* about speaking up or disagreeing.
- Are too *sensitive* to hurting others.
- Won't *push* their points of view, nor will they push back effectively.
- *Enjoy* more compliments.
- *Fear* corrective criticisms.
- *Stew and brood* when talks aren't going well.
- "It's only business, it's nothing personal!" rings untrue.
- Are *de-motivated* by criticism over the long haul.
- See sincere compliments as being *motivational.*
- Are *person* vs. policy focused.
- Are behind-the-scenes *workhorses* who may feel underappreciated.
- Are *relationship*-centered.
- Worry that they aren't *achieving* enough.
- Find that, when their *mood* is down, *performance* goes down.
- Are *intimidated* by booming voices or facial signs of disapproval.
- Can't hear logical arguments when *emotions* run high.
- Find that public *scolding* leads to personal *stewing.*
- When *distressed*, will act up and do something *stupid.*
- Will *yield* when they should push back and stand their ground.
- Are good *listeners* to a fault.
- Can see the "elephant in the room."
- Have solutions to pesky problems, but may not be able to lead the charge toward change.

If you are an E-type, you have uncommon common sense and easily intuit solutions to vexing problems at work.

Changing the Flat Tire of
Bad Communication, Instigator Style

Here are a few key summary points about how Instigator-type communicators (O'Grady, 2005) drive and operate quite differently from E-types, on the two-way Communicator Highway . . . in the lanes of *Beliefs and Behaviors*.

Instigator-type communicators:

- Are intimidated by the E-types' relationship skills.
- Value protecting loved ones, their country, their company.
- By nature, are big thinkers who don't mind disagreeing.
- Dislike hurting others but are too insensitive to the others' feelings.
- Will push their points of view, and push back effectively.
- Enjoy talking confidently and persuasively.
- Act like they don't fear corrective criticisms.
- Give themselves huge challenges on a regular basis.
- Have the attitude of, "It's only business, it's nothing personal!" to keep resentment in check.
- Are fired up by unfair criticism resulting in, "Well, I'll show you. . . ."
- See compliments as unnecessary, perhaps insincere, and demotivational.
- Drive the mood of the office or household, for better or worse.
- Are comfortable being in the middle of the action but can feel weary.
- Are progress- and change-centered, and they tend to be smart workers.
- Are achievement-centered throughout life.
- Are impatient if results don't come quickly enough for them.
- Find that, when their energy is down, driving performance speeds up.
- Are bored by soft voices, drooping postures, or facial signs of disinterest.
- Will stick to repeating logical points when emotions run high.
- Are prone to excessive self-esteem but can feel insecure.
- When distressed, can't bite their tongues and will say something stupid.
- Will be stubborn like a mule when they should sit back and listen up.
- Are doers to a fault and have trouble being in a relaxing pose.
- Use a this-is-now approach: "Since I apologized for my mistake, let's move on and get moving down the road!"
- Can't see how only talking about the "elephant in the room" helps clean up the piles of dung or mess left.
- Are cool under pressure, putting out fires, but they may stir the pot.
- Rely on the mind and intellectual powers as prime driving forces. (pp. 148-149)

If you are an I-type, then you are a natural-born leader, willing and able to take charge any time. You understand that your words say as much as your actions.

THE COMMUNICATION MATRIX DIAGRAM:
NEGATIVE VS. POSITIVE EMPATHIZER AND
INSTIGATOR COMMUNICATOR STYLES

The following Communication Matrix© is a powerful, visual, summary tool to help you assess to whom you are talking, by communicator type and by type of energy attitude. As one previous seminar participant quipped, "It was my 'Aha!' moment of '*Now* I know why someone hates me!'" Just look at the adjectives and put your finger on the quadrant that best describes where you and your cocommunicator are and where you would like to be.

Moreover, the following *negative* traits can be either *effective* or *ineffective*, depending upon how the trait is applied. For example, being *demanding* can *improve* performance but *unreasonably tax* a relationship.

Additionally, the following *positive* traits can sizzle in one situation but sour in another, like milk left out of the refrigerator too long. For example, being *slow-moving*, like the Tortoise, can *tax* the patience of the Hare, while being a *hard driver* can make *robots* out of people, when a human touch is needed the most.

Negative E-Type Communicators	**Negative I-Type Communicators**
(-) Empathizer-Types	(-) Instigator-Types
Compliant	Demanding
Sap	Sarcastic
Modest	Arrogant
Implosive	Explosive
Imitator	Intimidator
Wishy-washy	Unbudging
Yes, agree-able	No, disagree-able
Doesn't push back	Debates
How you play the game	Winning is everything
Sad	Mad
Positive E-Type Communicators	**Positive I-Type Communicators**
(+) Empathizer-Types	(+) Instigator-Types
Slow movers	Hard-drivers
Followers	Leaders
Sensitive	Insensitive
Regard	Genuine
Emotional	Logical
Intuits solutions	Problem-solvers
Expert listeners	Expert mapmakers
Relationship-focused	Results-focused
Flexible	Unbending

The Communication Matrix*

GOOD COMMUNICATION ISN'T A FLUKE

Good communication isn't a fluke. It involves a simple system of enlightened moves, which are all laid out in the *Talk to Me©* textbook (O'Grady, 2005). Additionally, *Talk to Me©* system tools can be accessed, at no cost to you, in the more than 200 articles at www.drogrady.com. The typecasting and other skills you learned in this contribution are all you need to start talking more positively and effectively today at work and at home. Why plug

---

*Copyright © 2008 Dennis O'Grady, PsyD (www.drogrady.com; Tel.: 937-428-0724)

in to this system? The *Talk to Me©* system helps you better handle the fear of confrontation and conflict, while helping you avoid unnecessary miscommunications that could blow up in your face. *The best news:* Your clients will feel you truly *can* walk in their shoes and, based on this trust, accomplish needed changes faster, making everyone smile.

Communicator Prejudices*

Critiques of E-types by I-types

I-types think:

- You are too sensitive
- You are too generous
- You are too passive
- You are too codependent
- You are too conforming
- You worry too much
- You are too depressed
- You don't take very good care of yourself
- You talk but never put your ideas on the table
- You are too laid back
- You are too easy-going
- You are too prudent
- You are a perfectionist
- You are too wishy-washy
- You are too emotionally needy
- You are too downhearted
- You are too demanding
- You pout like a big baby
- You can't stand going it alone
- You are dense as a rock
- You get along with everyone
- You don't know what you want
- You can't ever be satisfied
- You can't let go of fear and relax
- You beat up on yourself
- You shut down when you're hurt
- You're too good for your own good
- You're drug down by guilt
- You don't let anything go
- You're too patient
- You're afraid of success
- You're afraid of conflict
- You can't stand being happy

Critiques of I-types by E-types

E-types assume:

- You are too insensitive
- You are too selfish
- You are too aggressive
- You are too independent
- You are too rebellious
- You don't worry about a thing
- You are too optimistic
- You only take care of yourself
- You talk too much
- You are too driven
- You are too critical
- You are too imprudent
- You are a workaholic
- You are stubborn as a mule
- You don't need anyone
- You don't feel anything
- You don't care
- You don't get mad, you get even
- You are a loner
- You are too smart for your own good
- You can't get along with those who disagree with you
- You only think about your wants
- You ought to be satisfied with what you've got
- You're mad and grumpy too much of the time
- You don't listen to corrective feedback
- You can't think straight when you're mad
- You think I'm bad when you're mad
- You don't feel guilty enough
- You want to get past the past or throw in the towel
- You're too impatient
- You're afraid of failure
- You love conflict
- You can't buy happiness

CONTRIBUTOR

Dennis O'Grady, PsyD, is a clinical psychologist specializing in communication. He has worked for more than 30 years with top executives and their teams to overcome barriers to ongoing success in their companies or organizations. He is the founder of New Insights Communication, a management consulting firm dedicated to the advancement of organizational development, and professional and personal growth. His executive coaching and business consulting programs focus on the areas of communication, leadership development, change management, and conflict resolution. Dr. O'Grady is the author of three works which include *Taking the Fear Out of Changing, No Hard Feelings*, and *Talk to Me: Communication Moves to Get Along With Anyone*. He is a psychology media expert to TV, radio and newspapers and has been sourced in the *Dayton Daily News*, *Dayton Business Journal, USA Today, Columbus Dispatch, Cincinnati Enquirer* and the *Detroit Free Press*, among others. He is a Clinical Professor at Wright State University School of Professional Psychology and has been a workshop presenter for such educational agencies as Sinclair Community College, the University of Dayton, and Miami University Middletown Campus. He is President of the Dayton Area Psychological Association. Dr. O'Grady may be contacted at 7501 Paragon Road, Suite 200, Dayton, OH 45459. E-mail: newinsights@drogrady.com

RESOURCES

Cited Resources

Horovitz, B. (2007, March 27). Alpha Moms leap to top of trendsetters. Retrieved September 15, 2008 from http://www.usatoday.com/money/advertising/2007-03-26-alpha-mom_N.htm

O'Grady, D. E. (2005). *Talk To Me: Communication Moves To Get Along with Anyone*. Dayton, OH: New Insights Communication.

Additional Resources

Donaghue, E. (2007, July 19). Communication now part of the cure: Movement has begun to help doctors listen and patients understand. *USA TODAY*, D.7, 8.

Goldberg, H. (2007). *What Men Still Don't Know About Women, Relationships and Love*. Fort Lee, NJ: Barricade Books.

Gottman, J. M., & Silver, N. (1999). *The Seven Principles for Making Marriage Work: A Practical Guide From the Country's Foremost Relationship Expert*. New York: Three Rivers Press.

Gottman, J. M., Gottman, J. S., & DeClaire, J. (2007). *Ten Lessons To Transform Your Marriage: America's Love Lab Experts Share Their Strategies for Strengthening Your Marriage*. New York: Three Rivers Press.

Gray, J. (1992). *Men Are from Mars, Women Are from Venus: The Classic Guide to Understanding the Opposite Sex*. New York: HarperCollins.

Hogan, R. (2007). *Personality and the Fate of Organizations*. Mahwah, NJ: Lawrence Erlbaum.

Jung, C. G. (1923). *Psychological Types*. London: Routledge.

Kurdek, L. A. (1984). Nature and correlates of relationship quality in gay, lesbian, and heterosexual cohabiting couples. In B. Greene & G. Herek (Eds.), *Contemporary Perspectives on Gay and Lesbian Psychology: Theory, Research, and Applications* (pp. 133-155). Beverly Hills, CA: Sage.

Laney, M. O. (2002). *The Introvert Advantage: How to Thrive in an Extrovert World*. New York: Workman Publishing.

O'Grady, D. E. (1992*). Taking the Fear Out of Changing: Guidelines for Getting Through Tough Life Transitions*. Boston: Bob Adams Media.

O'Grady, D. E. (1997). *No Hard Feelings: Managing Anger and Conflict in Your Work, Family, and Love Life*. (Cassette Recording Series). Dayton, OH: New Insights Communication.

O'Grady, D. E. (2008a). *The Talk 2 Me© Communicator Driver Manual for Dayton Freight Lines*. Dayton, OH: New Insights Communication.

O'Grady, D. E. (2008b). *Just Talk: Building Trust Through Positive and Effective Communication*. Workshop communications training manual for Motoman, Inc. Retrieved January 1, 2008, from http://www.drogrady.com/motoman/JustTalk_rev111207.pdf

Tannen, D. (1990). *You Just Don't Understand: Women and Men in Conversation*. New York: Ballantine Books.

Tannen, D. (2006). *You're Wearing That?: Understanding Mothers and Daughters in Conversation*. New York: Ballantine Books.

Introduction to Section II: Practice Management and Professional Development

The PRACTICE MANAGEMENT AND PROFESSIONAL DEVELOPMENT section includes contributions that assist practitioners in building and managing their practices in effective ways. In the first contribution, Martyn Whittingham and Gregory T. Capriotti address ethical issues relating to group work. The authors identify key issues regarding applications of ethical standards and address clarification of legal and ethical obligations. Specific ethical codes relating to group work are highlighted, as well as issues relating to confidentiality. Dual relationships are addressed, as well as issues relating to concurrent therapy in which a client is treated in group and individual treatment at the same time. Ethical issues relating to experiential training groups and cyber counseling are addressed. The contribution ends by addressing the ethical imperative for cultural competence in group work.

In the second contribution, Samuel Knapp and Leon VandeCreek address risk management and positive ethics. Rather than viewing an ethics code as a way to prevent doing harm, the authors suggest a conceptual shift to maximizing benefits to others. In addressing risk management from this positive perspective, the authors identify a series of positive risk-management strategies including well-informed consent, high standards for documentation, the use of consultation, and redundant protection. The contribution concludes with an excellent case example which illustrates positive risk management principles.

The Ethics of Group Therapy

Martyn Whittingham and Gregory T. Capriotti

Before reading this contribution, please answer the questions below.

GUIDED QUESTIONS

- What ethical code or codes are you beholden to with respect to *group work*?

- Is it unethical to skip group screening?
  (Yes / No / It depends [please state])

- Is it unethical to *not* highlight cultural differences in conflict style during conflicts between members of different cultural backgrounds?
  (Yes / No / It depends [please state])

- Is it ethical to run a group online?

- Is it unethical for the instructor of the course to also lead experiential training groups for students being trained in group work?
  (Yes / No / It depends [please state])

OVERVIEW

The need to revisit the area of group work ethics is timely. Innovations are in part driven by a response to the lessons of the past, the needs of the present, and an anticipation of the needs of the future. In the case of the ethics of group work, all factors and more are present. This contribution is not intended to be a comprehensive review of group work ethics. Rather, it will explore group work along time lines and important issues. Some issues, such as the notion of "To what group ethics am I beholden?" are revisited and not taken as a given assumption. In fact, readers are asked to challenge themselves on that question. We will revisit "old" issues in ethics and group that are still relevant and contentious today. This will include revisiting the issue of experiential training groups. We will seek to reposition multicultural issues along a different time line, moving it from the future to the present. Finally, the issue of cyber counseling will be addressed with respect to its rapidly emerging present and future.

These ethical challenges, while sharing some similarities to those faced a decade ago, are increasingly moving into uncharted waters. However, this contribution will begin with a question that has already been implicitly asked: What are the relevant ethical guidelines for group workers, and why are some guidelines being used in this contribution that do not seem relevant to me?

WHAT ORGANIZATIONS DO GROUP WORK SPECIALISTS BELONG TO?

The field of group work encompasses many different disciplines, including but not limited to social work, counseling, psychiatry, clinical and counseling psychology, and others. Each "parent" organization (e.g., American Psychological Association [APA], for psychologists) often includes subdivisions that specialize in group work (e.g., Division 49 for APA; Association for Specialists in Group Work [ASGW] for American Counseling Association [ACA]). In some cases, these organizations have their own ethics codes or best practices guidelines that *augment* the ethics code of the parent organization (e.g., ASGW's Best Practice Guidelines are meant to augment ACA's ethics code). In some cases there are also special interest groups within organizations (such as APA Division 17's Special Interest Group in Group Work). There are also freestanding organizations (such as American Group Psychotherapy Association [AGPA]) that serve to link up different professions (such as social work, counseling, etc.) through a mutual interest in group work. It is therefore possible to be a member of multiple organizations and therefore be beholden to several different ethical codes, guidelines, and best practices. Figures 1 and 2 (p. 175) illustrate some of the different group-related ethical codes and guidelines available to members of ACA and APA, together with their subspecialties and divisions.

It is worth noting that for these organizations, in some circumstances a supervisor may be, for example, a psychologist, working with employees who are counselors, but whose APA ethics code offers somewhat less clear guidance and requirements than does the ACA code used by a supervisee. This example highlights the difficulties associated with working within a multidisciplinary team that is beholden to different ethical codes.

WHICH ETHICAL STANDARDS APPLY?

As several authors (G. Corey, M. S. Corey, & Callanan, 2003; Gladding, 2003; Herlihy & Remley, 1995) indicate, the presence of so many, sometimes overlapping but sometimes contradictory, standards of ethics provide for a confusing ethical landscape. This is further compounded with respect to group work. Gladding (2003) states: "In a field such as group work, in which practitioners come from varied backgrounds, often some question arises as to which code of ethics to follow and when" (p. 225). This may at first glance seem less like a confusing issue than a prompt for a very obvious answer: "I am answerable to the ethics of the parent organization (e.g., APA) that licenses me, while also being beholden to federal and state laws and codes and organization policies and procedures." However, there are multiple organizations that practice group work, each with ethical guidelines that in most cases agree, but in some cases diverge with respect to what is or is not ethical (G. Corey et al., 2003).

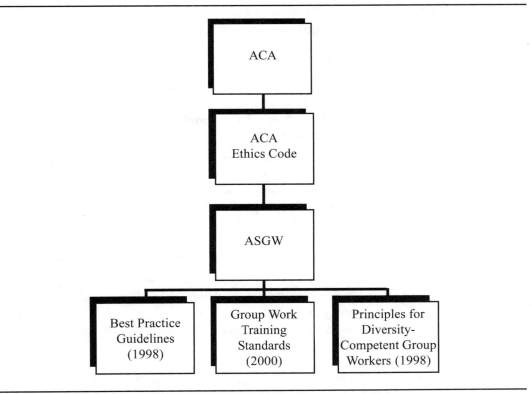

Figure 1. American Counseling Association.

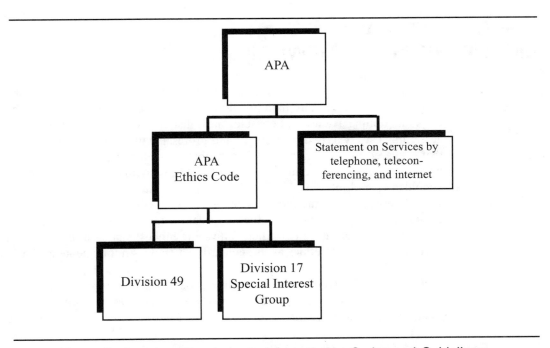

Figure 2. American Psychological Association Codes and Guidelines.

An example of a Clarification of Legal and Ethical Obligations

Equally, in following an ethical standard from their parent organization, therapists might in some cases place themselves at odds with legal statutes or organizational procedures. APA (2002) offers specific guidance on both these issues, stating:

1.02 Conflicts Between Ethics and Law, Regulations, or Other Governing Legal Authority

If psychologists' ethical responsibilities conflict with law, regulations, or other governing legal authority, psychologists make known their commitment to the Ethics Code and take steps to resolve the conflict. If the conflict is unresolvable via such means, psychologists may adhere to the requirements of the law, regulations, or other governing legal authority.

1.03 Conflicts Between Ethics and Organizational Demands

If the demands of an organization with which psychologists are affiliated or for whom they are working conflict with this Ethics Code, psychologists clarify the nature of the conflict, make known their commitment to the Ethics Code, and to the extent feasible, resolve the conflict in a way that permits adherence to the Ethics Code.

Close examination of both these guiding statements shows that the "answer" is a complex one with many factors to take into account in each case, many of them process-based in nature. However, what this highlights is that ethics for group workers can be potentially confusing and, though mostly overlapping, also contradictory.

THE CASE FOR A MULTIETHICAL FRAMEWORK

However, as G. Corey, Williams and Moline (1995) state: "Becoming an ethical group practitioner involves more than merely avoiding the breaking of laws or ethical codes. It implies functioning at a level of consciousness geared toward doing whatever it takes to function at the highest level, both personally and professionally" (pp. 161-162). This position is one that is shared by the authors of this contribution with respect to group ethics. In establishing what group ethics to use in any given situation, particularly in one where group workers are beholden to multiple sets of ethics, care should be taken to seek out the *highest* ethical standard. Although each practitioner is beholden to the ethics of his or her respective parent organization, a case could be made that an organization should examine all sets of group ethics and, when they are not in conflict, follow the highest standard of practice. For example, an agency may use APA ethics as its standard, which does not mandate group screening.

FOCUSED QUESTION: When is the next possible meeting time you could sit down and compare ethical codes of your group workers' respective parent organizations to ensure you are meeting the highest ethical standard of group work practice for your organization?

The Case of Group Screening

One such example of a possible ethical mismatch is the aforementioned case for group screening. Screening is described by Gladding (2003) as a three-part process, involving (a) the leader selecting a group he or she is qualified and able to run; (b) recruiting members by letting them know the goals of the group, procedures to be used, expectations of them and the leader(s), and major risks and rewards that might be expected; and (c) conducting one-to-one or small group interviews to ensure compatibility. Although it is not clearly articulated in APA standards of ethics for group work, it is present in ACA guidelines (2005) as a mandate:

Group Work A.8.a. Screening

Counselors screen prospective group counseling/therapy participants. To the extent possible, counselors select members whose needs and goals are compatible with goals of the group, who will not impede the group process, and whose well-being will not be jeopardized by the group experience.

A group leader following a minimal standard of care and practice for APA might determine that group screening, though desirable and "aspirational," is not an ethical imperative and therefore might be sacrificed for the sake of expediency when other professional tasks seem more pressing. For another professional within that same organization, following a different set of professional ethics (such as ACA's code of ethics), this failure to screen is in direct violation of an ethical mandate. Hence an organization might be inadvertently placing one of its members in violation of his or her ethical code by not adhering to the ethical standard of group screening. The onus is therefore on the organization to ensure that its policies and day-to-day organizational needs do not place its employees in an ethical bind.

QUESTION: Does your parent organization mandate group screening in its ethical code?

QUESTION: Does your group work specialty mandate group screening in its ethical code (e.g., Division 49; AGPA; ASGW)?

QUESTION: Does your agency mandate screening? If not, is harm being caused?

SPECIFIC ETHICAL CODES RELATED TO GROUP WORK

Other ethical guidelines could also be addressed in such an organizational review of practice. Although of course there are multiple relevant ethical codes and principles that can be brought to bear on group therapy, several are more frequently mentioned in the literature of this field, namely (a) confidentiality, (b) dual relationships, (c) voluntary and involuntary membership of groups, (d) member screening and orientation, (e) informed consent, and (f) record keeping.

Of these, the first ethical issue, confidentiality, has one of the most significant differences when compared to the ethics of individual therapy. This is demonstrated by the reference to it within APA's ethics code. Despite several other mentions of group therapy in the ethics codes mentioned elsewhere in this contribution, it is interesting to note that the only specific code named "group therapy" in APA's code of ethics (2002) is **10.03 Group Therapy**, which states:

When psychologists provide services to several persons in a group setting, they describe at the outset the roles and responsibilities of all parties and the limits of confidentiality.

Although roles and responsibilities speak to the previously referenced idea of a need for orientation and group screening, the inclusion of confidentiality noting "limits" speaks to the special status of this construct within group work.

THE SPECIAL CASE OF CONFIDENTIALITY

Confidentiality is an issue with a particularly different meaning to the group worker and client. Because the therapy relies on self-disclosure to be successful, and because other group members are not legally or ethically bound by confidentiality, there is a risk to group members that their confidentiality may not be upheld. Although the therapist is bound by an ethical code, other group members are not.

In an excellent and comprehensive article, Lasky and Riva (2006) outlined many issues related to confidentiality. As they point out, informed consent around confidentiality in groups is key. Group members must be informed of this, and it is typical for groups to enter into prolonged discussion about what this means to them and how they can navigate through this uncertainty and lack of guarantee.

As Lasky and Riva (2006) also point out, there is also a serious concern around the issue of many states not seeing content of therapy as privileged because it falls under the third-party rule – that is, if an utterance is made in the presence of a third party, the rules of confidentiality are not seen to apply because the third party presence implies it was "in public." Hence, from a legal standpoint, the communication is not privileged. Smokowski, Rose, and Bacallao (2001) point out that group casualties (those who have felt psychological distress as the result of a group experience) are most defined by their self-report that their confidentiality was breached. As Lasky and Riva (2006) further point out, it is common for group members to breach each other's confidentiality. They suggest that for group members, this may be due to two reasons: first, that there are no clear consequences, and second, because they do not understand the specifics of how confidentiality is enacted outside of therapy. This second issue suggests group leaders need to address with group members possible circumstances under which they might be tempted and offer suggestions on how to manage this. This issue is one not dissimilar to that experienced by therapists – for example, after a particularly difficult session, the client is left upset and this is noticed by a spouse who asks "what is wrong?" Without guidance, clients are then caught in a no-win situation where they must either repress and deny and feel no release from their upset while simultaneously blocking a needed support network, or face the guilt of breaching a group member's confidentiality. One possible option is for the group leader to prepare members to share their own feelings and reactions without naming the person involved.

However, this set of factors is not limited to "unaware" group member clients. Anecdotal information suggests these risks also apply to graduate students taking part in experiential groups as part of their group therapy training. In discussions with colleagues and students, the authors of this contribution encountered many instances of students breaching each other's confidentiality, in some cases with serious consequences. Hence, lack of knowledge of ethical codes may not be the only factor in breaches; rather, processes for self-regulating affect via gossip, and memory effects related to context in which information was given, may be far more difficult to inhibit than is sometimes imagined, even when admonishments are clear and consequences serious.

Confidentiality Options

There is a wide range of options with respect to confidentiality and an equally wide dispersion of therapist approaches to this issue, with no one approach showing as a clear "favorite" among group workers (Lasky, 2005). The options included in Lasky's (2005) study are (a) asking for "complete" confidentiality, (b) distinguishing between your own confidentiality and that of others, (c) outlining general consequences of a breach of confidentiality, (d) the need to maintain confidentiality even after group has ended, (e) outlining of specific consequences (e.g., termination from group), and (f) informing of limits of confidentiality – that it cannot be "guaranteed." However, regardless of the position each group worker takes, it is certainly a key part of informed consent and needs careful monitoring. The question of confidentiality is also compounded when running groups for children and adolescents or in settings where clients are incarcerated. In these and other cases, specific questions regarding limits of confidentiality need particularly careful thought and attention.

QUESTION: What is your typical statement on confidentiality? Is this the same for every group in your organization or does it depend on each individual therapist?

QUESTION: What special issues are involved in confidentiality in groups for your organization (e.g., age of client, incarcerated, etc.)?

DUAL RELATIONSHIPS

Dual relationships are also of considerable concern to group therapists. It is a common question to ask whether someone who is an individual therapist should also act as the group therapist for the client. Clearly, the answer to this is complex and involves many factors, including, but not limited to (a) setting issues (policy and procedure, specific issues of the population), (b) the ability of the therapist to manage two "different" sets of information without accidentally breaching confidentiality in group, (c) the advisability or otherwise of extra-group contact (ranging from the ethically required, such as ensuring safety of a group member, to the ethically forbidden, such as having sexual contact with a client), and a wide range of other concerns. One such special case of dual relationships and "extra-group" contact lies in the case of concurrent therapy.

Concurrent Therapy

Concurrent therapy consists of a specific client being treated in group therapy and individual therapy at the same time (Taylor & Gazda, 1991). Concurrent therapy can take several different forms, with some evoking more ethical concerns than others.

Yalom (2005) makes the distinction between *combined therapy* and *conjoint therapy*. Combined therapy involves the same therapist providing individual therapy and group therapy to the same client. Conjoint therapy involves the client receiving group therapy from one or two therapists and at the same time receiving individual therapy from a different therapist

According to Taylor and Gazda (1991), a primary ethical concern faced in concurrent therapy is confidentiality and the transfer of information from one setting to the other. This can be an especially challenging situation in combined therapy, because the same therapist is offering both services and it can be extremely difficult for that therapist to remember what information the client volunteered in individual and what was proffered in group. Hence, the therapist risks inadvertently breaching the client's confidentiality in group by revealing information garnered in individual. However, this need to hold back information may also serve to impede group workers' abilities to intervene effectively if they are constantly "double checking" themselves, thereby at times missing the chance to work in the here-and-now more effectively. There is a high probability that the therapist will experience difficulty remembering what information was received in which format, and which information is appropriate to disclose in front of the therapy group (Taylor & Gazda, 1991).

Taylor and Gazda (1991) recommend that concurrent therapy be avoided when there are multiple therapists working with one individual client. If this is unavoidable, then a high degree of communication is necessary between therapists. They also discuss the importance of informed consent from the client that gives the therapists permission to discuss protected information about the client. For example, a client may permit the individual therapist to focus on interpersonal issues and use knowledge of these from individual therapy in group. However, he or she may wish to keep a past trauma incident hidden from the group and not wish the therapist to divulge this. The need for prior discussion and granting of informed consent here is paramount. In such cases, it may also behoove the therapist to keep a written contract of such an agreement.

QUESTION: What are the rules you and your agency or setting have around extra-group contact? Concurrent or conjoint therapy?

Of course, the issues of concurrent and conjoint therapy, dual roles, and confidentiality come sharply into focus when considering one of the most contentious and ethically fraught areas of group work, the use of experiential training groups in training programs.

EXPERIENTIAL TRAINING GROUPS

Training of group leaders also carries with it ethical challenges. As with much therapist training, a dynamic tension exists between the need to train, allowing for mistakes to be made and learned from, and the coexisting need for the gatekeeping function.

This tension comes sharply into focus for training of group leaders when considering the use of experiential training groups.

Pros and Cons

The Council for Accreditation of Counseling and Related Training Programs (CACREP) states that group work trainees should participate in at least 10 clock hours of planned group experience.

Although APA does not share this minimum clock hours of experiential group mandate, it does have ethical codes pertaining to this practice. The consensus around this issue is rapidly changing. Historically, the group experience was professor-led, with students expected to engage and disclose fully, a practice dating back to the origins of group in the psychoanalytic tradition. In the mid-1990s, Hetzel, Stockton, and McDonnell (1994) reported that at least two thirds of training programs used experiential groups. However, despite a broad consensus, as far back as the early 1990s, Merta and Sisson (1991) stated that experiential group training, ". . . has recently become the focus of increasing criticism among counselor educators because of the existence of dual relationships (i.e., instructors serving as group leaders and students serving as group members) and their potential for unethical practices (e.g., invasion of privacy and abuses of power by the instructor)" (p. 236). This change in the early 1990s has been reflected more recently by Barlow (2004), who pointed out that concerns about dual roles meant that many programs do not require this at all. Hence this is an issue of great contention in the field of group work that has its advocates and its detractors.

However, it still receives broad-based support among therapists on theoretical grounds (Dies, 1994; Dies & MacKenzie, 1983; Fuhriman & Burlingame, 1994, 2001), with Barlow (2004) pointing out the "importance of combining skills – experiential, supervision, observation, and academic – in the training of group therapists" (p. 114). Kline and colleagues (1997) engaged in qualitative research in which students reported finding that experiential groups improved their ability to understand the client's experience, allowed greater awareness of knowledge and skills around feedback delivery, and increased awareness of their own and others' interpersonal behaviors. However, there has been little else in the way of systematic research on this teaching technique that establishes its efficacy, suggesting that this belief in the efficacy of experiential groups is based more on anecdotal evidence and teaching experience than on empirical data. Moreover, as Merta and Sisson (1991) acknowledged in the early 1990s, ". . . counselor educators are ethically 'at risk' when using this popular learning experience" (p. 236). Despite this warning and APA (2002) guidelines, the issue remains problematic. APA guidelines on group leadership are clear:

7.05 Mandatory Individual or Group Therapy

(a) When individual or group therapy is a program or course requirement, psychologists responsible for that program allow students in undergraduate and graduate programs the option of selecting such therapy from practitioners unaffiliated with the program.

(b) Faculty who are or are likely to be responsible for evaluating students' academic performance do not themselves provide that therapy.

Yet despite this clear guideline, a recent article (Pepper, 2007) reported the continued practice of some psychoanalytic institutes mandating that ". . . trainees *must* be in group treatment with members of the senior staff with whom they have other professional or social ties" (p. 15). This speaks to perhaps several issues within our field. Although it is not clear from this article whether these institutions adhere to APA guidelines within their program, it can be seen that different programs of group training can have widely differing standards of practice around this area. As Davenport (2004) states, "Corey (2000) argues that if students know of the requirement before they enter, the practice is ethical; others (e.g., Remley & Herlihy, 2000) recommend strongly that some other professional run the group, not the professor" (p. 44). However, that being said, the ethical and professional issues around this issue are particularly complex. The ethical issues to balance include student right to privacy, informed consent, gatekeeping, achieving an unbiased evaluation of student performance, and offering a training experience that develops competence.

Leadership Options

Leadership options for running such groups include Furr and Barret (2000) at the University of North Carolina at Charlotte, who describe using adjuncts to lead their experiential groups. However they mention that "students are told that if the adjunct faculty member has concerns about their appropriateness for the counseling profession, such concern will be communicated to the faculty" (p. 96), therefore retaining the gatekeeping role. Other programs utilize advanced doctoral students to run the groups, and sometimes add another layer of confidentiality by having them be supervised by an adjunct or outside therapist. However, Davenport (2004) cautions that when doctoral led, ". . . may we be expecting some of them to practice beyond their competency, a violation of ACA ethics code C.2 (Professional Competence)?" (p. 45). Further models include using adjunct faculty or external therapists unconnected to the program to avoid the possibility of later teaching responsibilities placing them in a dual role.

The program here at Wright State University offers students the chance to role play a part given by the instructor (or one of their choosing), thus also allowing them an "out" so they can participate and learn from the experience but still retain their personal privacy. Further safeguards include allowing members to self-select group membership to avoid other students they are either intimately involved with or have strong negative feelings against. This then somewhat mitigates subgrouping as well as the possibility of someone with an "axe to grind" bringing this into the group and confusing both members and the leader with "unprovoked" attacks.

Apples and Oranges?

One of the unstated issues relating to the experiential group is this: The training is meant to mimic a therapy experience. However, it could be argued that the experience is significantly different than that. For example, it is not a continuous, discreet experience where members bring real problems, do not meet outside of group, and do not see each other after the end of the group process. Problems can include preexisting resentments and power struggles that sometimes persist during and then after the life of the group has ended. For example, doctoral students mixed with masters level students and any rivalries and resentments that sometimes emerge; preexisting conflicts (perceived slights, power struggles, casualties of gossip, scapegoats, divisions within the group due to issues arising around diversity [age, ethnicity, spirituality, sexuality, etc.]); or just members choosing very different levels of self-disclosure during the life of the group and the problems this creates.

These and other issues can lead to a continuance of problems, particularly if there is a lack of resolution of the conflict that can lead to deep-felt divisions that continue throughout the life of that cohort. Although some have a group experience that is powerful for all the right reasons, others may report feeling deeply damaged by their experience.

It could be argued, in fact, that the group experience has as much in common with a work group as it does with a therapy group – it has a preexisting membership, preexisting history, a life that continues after the end of the therapy, dual relationships, subgrouping, and is set in a common environment/ecological space. Therefore questions remain on both sides of the risk-benefit equation regarding this model of training.

QUESTION: In my training program, does my use of experiential training groups meet the needs for gatekeeping, training, student privacy, and obligations of the accrediting agency for my institution?

The question of whether experiential groups will continue and if so, in what form, suggests a reconsideration by training programs regarding what and how they choose to teach. With respect to multicultural group work, this training consideration is arguably even more urgent and will now be considered.

MULTICULTURAL GROUP WORK: COMPETENCE AS AN ETHICAL IMPERATIVE

The field of multicultural competence has only relatively recently begun to enter into formulations of best practices in group work. However, in doing so, it has moved forward rapidly, albeit unevenly. Arguably, the standard bearer for group multicultural *practice* has been the ASGW, who has produced the Principles for Diversity-Competent Group Workers (1998). Many key figures in group work (Delucia-Waak, 1996; A. E. Ivey, Pedersen, & M. B. Ivey, 2001; Merta, 1999; Trotzer, 1999) have expressed sentiments similar to those of Arredondo (1994), who stated that *all* counseling practice, including group work, must be conceptualized and reframed as multicultural counseling. However, this is a standard that many therapists still perceive as "aspirational" rather than related to basic competence.

However, for many group workers in ethnically diverse cities, the need for multicultural competence is less of an aspiration than a necessity. Table 1 (p. 183) shows the ethnic makeup of several metropolitan cities from the U.S. Census of 2000 (U.S. Census Bureau, 2000). For the practitioner working in Miami, for example, the need to understand issues pertaining to diversity is nothing short of an ethical imperative. It would be close to impossible to practice in a competent manner, much less an expert one, without a strong grasp of the complex relationships between cultural identities, gender, sexuality, and socioeconomic status, to name but a few variables.

TABLE 1: U.S. Census of 2000*

	Hispanic	African-American	Asian-American	Total%
Los Angeles	47%	11%	10%	68%
New York	27%	25%	10%	62%
Miami	66%	20%	1%	87%
San Francisco	14%	8%	31%	53%
Chicago	26%	36%	4%	66%
Houston	37%	25%	5%	67%
San Antonio	59%	7%	2%	68%
Dallas	36%	26%	3%	65%

*Source: U.S. Census Bureau (2000)

Although this previous assertion draws attention to key cities, the demographics of America are also changing more widely. Breaking American demographics down further into ethnicity by age, it can be seen that young Americans are approaching a 1:1 ratio of Caucasian to ethnic minorities (See Figure 3 below). What this means is that the reality for younger age groups is that they will be encountering diversity very differently from those one and two generations ahead of them. These figures add weight to D. W. Sue & D. Sue's (2008) assertion that "cultural competence is superordinate to counseling competence" (p. 35). These rapidly changing demographics are moving what hitherto have been considered "aspirational" and "best practices" guidelines into the realms of basic competence and a necessity for effective practice.

Debiak (2007) also makes a compelling case for the necessity of multicultural competence in attending to GLBTQ (Gay Lesbian Bisexual Transgendered and Questioning) issues in a group. He also defines this not as an aspiration or best practice, but as an ethical *imperative*.

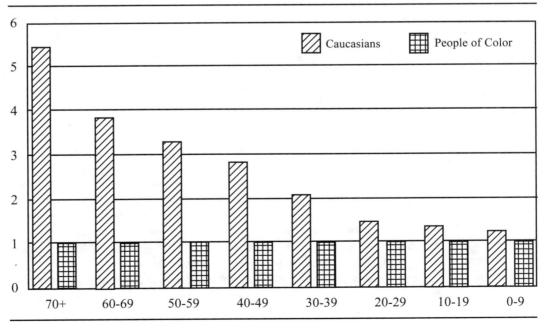

Figure 3. Ratio of Caucasians to People of Color in Successive Age Groups
(Source: U.S. Census Bureau, 2000)

He describes the process of ethically competent decision making in deciding whether a gay male is an appropriate referral to an otherwise homogenously heterosexual group.

MULTICULTURAL GROWTH AS BASIC COMPETENCE

ASGW Multicultural Group Competencies

As D. W. Sue, Arredondo and McDavis (1992) point out in their discussion of multicultural counseling competencies, there are three main characteristics a counselor must possess: Counselors must (a) understand their own biases, values, and beliefs; (b) understand the world view of clients who may be culturally different; and (c) develop intervention strategies that are culturally appropriate.

They also indicate that there are three main *domains* that combine with these characteristics. They are (a) attitudes and beliefs, (b) knowledge, and (c) skills. To be an ethical group therapist, the issue of developing competence in all these areas is now increasingly an imperative. Although the implications for these domains are wide ranging, there are specific negative and positive outcomes related to these competencies.

Example of Multicultural Competencies: Screening Revisited

The implications for competence in diversity are broad; however, to return to the earlier example of group screening, it can be seen that this is an area that has implications for all aspects of therapy *competence* rather than just *aspiration*. For example, an African-American male client in distress is referred to a group run by two Caucasian therapists and comprising exclusively Caucasian male and female clients. The client attends once and never returns. Months later, unbeknownst to the group worker, the client has deteriorated considerably.

Although the research on group dropout is weak (McCallum et al., 2002), the research on the contribution of multicultural variables to group dropout is almost nonexistent. However, Merchant and Butler (2002), in working in a residential setting with adolescent African-American males, outlined their pregroup screening as consisting of the following questions:

1. Can you tell us about your cultural/racial heritage?
2. How would a group like this be helpful to you?
3. Would you feel comfortable sharing in a group like this?
4. What is your experience of being *a person of color* (use term preferred by individual) at this residential treatment center?

Although this questionnaire was highly context specific to that treatment setting, it does speak to the need for assessment tools that help screen for cultural variables of import to the selection of clients. This kind of instrument as part of a group screening might in combination with other screening questions, serve to better address the issue of premature dropout. Other suggestions might include questions that address Helms's (1984) stages of racial identity model as a possible predictor of group dropout or negative climate.

However, diversity questions also present a wide range of other possible ethical dilemmas. For example, a client might express that she would only join a group if another homosexual client was also present. This then presents the therapist with the dilemma of breaching the confidentiality of the other group member. Therefore, any group screening must take into account the biases, multiple identities, and likelihood that a group member might feel excluded or unsafe due to cultural or other diversity-related variables. Group workers must take care to consider the competing needs of a wide variety of ethical dictates in doing so.

Other multicultural considerations include but are not limited to (a) differing notions of confidentiality (particularly with family and extended family); (b) ideas and values around self-disclosure (and the shame associated with self-disclosure or taboos against speaking negatively about family); (c) differing interpersonal styles (and cultural beliefs behind them); (d) conflicting cultural styles of expression (e.g., conflict avoidant vs. confrontational); and (e) differing values of therapists and clients with respect to issues such as autonomy, individualism vs. collectivism, and religiocultural differences related to belief systems.

The next decades will involve increasing focus on these and other group-related diversity issues. In fact, it could be argued that group therapy offers rich potential (provided that therapists are sufficiently well trained or retrained) to offer the kind of services that might be well suited to the problems of interaction in a changing world.

QUESTION: What type of training have you had in multicultural practice? What gaps in your training exist? Where are places to get those trainings?

ETHICS IN CYBER COUNSELING WITH GROUPS

In this rapidly changing world, there has also now entered into the world of group work an issue that is racing even further ahead of ethics and best practices guidelines: cyber counseling.

As Yalom and Leszcz (2005) state: "Just a few years ago, the idea of Internet virtual group therapy seemed the stuff of fantasy and satire" (p. 520). However, as they point out, there is a developing body of research suggesting positive outcomes for technology-assisted group work. Yalom and Leszcz (2005) make a strong case for the potential efficacy of using the Internet and other technology-based applications to perform group work. They cite studies (e.g., Hopss, Pepin, & Boisvert, 2003; Luce, Winzelberg, & Zabinski, 2003) suggesting positive outcomes for clients using group cybercounseling. However, they also point out the ethical concerns related to group work utilizing technology. Page (2004) suggests that the National Board of Certified Counselors (NBCC) and ACA provide guidelines to aid clinicians in ethical decision making when conducting Internet counseling; the guidelines do not specifically refer to group counseling.

Yalom and Leszcz (2005) mention the nature of the contract, payment issues, the limits of responsiveness to online emergencies, and other key ethical issues such as those related to informed consent, confidentiality, and the requirements for a secure and reliable communication. All of these issues take on a distinctly different "flavor" when addressing group work, but group work ethical guidelines have yet to clearly elucidate what these are and how they should be handled. Adhering to the previous maxim of finding the highest ethical standard, the NBCC (2007) has guidelines for Internet counseling that includes various ways to address each of these issues. However, group will add its own unique permutation to each, with, for example, the aforementioned issue of confidentiality now including the risk that a group session or disclosure ends up somehow in the public arena.

For example, the NBCC (2007) guidelines state: "As part of the counseling orientation process, the Internet counselor explains to clients how to cope with potential misunderstandings when visual cues do not exist." However, though this is laudable, this calls into question how members can generalize interpersonal learning since so much of what we communicate is interpersonal and relies on visual cues both received and given. These and other questions have yet to be successfully resolved. That being said, as D. Robson and M. Robson (2000) indicate, this may be a very practical method of obtaining psychological services for individuals who live extremely far from mental health settings and/or those with disabilities that make it difficult for them to leave their homes.

Page (2004), however, also indicates that Internet counselors are supposed to adhere to the ethical codes and ethical standards of the location of their client and their own location. If the client is in another country, other international laws and codes may also need to be honored. Further, the author suggests that if a therapist is going to refer an individual to an Internet group, it is important that the therapist assess the individual's computer skills and his or her access to and quality of Internet services. There are many such issues and questions arising from this fledgling field and innovative practice will need equal energy devoted to maintaining the highest standards of ethical practice.

QUESTION: What ethical codes and best practice guidelines am I using as I consider cyber-counseling?

CONCLUSION

The field of group work is at a critical ethical juncture. With demographics rapidly changing, the increasing availability of technological opportunities (and their concomitant risks) and the continued challenges of training, the ethical group worker and organization must remain vigilant in maintaining the highest ethical standards. This contribution offers some guidance on current issues in ethical practice but in reality is only a starting point to stimulate discussion on what is the most ethical level of practice to aspire to. The ethical challenges facing group workers over the next few years will require the kind of action from practitioners that only begins with closing this contribution and considering, "How does this impact me and my organization?"

Now please answer the questions from the beginning of the contribution again and compare your answers.

GUIDED QUESTIONS

- What ethical code or codes are you beholden to with respect to *group work*?

- Is it unethical to skip group screening?
  (Yes / No / It depends [please state])

- Is it unethical to *not* highlight cultural differences in conflict style during conflicts between members of different cultural backgrounds?
  (Yes / No / It depends [please state])

- Is it ethical to run a group online?

- Is it unethical for the instructor of the course to also lead experiential training groups for students being trained in group work?
  (Yes / No / It depends [please state])

CONTRIBUTORS

Martyn Whittingham, PhD, is an Assistant Professor at Wright State University, where he teaches group work classes and social psychology. Dr. Whittingham supervises students in the University's Counseling and Wellness Services. He has research and practice interests in multicultural group work, uses of the interpersonal circumplex as a clinical tool, and allying science more closely to practice. Dr. Whittingham may be contacted at 053 Student Union, 3640 Colonel Glenn Highway, Dayton, OH 45435. E-mail: martyn. whittingham@wright.edu

Gregory T. Capriotti, BS, is currently a doctoral student in clinical psychology at Wright State University School of Professional Psychology in Dayton, Ohio. Prior to entering his graduate training, he received his Bachelor of Science degree at Juniata College in Huntingdon, Pennsylvania. He currently serves on the board for the Student Committee of Divisoin 49 (Group Psychology and Group Psychotherapy) of the American Psychological Association. Mr. Capriotti may be contacted by E-mail: capriotti.2@wright.edu

RESOURCES

American Counseling Association. (2005). *Code of Ethics and Standards of Practice as Approved by Governing Council, April 1997.* Alexandria, VA: Author.

American Group Psychotherapy Association. (1991). *Guidelines for Ethics.* New York: Author.

American Psychological Association. (2002). *Ethical Principles of Psychologists and Code of Conduct.* Washington, DC: Author.

Arredondo, P. (1994). Multicultural training: A response. *Counseling Psychologist, 22,* 308-314.

Association for Specialists in Group Work. (1998). Association for specialists in group work best practice guidelines. *Journal for Specialists in Group Work, 23,* 237-244.

Association for Specialists in Group Work. (1998). Association for Specialists in Group Work principles for diversity-competent group workers. *Journal for Specialists in Group Work, 24,* 7-14.

Association for Specialists in Group Work. (2000). *Professional Standards for the Training of Group Workers.* Alexandria, VA: Author.

Barlow, S. H. (2004). A strategic three-year plan to teach beginning, intermediate, and advanced group skills. *Journal for Specialists in Group Work, 29*(1), 113-126.

Corey, G., Corey, M. S., & Callanan, P. (2003) *Issues and Ethics in the Helping Professions* (6th ed.). Pacific Grove, CA: Brooks/Cole.

Corey, G., Williams, G. T., & Moline, M. M. (1995). Ethical and legal issues in group counseling. *Ethics & Behavior, 5*(2), 161-183.

Davenport, D. S. (2004). Ethical issues in the teaching of group counseling. *Journal for Specialists in Group Work, 29*(1), 43-49.

Debiak, D. (2007). Attending to diversity in group psychotherapy: An ethical imperative. *International Journal of Group Psychotherapy, 57*(1), 1-12.

Delucia-Waak, J. (1996). Multicultural group counseling: Addressing diversity to facilitate universality and self-understanding. In J. Delucia-Waak (Ed.), *Multicultural Counseling Competencies: Implications for Training and Practice.* Alexandria, VA: American Counseling Association.

Dies, R. R. (1994). *The Therapist's Role in Group Treatments.* New York: Guilford.

Dies, R. R., & Mckenzie, K. R. (1983). *Advances on Group Psychotherapy.* New York: International Universities Press.

Fuhriman, A., & Burlingame, G. M. (1994). Measuring small group process: A methodological application of chaos theory. *Small Group Research, 25*(4), 502-519.

Fuhriman, A., & Burlingame, G. M. (2001). *Handbook of Group Psychotherapy: An Empirical and Clinical Synthesis.* New York: Wiley.

Furr, S. R., & Barret, B. (2000). Teaching group counseling skills: Problems and solutions. *Counselor Education and Supervision, 40*(2), 94-104.

Gladding, S. (2003). *Group Work: A Counseling Specialty* (4th ed.). Upper Saddle River, NJ: Merrill Prentice Hall.

Helms, J. E. (1984). Toward a theoretical explanation of the effects of race on counseling: A black and white model. *The Counseling Psychologist, 12,* 153-165.

Herlihy, B., & Remley, T. P. (1995) Unified Ethical Standards: A Challenge for Professionalism. *Journal of Counseling & Development, 74*(2), 130-133

Hetzel, R., Stockton, R., & McDonnell, K. (1994, April). *Trends in Training Group Counselors.* Paper presented at the American Counseling Association Annual Convention, Minneapolis, MN.

Ivey, A. E., Pedersen, P., & Ivey, M. B. (2001). *Intentional Group Counseling: A Microskills Approach.* Belmont, CA: Brooks/Cole.

Hopss, S., Pepin, M., & Boisvert, J. (2003). The effectiveness of cognitive behavioral group therapy for loneliness via inter-relay chat among people with physical disabilities. *Psychotherapy: Theory, Research, Practice, Training, 40,* 136-147.

Kline, W. B., Falbaum, D. F., Pope, V. T., Hargraves, G. A., & Hundley, S. F. (1997). The significance of the group experience for students in counselor education: A preliminary naturalistic inquiry. *Journal for Specialists in Group Work, 22*(3), 157-166.

Lasky, G. B. (2005). Confidentiality in groups: Rate of violations, the consent process, and group leader level of experience. *Dissertation Abstracts International: Section B: The Sciences and Engineering, 66*(5-B).

Lasky, G. B., & Riva, M. T. (2006). Confidentiality and privileged communication in group psychotherapy. *International Journal of Group Psychotherapy, 56*(4), 455-476.

Luce, K., Winzelberg, A., & Zabinski, M. (2003). Internet-delivered psychological interventions for body image dissatisfaction and disordered eating. *Psychotherapy: Theory, Research, Practice, Training, 40,* 148-154.

McCallum, M., Piper, W. E., Ogrodniczuk, J. S., & Joyce, A. S. (2002). Early process and dropping out from short-term group therapy for complicated grief. *Group Dynamics: Theory, Research, and Practice, 6*(3), 243-254.

Merchant, N., & Butler, M. K. (2002). A psychoeducational group for ethnic minority adolescents in a predominantly white treatment setting. *Journal for Specialists in Group Work, 27*(3), 314-332.

Merta, R. (1999). Multicultural group work. In J. P. Trotzer (Ed.), *The Counselor and the Group: Integrating Theory, Training and Practice* (3rd ed.). Philadelphia, PA: Taylor & Francis.

Merta, R. J., & Sisson, J. A. (1991). The experiential group: An ethical and professional dilemma. *Journal for Specialists in Group Work, 16*(4), 236-245.

National Board of Certified Counselors. (2007). *The Practice of Internet Counseling.* Retrieved August 15, 2008 from http://www.nbcc.org/webethics2

Page, B. J. (2004). Online group counseling. In J. DeLucia-Waak, D. Gerrity, C.R. Kalodner, & M. Riva (Eds.), *Handbook of Group Counseling and Psychotherapy* (pp. 309-330). Thousand Oaks, CA: Sage.

Pepper, R. (2007). Too close for comfort: The impact of dual relationships on group therapy and group therapy training. *The International Journal of Group Psychotherapy, 57*(1), 13-23.

Rapin, L. (2004). Ethical and legal practice in groups. In J. DeLucia-Waak, D. Gerrity, C. R. Kalodner, & M. Riva, *Handbook of Group Counseling and Psychotherapy* (pp. 151-165). Thousand Oaks, CA: Sage.

Robson, D., & Robson, M. (2000). Ethical issues in internet counseling. *Counselling Psychology Quarterly, 12*(3), 249-257.

Smokowski, P. R., Rose, S. D., & Bacallao, M. L. (2001). Damaging experiences in therapeutic groups: How vulnerable consumers become group casualties. *Small Group Research, 32*(2), 223-251.

Sue, D. W., Arredondo, P., & McDavis, R. J. (1992). Multicultural counseling competencies and standards: A call to the profession. *Journal of Multicultural Counseling & Development, 20*(2), 64-89.

Sue, D. W., & Sue, D. (2008). *Counseling the Culturally Diverse: Theory and Practice* (5th ed.). Hoboken, NJ: Wiley & Sons.

Taylor, R. E., & Gazda, G. M. (1991). Concurrent individual and group therapy: The ethical issues. *Journal of Group Psychotherapy, Psychodrama, and Sociometry, 44*(2), 51-59.

Trotzer, J. P. (1999). *The Counselor and the Group: Integrating Theory, Training and Practice* (3rd ed.). Philadelphia, PA: Taylor & Francis.

U.S. Census Bureau. (2000). United States Census 2000. Retrieved August 15, 2008 from http://www.census.gov/

Yalom, I., with Lesczc, M. (2005). *The Theory and Practice of Group Psychotherapy* (5th ed.). Cambridge, MA: Basic Books.

Risk Management: A Perspective Based on Ethical Principles

Samuel Knapp and Leon VandeCreek

The difficulties inherent in mental health practice can be compounded when the practitioner is the subject of a disciplinary complaint, whether it is a licensing board complaint, ethics charge, malpractice suit, or another disciplinary action. Although the risk of being disciplined is relatively low, it still creates a great deal of anxiety among many practicing mental health professionals.

The purpose of this contribution is to describe practices designed to reduce the risk of being the subject of a disciplinary complaint and, at the same time, ensure close adherence to fundamental ethical principles. Our perspective is that risk management procedures, like all of professional conduct, should be based upon a solid ethical foundation. With that perspective in mind, we endorse the risk management perspective developed by the American Psychological Association Insurance Trust (Bennett et al., 2006), amplify on certain features of that risk management perspective, and give an illustration based upon a case example involving a suicidal patient.

RISK MANAGEMENT AND POSITIVE ETHICS

Many mental health professionals today conceive of ethics primarily or exclusively as a set of laws regulating a profession, as an ethics code that includes a set of proscribed behaviors, or as the adjudicatory procedures of disciplinary bodies. Consequently, the study of ethics, defined in terms of rules and punishments, often becomes anxiety producing. This reflects a "Ten Commandments" approach wherein ethics represents a fixed entity of prohibitions or commandments that must be followed. The spirit or underlying philosophy behind these commandments is seldom considered. This "dark underside" of ethics generates anxiety, defensiveness, and the potential for emotional distance from patients or others. This limited view of ethics fails to inform mental health professionals of the ways that ethics can be uplifting for those who try to function effectively. It unnecessarily presents ethics in an unpleasant manner.

Ethics could better be viewed as a way to help mental health professionals fulfill their highest potential. It could mean relying on an underlying philosophical system of thought to guide day-to-day decision making and to help mental health professionals think through thorny and complex ethical dilemmas. Ethics should not focus just on how to avoid harming others, but also on the best ways to help others (Knapp & VandeCreek, 2006). Similarly, risk management should not focus on just how to avoid harming others, but also on how to maximize benefits to others. The risk management approach of Bennett et al. (2006) does that to the extent that it presents three major risk management strategies (informed consent, consultation, and documentation,) that both protect the professional and, at the same time, promote patient or public welfare.

BASICS OF RISK MANAGEMENT

Generally the relationship between professional incompetence and the likelihood of being the subject of a disciplinary complaint or malpractice suit is positive, but in the low range of probability. That is, mental health professionals who miss the mark in their work are more likely to be subject to those complaints. However, there is an element of arbitrariness in the disciplinary process, and occasionally competent and ethical mental health professionals have complaints filed against them.

Some patients and contexts are more likely to generate a risk of being accused of ethical misconduct. Patients who are more likely to file disciplinary complaints or lawsuits are those who have difficulty forming productive relationships, such as those who have a background of being abused, who have Cluster B personality disorders (borderline, narcissistic, etc.), who are wealthy and have a sense of entitlement, or who are seriously suicidal or homicidal. The contexts in which disciplinary actions are more likely to occur include those in which there is an assessment with external implications (such as a child custody evaluation), when the patient is involved in some kind of litigation (such as being involved in an automobile accident and claiming psychological damage), or when the patient is showing life-endangering features. The characteristics of the patients interact with the context. For example, patients with serious personality disorders may be more likely to settle disagreements through litigation as opposed to working them out directly.

Although quality of services given is an important factor in whether a patient files a complaint, the quality of the relationship with the patient is also important. Data from physicians may be instructive here. Primary care physicians who have fewer claims are more likely to use more orienting statements (explaining procedures to patients), humor in their conversations, and facilitating statements (statements that encourage patients to express their concerns; Levinson et al., 1997). When asked about their reasons for filing lawsuits, patients often report that the lack of good communication helped drive their decision. They reported that they felt that the physician had devalued their opinions, delivered information poorly, failed to understand their point of view, or tried to withhold information (Beckman et al., 1994; Levinson et al., 1997). Along those lines, Brown (1994) warned against turning ethics into "a concrete wall" that separates us "from human connections" (p. 276).

NEGATIVE OR FALSE RISK MANAGEMENT PROCEDURES

Unnecessarily defensive or insensitive risk management strategies increase the vulnerability of mental health professionals to an allegation of misconduct, to the extent that they distance professionals from authentic and meaningful relationships with their patients. Of course, mental health professionals need to be cognizant of the possibilities of disciplinary consequences and to have a certain healthy amount of anxiety about liability. However, proper risk management should be driven primarily by a concern to be consistent with overarching moral principles and be designed to promote patient or public welfare. Professionals should not let their care be driven by excessive anxiety or distrust of patients.

Fear-based risk management strategies are not founded on moral principles but rather can be described as "false risk management strategies." Bennett et al. (2006) identified several of these, such as "always get a suicidal patient to sign a safety contract," or "never keep detailed records when patients present a threat to harm themselves or others" (p. 33). They also warned that "any purported risk management strategy that tells you to do something that appears to harm a patient or violates a moral principle needs to be reconsidered" (p. 32).

POSITIVE RISK MANAGEMENT STRATEGIES

Bennett et al. (2006) have identified three such positive risk-management strategies (informed consent, consultation, and documentation) that are consistent with good patient care and are based on sound ethical principles. Our model adapts and builds upon those perspectives, although we are adding a fourth strategy (redundant protections). Generally speaking, these strategies should be used openly with the goal of being as transparent as possible. These risk management strategies and their implementation principles are shown in Table 1 (below) along with their relationship to transparency and their basis in overarching ethical principles.

TABLE 1: Strategies and Their Moral Foundations

	Transparency	Overarching Moral Foundation
Informed Consent	Be as clear as possible about what you want to do together, how you propose doing it, and why.	Respect for patient autonomy and decision making
Consultation	When seeking consultation, be honest with yourself about your strengths and limitations. The best source of accurate information about yourself is others.	Beneficence
Documentation	Be accurate, honest, and diplomatic in documentation.	Beneficence
Redundant Protections	Be clear as to the purpose of the redundant strategy.	Beneficence, nonmaleficence

These strategies can be used in conjunction with each other and can be synergistic. That is, the strengths of these strategies increase when they are used together. For example, a consultation may lead a treating professional to institute more redundant protections with a patient, modify the manner of documenting treatment, or revisit elements of the informed consent process with the patient. The overlap of these risk management strategies is shown in Table 2 (p. 192).

TABLE 2: Synergy of Risk Management Strategies

	Informed Consent	Consultation	Documentation	Redundant Protections
Informed Consent		One of the goals of consultation may be to determine how to maximize patient participation in the treatment process.	The very act of documenting may generate ideas on how to maximize patient participation in the treatment process.	Periodically check with patient to ensure congruence on goals, methods, and perceptions of progress.
Consultation	Informed consent can be viewed as a consultation with the patient.		The very act of documenting may be viewed as self-consultation.	Consultations may be a redundant protection to the extent that they provide a second source of data on a patient.
Documentation	Informed consent needs to be documented.	Document all consultations.		Document redundant protections.
Redundant Protections	Patients who fully participate in treatment are more likely to provide additional data that can confirm, contradict, or modify clinical impressions.	Consultation can be viewed as a second source of data on a patient.	The very act of documenting may generate self-reflections on the patient and generate additional ideas to guide treatment.	

Mental health professionals should increase their attention to these risk management strategies whenever the risk of harm to the patient or the public increases or a deeply held moral principle is threatened. High-risk situations require the mobilization of all resources including those of the patient, other professionals, and the full resources of the treating professional. Risk management strategies have a goal of mobilizing these resources to their fullest. The goal of the informed consent process, as broadly defined, is to *maximize patient participation* in the treatment process; the consultation process, as broadly defined, is used to *engage another professional* in the treatment process; and documentation, among other things, is designed to *increase the clinician's acuity and self-awareness* of the treatment process.

INFORMED CONSENT

As much as is clinically indicated, it is desirable to maximize patient involvement in designing the goals and procedures of treatment. The most obvious way in which this occurs is through the informed consent process, although psychotherapists can maximize patient involvement in other ways as well. It is another overarching moral principle that mental health professionals should attempt to respect the decision-making autonomy of patients about whether to enter treatment, the goals of treatment, and the procedures that are used during treatment.

Good informed consent procedures involve more than just obtaining signatures on paperwork. Informed consent is an ongoing process whereby the goals and procedures of therapy are revisited as necessary. At times, the provider may need to remind the patient of certain parameters of treatment that were agreed upon when services started. At other times, new clinical information may suggest a modification in the original treatment plan. At all times, it is desirable to have a good working relationship so that patients can feel free to bring up issues of concern to them.

We use the term maximizing patient participation to emphasize that patient involvement should occur throughout the treatment process, not just at the beginning. Of course, a strong informed-consent process is very important as it sets the stage for future efforts to maximize patient participation in the treatment process.

The general rule throughout the informed-consent process is to be as transparent as possible with the patient about clinical impressions and treatment recommendations. Of course, these need to be presented tactfully. For example, telling a patient that she is a borderline is unlikely to be helpful. However, telling a patient that you are seeing fluctuating moods, disruptive interpersonal relationships, and impulsiveness may help the patient to define her problems. Nonetheless, in some high-risk situations when the life of the patient or another is at risk or another moral value is in jeopardy, it may be justified to withhold information from a patient.

Involving patients in treatment decisions may act as a second source of information about the effectiveness or course of treatment. If patients appear to be doing poorly or not responding to treatment as expected, it may be desirable to revisit the treatment goals or the informed-consent process with them again. Some questions to consider include: Are you addressing the goals that are most important for them? Is your process of treatment helpful for them? Do they wish to try another set of techniques?

CONSULTATION

Of course, it is desirable that mental health professionals act competently in their treatment of others. Competence is based on the overarching ethical principle of beneficence or promoting patient welfare. Mental health professionals can enhance their competence in many ways, such as readings, attending continuing education programs, or other formal educational programs. However, when in the middle of treatment with an actual patient, the optimal way to ensure competence is through consultation.

Consultation needs to be distinguished from supervision. Consultation is a process whereby one peer requests information or feedback from another concerning the quality of the professional service. By its very nature, consultation involves an exchange between legal equals. The mental health professional who receives the consultation still retains the right to decide what course of action to take. In contrast, supervision is an arrangement between persons who are legally unequal. The supervisee does not have independent decision-making ability. Legally, the supervisee represents an extension of the supervisor (his or her arms and legs).

Consultation is more effective when persons seeking the consultation are transparent, nondefensive, and open about their actions and feelings. The authors have had situations where, in hindsight, it seemed that the person seeking the consultation was attempting to gather support for a predetermined treatment plan. Of course, in high-risk situations there may be times when mental health professionals have a general idea of how they would like to proceed and seeking consultation as a redundant protection. Nonetheless, the consultation will be more helpful if there is openness to other ideas or perspectives.

Consultation has at least three benefits. First, the person receiving the consultation may receive new information about the clinical situation being considered. Second, the very process of seeking a consultation may help reduce high emotional arousal and help the person getting the consultation to think through situations more clearly. Finally, the consultant may be able to give feedback on the process or thinking, feelings toward the patient, or other aspects of progress with this patient.

In high-risk situations, it is recommended that the professional receiving the consultation document in writing the fact of the consultation and the general issues discussed. The legal liability to the consultant is minimal; that is, consultants who have not met the patient of interest are not likely to be subject to disciplinary action triggered by the patient. On the other hand, the consultant could be challenged by the provider who believes the consultation was faulty.

DOCUMENTATION

Documentation serves many purposes. It may be required in order to ensure compliance with insurance policies, meet legal or accreditation requirements, or used as a source of archival information for research. In addition, documentation can help promote patient welfare in that it helps mental health professionals refresh their memories and creates a record that can be sent to future or current health providers. Furthermore, many mental health professionals find that the process of creating thoughtful and well-written records can help them think through a clinical problem. To the extent that they do, good documentation is based on the overarching moral principles of beneficence (promoting patient welfare).

Of course, good records also are important for risk management purposes in that they protect mental health professionals in the event that there are allegations of misconduct. From a legal perspective, the general rule is, "if it isn't written down, it didn't happen." The authors have known malpractice attorneys who reported that they have had great difficulty defending mental health professionals who have poor records, even though they believe that the quality of care was acceptable or, at times, even commendable. On the other hand, nothing deters a frivolous or marginal suit quicker than documentation that shows how the clinical decisions were based on reasonable clinical judgments.

Good records should reflect a provider's willingness to be transparent, in that the provider should record information accurately and thoroughly enough to justify the clinical decisions made. Of course, honesty needs to be balanced with diplomacy, and there is no need to include gratuitous information that could harm or embarrass the patient unless it is essential to fulfill a clinical need. For example, the fact that a patient may be unattractive physically should not be recorded unless it is directly related to a clinical problem (e.g., a patient was depressed following comments about his physical appearance).

Harris (Bennett et al., 2006) has used the analogy of writing notes in the same manner in which his 8th-grade teacher graded algebra homework. That is, the teacher gave partial credit if the students wrote down their work and thereby documented that the decision-making processes that they used were reasonable even if the final answer was not correct. Similarly, mental health professionals should write their decision-making processes in their notes, especially in high-risk situations. The general goal is to be as transparent as possible in decision making. If it ever became necessary to review the work of the psychotherapist, the reviewer should be able to understand the information used and the reasoning of the psychotherapist for the decisions made. Even if a tragedy were to occur and, for example, a patient died from a suicide, ideally the reviewer would be able to say that, given the information that was available at the time, the decisions of the psychotherapist were reasonable.

Good psychotherapy notes are legible, comprehensive, and internally consistent. In addition, according to Rudd (2006), one rule of thumb in dealing with suicidal patients is to never raise a high-risk issue without addressing it in the notes. For example, do not write about such an issue (e.g., "Patient expressed interest in harming his roommate") without addressing or closing the issue in a subsequent note (e.g., "Patient realizes that he overreacted to his roommate and they are getting along a lot better now"). Good record-keeping habits that help mental health professionals keep patient welfare in mind act as a "redundant protection," or a check on the provider and the treatment of the patient.

The general rule of Bennett et al. (2006) is to increase the level of documentation as the degree of risk (to the patient, others, or to the mental health professional) increases. As noted above, some patients or contexts create a higher risk to mental health providers. Whenever patients show life-endangering qualities, it is useful to increase the detail and quality of the documentation.

REDUNDANT PROTECTIONS

Redundant protections may not be indicated in all high-risk situations, but they provide an invaluable source of protection. They are what one workshop participant called "the belts and suspenders" approach. The concept of redundant protections is informed by medical errors and safety research. For example, when going to a hospital for a medical procedure such as surgery, it is typically required that every person who has an interaction with the patient verify the patient's name and procedure to be performed. Consequently, if one health care professional errs and gets the wrong name or the wrong procedure, the next health care professional dealing with the patient will catch the error. Redundant protections are also found in transportation safety and other arenas. Commercial airplanes, for example, are required to have a pilot and a co-pilot. In the event that an adverse event happens to one of them that prevents the person from handling the controls, the other will be able to take over the plane.

For example, when dealing with a depressed patient, it may be desirable to have a source of information about the patient's well-being in addition to the self-report of the patient. The second source of data could include access to a spouse or other family member, or even a brief screening instrument given to the patient before a psychotherapy appointment. The general rule is to be transparent with the patient about the reason that a second source of data is being sought.

In a sense, all risk management strategies involve a certain amount of redundant protections, in that informed consent ensures that the patient's perspective is more fully represented, consultation ensures that the perspective of an outside professional is present, and documentation helps ensure that treating professionals themselves are attending to the salient assessment and treatment issues.

CASE EXAMPLE: A SUICIDAL PATIENT

The suicide of a patient is an occupational risk for all psychotherapists. The odds for losing a patient to suicide are 1 in 2 for psychiatrists, 1 in 5 for psychologists (Chemtob et al., 1989), and 1 out of 9 for psychology trainees (Kleespies, Penk, & Forsyth, 1993). In addition, 16% of the members of the Pennsylvania Psychological Association reported having at least one patient suicide in a 12-month period (Knapp & Keller, 2004).

Suicides take an emotional toll on treating professionals as well as the patient's family. It is not uncommon for psychotherapists to undergo a grieving process or even a depression after the suicide of a patient. The authors know of psychotherapists who have left the field or retired after a patient suicide, even though there were no indications of negligent conduct on their part.

In addition to the personal tragedy for the family and the pain caused to the treating psychotherapists, patient suicides or attempted suicides are a frequent cause of malpractice suits (5.4% for psychologists and 17% for psychiatrists; Bender, 2005). However, they are far less likely to be a cause of a suit for an individual being treated as an outpatient. The general legal view is that outpatient therapists have far less control over the behavior of their patients and therefore cannot be held to the same standards as inpatient units, where the behavior of the patients can be more closely monitored.

Most psychotherapists will treat many suicidal patients throughout their careers. It is not uncommon for psychotherapists to have at least one patient with strong suicidal ideation at any given time in their practices. Among respondents to the National Comorbidity Survey (a study of the prevalence of mental disorders), 13.5% reported suicidal ideation, 3.9% had a plan, and 4.6% had made an attempt sometime during their lives (Kessler, Borges, & Walters, 1999).

Consider the following case example* and how a psychotherapist might respond to it using the ethically based risk management strategies.

Calvin, a 21-year-old college senior who recently has broken up with his long-standing girlfriend presents for treatment with major depression, strong suicidal ideation, and access to weapons in his apartment. In an effort to self-medicate himself he is abusing prescription and nonprescription medication.

He is assigned as a patient to Dr. Hirokotu.

Dr. Hirokotu starts the treatment the same as she does for most clients. That is, she listens to Calvin's description of his presenting problems, conducts a mental status examination, and completes a social history. When she learns of the extent of his suicidal ideation, she immediately considers the three processes for treating suicidal and life-endangering patients described by Appelbaum (1985): assessment, development of a treatment plan, and implementation of the treatment plan. Each of these processes is crucial, and an error in any of these stages could be fatal. Of course, these processes are not always sequential, as information may be acquired during the implementation of the treatment plan that influences the assessment of the degree of dangerousness, and so on. The application of these risk management processes across Appelbaum's three processes is shown in Table 3.

TABLE 3: Risk Management Across the Processes of Assessing and Treating Dangerous Patients

	Assessment	Development of Treatment Plan	Implementation of Treatment Plan
Informed Consent	In addition to the regular informed consent process, does the patient understand the goals of the assessment? Are efforts made to enlist the cooperativeness of the patient in the process?	Is the patient involved in the development of the treatment plan as much as possible? If a safety agreement is used, does the patient participate in its development?	Is the patient involved in the implementation of the treatment plan as much as possible? Is the patient involved in modifying the plan? Is the patient involved in any revisions to the safety plan?

---

*Names and characteristics in all case examples have been changed to protect confidentiality.

TABLE 3: Risk Management Across the Processes of Assessing and Treating Dangerous Patients *(Continued)*

	Assessment *(Continued)*	Development of Treatment Plan	Implementation of Treatment Plan
Consultation	Although a preliminary determination of dangerousness needs to be made on the spot, does the provider incorporate data from consultants, especially if life-endangering features are areas outside of his or her expertise?	Does the treatment plan reference the recommendations of consultants?	If there are problems in compliance, or the patient otherwise fails to respond to treatment, is consultation sought and documented?
Documentation	Increase the level of documentation as the degree of threat increases. Does the documentation include the methods used and form a basis for the conclusions reached? Are the results of consultations included in the documentation? If disagreements with consultants occur, are they documented and accounted for? If discrepancies occur in the sources of data, are they noted and accounted for?	Does the documentation link the assessment to the treatment plan? Are the results of consultations included in the documentation? If disagreements with consultants occur, are they documented? Document all major treatment decisions: to hospitalize or not; to refer for medications or not, and so on.	Does the documentation include compliance with and responsiveness to treatment? Are any issues raised in the assessment and development of the treatment plan addressed? Are the results of consultations included in the documentation? If disagreements with consultants occur, are they documented? As treatment progresses, document all major treatment decisions: to hospitalize or not; to refer for medications or not, and so on.
Redundant Protections	Is the determination of dangerousness made on the basis of multiple measures? Can the discrepancies in the measures be accounted for? Are collateral contacts used as much as is clinically indicated?	Are multiple sources of data used in developing the treatment plan?	Are there ongoing assessments of the responsiveness to treatment? Are mechanisms in place to check clinical intuition? Are collateral contacts used as much as is clinically indicated?

APPLICATION OF RISK MANAGEMENT STRATEGIES

The common risk management strategies are informed consent, consultation, documentation, and redundant protections. Each of these strategies will be reviewed with application to this patient.

Informed Consent

Dr. Hirokotu knew that Calvin was depressed, but nonetheless took great pains to describe the treatment process to him. She tried to involve him in all treatment decisions. She asked: Do you want a collateral contact present? Do you want your parents to be involved? Do you want to consider medications? In each of these decisions, she encouraged Calvin to consider the advantages and disadvantages.

Recognizing that Calvin was depressed and in emotional turmoil, and was therefore poor at generating options for himself, she was more active with suicide prevention suggestions at first, but with the general goal of moving Calvin from external to internal control. She tried to maximize Calvin's involvement in treatment as much as was clinically indicated. This was especially important when dealing with Calvin so that he understood the crisis management systems in place, what to expect if there were a referral to a psychopharmacologist, and so on.

She involved Calvin in treatment through a safety agreement that was created collaboratively. As noted above, it is a false risk management strategy to believe that safety contracts are always indicated. In fact, under some circumstances, they can be clinically contraindicated. To date, there is no evidence indicating that safety agreements are effective in reducing patient suicides (Kroll, 2000). In addition, safety agreements can be clinically contraindicated if they are used primarily to reduce the anxiety of the provider or if they are imposed without input from the patient. A safety agreement is no substitute for a comprehensive evaluation and treatment plan. The mere fact that Calvin might have acquiesced to a safety contract provides little assurance that he will be safe.

Here is Calvin's safety agreement:

Sometimes when I feel depressed I begin to catastrophize my problems, forget about the people who love me, and become overly pessimistic. When I start feeling really depressed, I can read this reminder that I am gradually getting better, that I have friends and family to call when I feel low, and I have activities that I really enjoy. If the suicidal thoughts appear especially strong, I will call the clinic at xxx-xxxx.

Of course the actual agreement needs to vary depending on the wishes of patients and the use of language that is unique to them.

Consultation

Dr. Hirokotu, like other mental health professionals, routinely asks every patient about present and past suicide ideation or attempts during the first meeting. She knows that no patient is too healthy to be asked. She also follows the general rule of thumb to never treat a highly suicidal or seriously depressed patient without consultation. In addition, Dr. Hirokotu routinely seeks consultations when seeing individuals with coexisting serious personality disorders or substance abuse disorders. Calvin did not appear to have a personality disorder, but she did seek consultation on how to interpret and intervene with his heavy drinking.

Documentation

Dr. Hirokotu increases the level of her documentation when she learns of the extent of Calvin's suicidal ideation. Among other things, she is precise and clear about decision making. For example, when she describes a suicidal "gesture," she operationally defines it as an act that Calvin did in the absence of a clear intent to kill himself (in this case it was most likely to obtain some psychological relief). She described the means used, extent of injuries, and the medical attention received. She also reported her method of acquiring information about suicidality (self-report, report from others, tests or screening inventories). She described suicidal ideation clearly, including its frequency, intensity, and duration (whether it was chronic or acute) and its relationship to external stressors or events that tended to precipitate it.

Although Calvin was consistent in his description, Dr. Hirokotu was prepared to describe apparently contradictory information and attempt to reconcile or explain it (such as a divergence between information in the interview and that obtained in a screening inventory or from a third party). As recommended by Rudd (2006), she would not open a risk factor without closing it. That is, she would not identify a stressor or trait as creating risk without having future notes indicating how she addressed it. For example, she would not write, "Calvin says he will commit suicide if he cannot start getting dates" without indicating in her notes how she was addressing his reactions to those relationship issues. Protective features were documented.

Dr. Hirokotu described her treatment plan using the "8ᵗʰ-grade algebra teacher model"; that is, she described how she reached her decision about treatment methods and why it was clinically indicated. In Calvin's case, this meant obtaining a supplementary assessment from a drug and alcohol expert to determine if there was a coexistent drug or alcohol problem.

The extent to which the patient complied with treatment was documented, as were efforts to improve compliance or address noncompliance.

Redundant Protections

Dr. Hirokotu documented the redundant protections she used. In this case, she used a brief screening instrument for suicidality before seeing Calvin for each session. She knew that it is common for depressed patients, when in the treatment room, to feel a temporary boost in their spirits and to minimize the intensity or frequency of their suicidal impulses. However, a brief screening instrument given at the start of treatment provided a second source of information and acted as a check on Calvin. For example, if Calvin were to indicate high suicidality on the form, she would make suicidality a greater focus of treatment than if Calvin were to deny or minimize suicidality at the beginning of the treatment session. Of course, these sources of information should be documented.

In some situations, family members or friends may be another source of data. With the patient's permission, they may act as a second source of eyes and identify potential problems or opportunities for interventions.

CONCLUSION

Risk management need not be an unpleasant topic that focuses on personal protections at the risk of patient welfare. On the contrary, this contribution has shown that patient welfare is enhanced when ethically based risk management procedures are used. With careful forethought, these risk management strategies can mobilize the resources of the patient, the professional, and consultants in ensuring that the highest quality of service is provided.

CONTRIBUTORS

Samuel Knapp, EdD, has been the Director of Professional Affairs of the Pennsylvania Psychological Association since 1987. He has written or coauthored 15 books, 10 book chapters, and 90 peer-reviewed publications, and conducted 180 professional workshops. His major area of interest is in ethical issues. Dr. Knapp may be contacted at the Pennsylvania Psychological Association, 416 Forster Street, Harrisburg, PA 17102. E-mail: sam@papsy.org

Leon VandeCreek, PhD, is a licensed psychologist who is the past dean and current Professor in the School of Professional Psychology at Wright State University in Dayton, Ohio. He has been awarded the Diplomate in Clinical Psychology and he is a Fellow of several divisions of the American Psychological Association. His interests include professional training and ethical/legal issues related to professional education and practice. Dr. VandeCreek has served as President of the Pennsylvania Psychological Association, Chair of the APA Insurance Trust, Chair of the Board of Educational Affairs of the APA, and Treasurer of the Ohio Psychological Association. In 2005 he served as President of the Division of Psychotherapy of the APA. He has authored and coauthored about 150 professional presentations and publications, including 17 books. From 1992 to 2007 he served as Senior Editor of the *Innovations in Clinical Practice: A Source Book* series, published by Professional Resource Press. Dr. VandeCreek may be contacted at the Ellis Human Development Institute, 9 N. Edwin C. Moses Boulevard, Dayton, OH 45407. E-mail: leon.vandecreek@wright.edu

RESOURCES

Appelbaum, P. (1985). *Tarasoff* and the clinician: Problems in fulfilling the duty to protect. *American Journal of Psychiatry, 142,* 425-429.

Beckman, H. B., Markakis, K. M., Suchman, A. L., & Frankel, R. M. (1994). The doctor-patient relationship and malpractice. Lessons from plaintiff depositions. *Archives of Internal Medicine, 154,* 1365-1370.

Bender, E. (2005). Cost of malpractice suits requires more than money. *Psychiatric News, 40,* 25.

Bennett, B., Bricklin, P., Harris, E., Knapp, S., VandeCreek, L., & Youngrenn, J. (2006). *Assessing and Managing Risk in Professional Practice: An Individualized Approach.* Rockville, MD: APAIT.

Brown, L. (1994). Concrete boundaries and the problem of literal-mindedness: A response to Lazarus. *Ethics and Behavior, 4,* 275-281.

Chemtob, C., Bauer, G., Hamada, R., Pelowski, S., & Muraoka, M. (1989). Patient suicide: Occupational hazard for psychologists and psychiatrists. *Professional Psychology: Research and Practice, 20,* 294-300.

Kessler, R., Borges, G., & Walters, E. (1999). Prevalence of and risk factors for lifetime suicide attempts in the National Comorbidity Survey. *Archives of General Psychiatry, 56,* 617-626.

Kleespies, P., Penk, W., & Forsyth, J. (1993). The stress of patient suicidal behavior during clinical training: Incidence, impact, and recovery. *Professional Psychology: Research and Practice, 24,* 293-303.

Knapp, S., & Keller, P. (2004). Survey reveals stressful events for psychologists. *The Pennsylvania Psychologist, 64,* 6, 8.

Knapp, S., & VandeCreek, L. (2006). *Practical Ethics: A Positive Approach.* Washington, DC: American Psychological Association.

Kroll, J. (2000). The use of no-suicide contracts by psychiatrists in Minnesota. *American Journal of Psychiatry, 157,* 1684-1686.

Levinson, W., Roter, D., Mullooly, J., Dull, V., & Frankel, R. (1997). Physician patient communication: The relationship with malpractice claims among primary care physicians and surgeons. *Journal of the American Medical Association, 277,* 553-559.

Rudd, M. D. (2006). *Assessment and Management of Suicidality.* Sarasota, FL: Professional Resource Press.

Introduction to Section III: Assessment Instruments and Client Handouts

The ASSESSMENT INSTRUMENTS AND CLIENT HANDOUTS section includes instruments and handouts that practitioners can use to collect and organize information. Although some of the items included here have been formally developed and normed, others were designed for informal application and should not be used as formal instruments or for making specific diagnoses.

The value of forms and instruments depends upon their application by the clinicians who use them. It is important to emphasize that these forms are not necessarily designed to generate the types of inferences often associated with more formalized tests that have a long history of use. Readers should recognize the potential as the stated limitations of these materials and use them in accordance with accepted ethical principles and practice standards. It is assumed that anyone who uses these instruments will have a general clinical knowledge of the areas being evaluated.

Given the limitations noted previously, we have attempted to ensure that the materials that follow include sufficient information to allow readers to evaluate their appropriate application. Certain basic information and instructions have been included with each contribution, and the Resource sections contain references to more detailed materials and studies. Readers who wish to use these materials are advised to obtain the additional resources. If there is a desire to use the material for research purposes, most authors would appreciate being contacted so that data may be shared.

Four assessment instruments have been included in this section. The first one, Suicidal Older Adult Protocol (SOAP) by William Fremouw and colleagues, presents a suicide assessment protocol which can be used by mental health workers to provide an initial objective assessment of suicide risk in individuals 65 years and older. The second instrument is a Mental Status Examination by William F. Doverspike, which provides an outline of major content categories along with a brief narrative description of the client's mental status. The third assessment instrument is a Rating of Cognitive and Behavioral Status in Older Adults (R-CABS-OA) by Jeffery B. Allen, which can be useful in gathering cognitive and behavioral symptom information from a variety of sources including the client, caregiver, and clinician. The final contribution to the assessment instrument section is a treatment plan worksheet. William F. Doverspike's treatment plan worksheet can be instrumental in assisting clients to transform presenting problems into goals, and to break down goals into specific objectives needed to attain them.

This section also includes two client handouts. The first handout provides information on sleep disorders including different types of sleep problems and tips for better sleep. The second handout addresses the definition and detection of elder abuse.

Suicidal Older Adult Protocol–SOAP

William Fremouw, Katrina McCoy, Elizabeth A. Tyner, and Robert Musick

Older adults, 65 years and older, comprise 12.4% of the United States population yet account for 16% of completed suicides. The rate of older adult suicide is 14.3 per 100,000 people as compared to the overall rate for adults: 11.1 per 100,000 people. Approximately 14 older adult suicides occur each day – approximately one every hour and a half. Males complete 84.6% of older adult suicides, a rate 7.7 times greater than females. White males over the age of 85 are at the highest risk for completed suicide of any demographic category: 48.4 per 100,000 individuals. Conversely, for women, the rate of suicide typically peaks during middle adulthood (ages 45-49) and declines after age 60 (Centers for Disease Control and Prevention [CDC], 2006; see Figure 1 below).

Although older adults attempt suicide less frequently than younger individuals, they complete suicide at a higher rate. Among individuals over the age of 65, there is approximately one completed suicide for every four attempts. In comparison, among all age groups combined, there is one completed suicide for every 25 attempts, and among individuals ages 15-24, every 100-200 suicide attempts yield only one completed suicide (CDC, 2006).

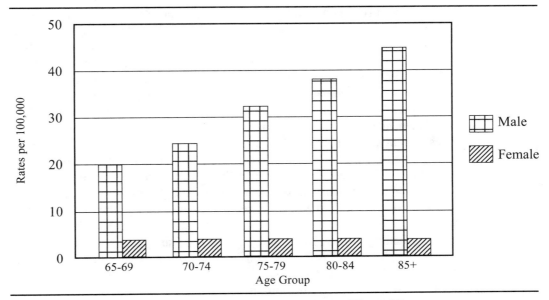

Figure 1. Suicide Rates for Ages 65 to 85 +
(Source: Centers for Disease Control and Prevention, 2006)

Conwell (2004) suggests that suicide attempts among older adults are more fatal as compared with younger individuals due to three factors: (a) the increased physical frailty of older adults, (b) the increased probability that they live alone, and (c) the increased likelihood that they use more lethal means. In fact, 72% of older adult suicides were completed using a firearm. Ninety-two percent of men completed suicide using a firearm, whereas 8% of women used this lethal means. Depression is the most important cause of older adult suicide, while alcohol or substance abuse plays a lesser function as compared with younger individuals (CDC, 2006).

RATIONALE FOR THE SOAP

Although the assessment and treatment of older adult suicidal behavior is extremely important, there is no current measure or procedure that is widely accepted. Luoma, Pearson, and Martin (2002) report that three quarters of older suicide victims had been seen by their primary care providers within 1 month, and almost one half were treated within 7 days of their suicides, yet the physicians did not detect the risk of imminent suicide. Therefore, the development of a protocol to assist in the screening for suicidal risk is clearly needed. The Suicidal Older Adult Protocol (SOAP) for ages 65+, described in this contribution, is the third guided clinical interview for assessment of suicide risk. The first was the Adolescent Suicide Assessment Protocol (ASAP; Fremouw et al., 2005) for ages 13 to 24, followed by the Suicidal Adult Assessment Protocol (SAAP; Fremouw et al., 2008) for assessment of individuals ages 25 to 65. All the measures are based on empirical research specific to the population. They began with a review of suicide risk assessment factors by Fremouw, De Perczel, and Ellis (1990) and have been updated with comprehensive reviews such as *Practice Guidelines for the Assessment and Treatment of Patients with Suicidal Behaviors* (American Psychiatric Association [APA], 2003). Because the SOAP is specific to older adults age 65 and older, the SAAP was revised based on the literature reviews by Conwell and Duberstein (e.g., Conwell, 2004; Conwell & Duberstein, 2001; Duberstein & Heisel, 2006) to focus on the unique and specific factors involved in suicide among older adults. In addition, the SOAP reflects the conceptual contributions of Bryan and Rudd (2006), who view suicide risk assessment as the combination of a baseline category of risk with identification of acute, short-term, exacerbating factors.

The SOAP integrates the above resources to form a guided clinical interview for the systematic assessment of adults aged 65 and above. It is organized into sections based on a general risk assessment model which includes both static and dynamic factors. The static factors are *demographic* and *historical* variables which cannot be changed by intervention. The dynamic factors include *clinical*, *contextual*, and *protective* variables which have potential for modification. The clinical factors are further divided into two categories based on relative permanence: clinical-stable variables such as physical illness, and clinical-acute variables such as current suicidal plans, which are more dynamic and can quickly change.

The SOAP is a guided clinical interview for adult suicide risk similar in format to the HCR-20 (Webster et al., 1995) and the ASAP (Fremouw et al., 2005), which assess risk of violence by psychiatric inpatients and risk of adolescent suicide, respectively. Based on interview, collateral information, and record review, an individual is evaluated on 18 items. Each item is rated as low, medium, or high, and 4 items have an additional level of extreme risk. As suggested by Simon (2004), the assessment of suicide risk is based on clinical judgment and not a total score. This permits consideration of unique or idiosyncratic factors that would be missed in a standard test or single number. After completion of the protocol, the number of items rated as low risk, medium risk, high risk, or extreme risk are tallied. Other unique factors are considered, and then the interviewer assigns an individual to one of three overall risk categories: low risk, medium risk, or high risk for suicide.

The operationalization of the items into low, medium, high, and extreme risk levels is partially based on research using Standardized Mortality Ratios (SMR). Harris and Barraclough (1997) conducted a metaanalysis of 249 studies which examined 44 medical and psychiatric disorders and suicide completions (not just attempts) with at least 2 years of follow-up data. They calculated a standardized mortality ratio (SMR) based on the relative risk of suicide for a particular disorder as compared to the expected rate of suicide in the general population. It reported, for example, that individuals with previous suicide attempts had an SMR of 38:1 and that individuals with a diagnosis of major depression had an SMR of 20:1 (as compared to the general population, where the value of the SMR is 1:1). Additional items not included in the Harris and Barraclough (1997) metaanalysis were coded in low, medium, high, or extreme risk based on other empirical literature which reported risk ratios. The four categories of risk are defined by increasing SMR odds ratios of suicide.

Categories	_Odds_	
Low Risk	1 - 2.9	:1
Medium Risk	3 - 4.9	:1
High Risk	5 - 14.9	:1
Extreme Risk	15+	:1

SOAP MANUAL

The SOAP is organized into six factors: *Demographic, Historical, Clinical-Stable, Clinical-Acute, Contextual,* and *Protective.* Demographic items are static, or unchangeable, and include gender, age, race, and marital status. *Historical* items are also static and consist of a history of suicide attempts and recent, planned serious suicide attempts (made in the last 3 months). *Clinical-Stable* items are Axis I diagnoses, physical illness, and functional impairment of activities of daily living (ADL). *Contextual* items are dynamic, or changeable, and include recent loss/stressors, access to lethal means, and social isolation. *Clinical-Acute* items include psychic distress, hopelessness, burdensomeness, and plans or preparations for suicide. These are rated by the client. *Protective* items are also dynamic and include moral objections, family-related concerns, and current mental health treatment. Additionally, an *Other Considerations* section is included to account for any idiosyncratic items, strengths, and vulnerabilities that may contribute to suicide risk of the individual.

The following sections describe the coding guidelines for the 18 items. The SOAP protocol is contained on pages 210-211. Unless otherwise noted, the American Psychiatric Association's *Practice Guidelines* (APA, 2003) and Conwell (2004) form the empirical basis for the coding of each item.

A. Demographic Factors

1. Gender/Race/Age. Females of any age or race are coded as Low Risk. Nonwhite males of any age are also coded as Low Risk. White males 65-80 years old are coded as Medium Risk, and white males above the age of 80 are coded as High Risk.

2. Marital Status. Married individuals are coded as Low Risk, and all others – single, divorced, or widowed – are coded as Medium Risk.

B. Historical Factors

3. Prior Suicide Attempts. A suicide attempt is any deliberate act of self-harm which has at least some probability of death. One previous attempt is coded as High Risk, while two or more previous attempts are coded as Extreme Risk. Spaces are provided to record the history of suicide attempts in terms of dates, means, and whether medical treatment (abbreviated Tx) was provided.

4. Recent, Planned Serious Attempt(s). A planned, nonimpulsive suicide attempt within the previous 3 months which had moderate lethality (i.e., requiring medical intervention) is coded as Extreme Risk.

C. Clinical Factors – Stable

5. Axis I Diagnosis. Diagnoses of dementia, anxiety disorders, and schizophrenia are coded as Low Risk. A diagnosis of substance abuse is coded as Medium Risk. A diagnosis of major depressive disorder or bipolar disorder is coded as Extreme Risk. Axis I diagnoses can be obtained from medical records or a comprehensive assessment.

6. Physical Illness. For females, the presence of illness does not elevate suicide risk and is therefore coded as Low Risk. For males, the presence of illness elevates suicide risk as mediated by depression (Conwell, 2004) and is coded as Medium Risk.

7. Functional Impairment of ADL. Activities of Daily Living (ADL) include, but are not limited to, tasks such as bathing, dressing, eating, cleaning, cooking, and traveling. Impairment of ADL elevates suicide risk as mediated by depression. Moderate impairment of ADL is coded as Medium Risk, and high impairment of ADL is coded as High Risk.

D. Contextual Factors

8. Recent Loss/Stressors. The death of a loved one within the last 4 years is coded as Medium Risk. Family discord (e.g., marital conflict), financial stressors (e.g., job loss, financial instability, and bankruptcy), and caregiving responsibilities (e.g., responsibility for a child or dependant adult) are coded as either Medium Risk or High Risk depending on the number of risk factors present. If only one of the three risk factors is present (i.e., family discord, or financial stressors, or caregiving responsibilities), code as Medium Risk. If more than one of the three risk factors is present (in any combination), code as High Risk.

9. Access to Lethal Means. Method of suicide is often selected on the basis of convenience and availability.

9a. If unlocked, loaded firearms are easily available (in residence or vehicle), code as Medium Risk. If a firearm has been recently purchased (within the last year), code as High Risk.

9b. If pills with potentially lethal dosages or poisons are easily available, code as Medium Risk. If pills with potentially lethal dosages or poisons are being stockpiled (accumulated and stored for future use), code as High Risk.

10. Social Isolation. Living alone in the absence of trusted friends or confidants is coded as Medium Risk. [Note: living alone, yet possessing trusted friends or confidants, does not elevate risk for suicide.]

E. Clinical Factors – Acute

The following items should be rated by the client on the 4-point scale provided in the protocol.

11. Psychic Distress. The client should rate her or his current level of psychological misery or distress.

12. Hopelessness. The client should rate her or his current belief that the future is hopeless; that life will not get better.

13. Burdensomeness. The client should rate her or his perception that she or he is a burden on other people.

14. Suicide Plan and Method. Client should rate the presence and, if applicable, the specificity of her or his plan to commit suicide and the methods available to do so.

F. Protective Factors

Protective factors are dynamic and significantly reduce the chance of an individual committing suicide. These factors lessen the risk of suicide by ameliorating existing risk factors. Because the absence of protective factors increases risk of suicide, reverse scoring is used for these items.

15. Moral Objections. The presence of moral or religious beliefs that suicide is a sin or immoral should be coded Low Risk.

16. Family-Related Concerns. Responsibility for family (including, but not limited to children) and recognition of belongingness to and connection with family members should be coded Low Risk.

17. Mental Health Treatment for Mood Disorder. The absence of mood disorder (major depressive disorder, or bipolar disorder) or current treatment of mood disorder should be coded as Low Risk. The presence of a mood disorder that is not currently being treated should be coded as Medium Risk.

18. Other Reasons for Living. Client should be asked to enumerate any additional reasons for living that may serve as protective factors for not attempting suicide. Lack of *any* reasons for living should be coded as Medium Risk.

Other Considerations

Suicide risk consists of an intricate combination of multiple risk factors. Checklists do not always account for idiosyncratic risk factors, strengths, and vulnerabilities. List anything here that should be considered as risk or protective factors for the individual.

Response Guidelines

After the interviewer rates each of the 18 items, the total number of items in each risk category should be totaled. The interviewer then determines the number of the nine High Risk and the four Extreme Risk items that were endorsed. If these High and Extreme Risk items were from the static demographic or historical factors, then the baseline level for risk is elevated to a "chronic high risk" (Bryan & Rudd, 2006). Next, the items endorsed under the Contextual, Clinical-Acute, and Protective factor are reviewed to determine if acute risk is elevated due to recent stressors, feelings of hopelessness, and so on, or absence of protective factors. Based on an overall review of the items, baseline of risk, plus current dynamic factors (and including any "other considerations"), the interviewer makes an OVERALL RISK APPRAISAL as Low, Medium, or High and proceeds with the appropriate responses to ensure the safety of the client.

Listed on page 2 of the SOAP protocol are 11 possible actions to be considered plus an "other" action. As first presented by Fremouw et al. (1990), these actions are listed in a hierarchical order for consideration but may be employed in any order provided the professional has a rationale for the action taken. It is necessary to document the actions taken and the rationale for each action. Furthermore, consultation with peers or supervisors is considered essential when dealing with High- or Extreme-Risk individuals. The use of the SOAP, consultation, and documentation will demonstrate that the mental health professional has exercised a high standard of professional judgment and has engaged in a "best practice" assessment and case management for patients.

If the individual is in the Low-Risk Category, then the original referral question should be pursued with lower concern about suicidal risk at the time. The evaluator should continue to monitor for change in risk factors such as recent loss, stressors, onset of depression or hopelessness, or social isolation, and reevaluate if acute changes have occurred.

If the individual is above the Low-Risk Category, several actions should be taken. First, strongly consider notifying family, caregivers, and significant others, as this extends care to a setting other than a clinician's office. These individuals often play crucial roles in continued monitoring of risk as well as taking specific precautions, such as the removal of firearms from the home. As outlined in the Actions Taken portion of the protocol, the evaluator should consider (a) referring for increased frequency of outpatient treatment, (b) referring for psychiatric consultation (and possible medications), and (c) consulting with a colleague or supervisor regarding the risk assessment. At minimum, these three steps are strongly encouraged for individuals in the Medium-Risk Category. Taking these actions would intensify treatment, provide additional resources such as medication, and ensure that the evaluator has consulted with another professional regarding this risk appraisal. Peer consultation demonstrates concern and sensitivity regarding the individual's risk and needs. Documenting the consultation is important to demonstrate appropriate professional action.

Additional actions that can be taken for clients in the Medium- or High-Risk categories are contracting for No Harmful Behaviors. These contracts are one of the many therapeutic strategies widely used; the contracts have strong clinical acceptance and demonstrate to the patient the concern of the therapist for the patient's welfare. However, the contract alone is not sufficient to ensure that the patient will not impulsively harm himself or herself.

Notifying the family, caregivers, and/or significant others is strongly encouraged. However, if the danger of harm is not imminent, it is desirable to ask the patient's permission to notify family, caregivers, and/or significant others prior to breaching confidentiality. If the danger to self is clear and imminent, guidelines for confidentiality do not apply, because the mental health professional must act to protect the life of the person at risk. Other parties could be informed of the patient's risk and asked to help with social support and assistance in obtaining treatment.

Reducing access to firearms and other lethal means, such as stockpiled medications or poisons, is imperative for clients at Medium or High risk. How this is accomplished would depend on where the firearms or medications/poisons are stored. Involving other parties to reduce this access or remove these potentially life-ending means would be the most conservative approach. Simply asking a patient to remove the harmful means would not be sufficient to assure that this major step is taken. In short, reducing access to lethal means requires the involvement of other parties.

Notifying legal authorities and/or Child Protective Services of risk to self or others should be considered if the suicidal risk is arising from current maltreatment through neglect or abuse or if the patient has angry/aggressive thoughts toward others in addition to himself or herself. Ethical guidelines require that the mental health professional carefully assess potential dangerousness to others and act with a "duty to protect" others who may be at risk. Notifying legal authorities and/or potential targets of risk are possible appropriate actions when danger extends to others (Fremouw et al., 1990). Finally, the mental health professional should consult with supervisors prior to notifying other agencies.

If an individual is in the High Risk category for suicidal behaviors, then increased therapeutic care is warranted. Referring the individual to day treatment or voluntary or crisis hospitalization is strongly recommended. Individuals at High Risk for suicidal behaviors are vulnerable to act on their suicidal ideation with little warning. Placing individuals in a more protected, intensive therapeutic environment would help monitor potential risk and provide treatment to lower that risk.

If an individual is unwilling to voluntarily commit to more intensive treatment, and he or she is demonstrating clear danger through suicidal planning, then involuntary hospitalization should be considered. The decision to seek involuntary hospitalization would require consultation with a supervisor. Although involuntary commitment may be necessary, it is sometimes countertherapeutic because the individual does not desire to be hospitalized. Therefore, this action is always considered the last resort and the most restrictive alternative for treatment.

CONCLUSION

The SOAP is an 18-item guided clinical interview for older adult suicidal risk based on the empirical literature of suicide completion risk factors. This protocol will provide a comprehensive evaluation of a person's current suicidal risk and guidelines for appropriate case management.

SOAP – Suicidal Older Adult Protocol (Ages 65-85)

Name_____ Age_____ Gender <u>M / F</u> Date_____ Rater_____

A. Demographic Factors

1. Gender/Race/Age

	L	M	H	E
Female/Nonwhite/65+ = L		░	░	
Female/White/65+ = L				
Male/Nonwhite/65+ = L				
Male/White/65-80 = M	░		░	
Male/White/80+ = H	░	░		░

2. Marital Status

Married = L, S/D/W = M

B. Historical Factors

3. Prior Suicide Attempts

	L	M	H	E
None = L, **1 = H** **2+ = E**		░	░	

Date _____
Means _____
Tx _____

4. Recent, Planned, Serious Attempt(s) (3 mo)

	L	M	H	E
No = L, **Yes = E**		░	░	

C. Clinical Factors - Stable

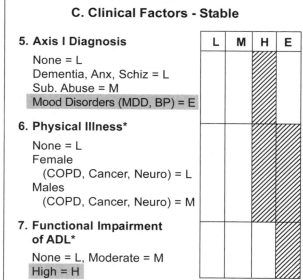

5. Axis I Diagnosis

	L	M	H	E
None = L			░	
Dementia, Anx, Schiz = L				
Sub. Abuse = M				
Mood Disorders (MDD, BP) = E				

6. Physical Illness*

	L	M	H	E
None = L			░	░
Female (COPD, Cancer, Neuro) = L				
Males (COPD, Cancer, Neuro) = M				

7. Functional Impairment of ADL*

	L	M	H	E
None = L, Moderate = M				░
High = H				

Total Factors: _____ _____ _____ _____

L (18) M (17) H (9) **E (4)**

*As mediated by Depression

D. Contextual Factors

8. Recent Loss/Stressors

	L	M	H	E
None = L				░
Bereavement (< 4 yrs) = M				
Family Discord, Financial, Caregiving = M or H				

9. Lethal Means Access

9a. Firearms
None = L, Yes = M
Recent Purchase = H
9b. Pills/Poisons
No = L, Yes = M
Stockpiled = H

10. Social Isolation

	L	M	H	E
No = L, Live Alone Without Confidants = M			░	

E. Clinical Factors – Acute
(To be rated by client)

11. Do you experience *psychic pain*, misery, or distress?

    (L) No **(L)** A little **(M)** Some **(H) A lot**

12. Do you feel *hopeless* regarding your life (life will not get better)?

    (L) No **(L)** A little **(M)** Some **(H) A lot**

13. Do you feel that you are a *burden* to others?

    (L) No **(L)** A little **(M)** Some **(H) A lot**

14. Do you have a *plan and/or method* to commit suicide?

    (L) No **(L)** General idea, no specific plans
    (M) Specific plan **(E) Specific plan with method available and scheduled**

F. Protective Factors

15. Moral Objections
Yes = L, No = M

16. Family Related Concerns
Yes = L, No = M

17. Mental Health Treatment For Mood Disorder
NA or Yes = L, No = M

18. Other Reasons for Living: _____

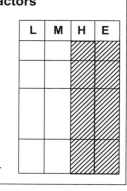

L	M	H	E
		░	░
		░	░
		░	░
		░	░

SOAP – Suicidal Older
Adult Protocol (Ages 65-85)

Other Considerations:

Risk Appraisal (check one):

Low ☐   Medium ☐   **High ☐**

Actions Taken (check all that apply):

1. Continue monitoring risk factors   _____
2. Notify/consult with supervisor   _____
3. Recommend/refer increased outpatient treatment   _____
4. Recommend/refer to psychiatric consult./med. evaluation   _____
5. Contract for NO HARMFUL BEHAVIORS   _____
6. Recommend elimination of access to firearms   _____
7. Notify legal authorities of risk to self or others (if applicable)   _____
8. Notify family (if applicable)   _____
9. Recommend/refer to day treatment   _____
10. Recommend/refer to crisis unit/voluntary hospitalization   _____
11. Initiate involuntary hospitalization   _____
12. Other _____   _____

_____   _____   _____
Interviewer   **Supervisor**   **Date**

CONTRIBUTORS

William Fremouw, PhD, received his doctorate from the University of Massachusetts in 1974. After an internship at the University of Rochester Medical School, he joined the West Virginia University faculty in 1975. He has been the Director of Clinical Training and the Chairman of Psychology. Dr. Fremouw earned a Diplomate in Forensic Psychology from the American Board of Professional Psychology (ABPP) in 1989. His current research interests include stalking and malingering. Dr. Fremouw may be contacted at 1226 Life Sciences Building, 53 Campus Drive, Morgantown, WV 26506. E-mail: William.Fremouw@mail.wvu.edu

Katrina McCoy, BA, received her bachelor's degree from West Virginia University. She is currently a doctoral student in the Clinical Psychology program at West Virginia University. Her research interests are in the areas of nonsuicidal self-injury and suicidal behaviors. Ms. McCoy may be contacted at 1224 Life Sciences Building, 53 Campus Drive, Morgantown, WV 26506. E-mail: Kmccoy@mix.wvu.edu

Elizabeth A. Tyner, MS, received her bachelor's degree from Western Michigan University and her master's degree at West Virginia University. She is currently a doctoral student in the clinical psychology program with a forensic emphasis at West Virginia University. Her research interests are in the areas of psychopathy, malingering, suicide risk assessment, forensic assessment, ethical/legal issues in clinical psychology, and criminal thinking styles. Ms. Tyner can be reached at 1124 Life Sciences Building, 53 Campus Drive, Morgantown, WV 26506. E-mail: etyner@mix.wvu.edu

Robert Musick, MSW, LCSW, is currently Director of Community Mental Health Services Development at Valley Health Care System in Morgantown, West Virginia. Mr. Musick also serves as the Executive Director of West Virginia's Counsel for the Prevention of Suicide. His background has been directing Crisis Service Programs, 24-hour crisis lines, walk-in crisis services, and Crisis Residential Unit. He is an adjunct instructor at West Virginia University's Division of Social Work. Courses taught have been in Management/ Supervision, mental health, and groups. In 2002 Mr. Musick was awarded the National Association of Social Worker's Management Person of the Year in West Virginia. Mr. Musick can be reached at 301 Scott Avenue, Morgantown, WV 26508-8804. E-mail: bmusick@valleyhealthcare.org

RESOURCES

American Psychiatric Association. (2003). *Practice Guidelines for the Assessment and Treatment of Patients With Suicidal Behaviors*. Washington, DC: Author.

Bryan, C., & Rudd, D. (2006). Advances in the assessment of suicide risk. *Journal of Clinical Psychology: In Session, 62,* 185-200.

Centers for Disease Control and Prevention. (2006). *Elderly Suicide Fact Sheet.* Retrieved December 28, 2006, from the American Association of Suicidology Website: http://www.suicidology.org/associations/1045/files/Elderly2004.pdf

Conwell, Y. (2004). Suicide. In S. Roose & H. Sackeim (Eds.), *Late Life Depression* (pp. 95-106). New York: Oxford University Press.

Conwell, Y., & Duberstein, P. (2001). Suicide in elders. In H. Hendin & J. Mann (Eds.), *The Clinical Science of Suicide Prevention* (pp. 132-150). New York: New York Academy of Sciences.

Duberstein, P., & Heisel, M. (2006). Suicide in older adults: How do we detect risk and what can we do about it? *Psychiatric Times, 23,* 46-50.

Fremouw, W., De Perczel, M., & Ellis, T. (1990). *Suicide Risk: Assessment and Response Guidelines.* Elmsford, NY: Pergamon.

Fremouw, W., Strunk, J., Tyner, E., & Musick, R. (2005). *Adolescent Suicide Assessment Protocol–20.* In L. Vandecreek & J. B. Allen (Eds.), *Innovations in Clinical Practice: Focus on Health and Wellness* (pp. 207-224). Sarasota, FL: Professional Resource Press.

Fremouw, W., Strunk, J., Tyner, E., & Musick, R. (2008). *Suicidal Adult Assessment Protocol–SAAP.* In L. Vandecreek & J. B. Allen (Eds.), *Innovations in Clinical Practice: Focus on Group, Couples, & Family Therapy* (pp. 179-189). Sarasota, FL: Professional Resource Press.

Harris, E., & Barraclough, B. (1997). Suicide as an outcome for mental disorders: A meta-analysis. *British Journal of Psychiatry, 170,* 205-228.

Luoma, J., Pearson, J., & Martin, C. (2002). Contact with mental health and primary care prior to suicide: A review of the evidence. *American Journal of Psychiatry, 159,* 909-916.

Simon, R. (2004). *Assessing and Managing Suicide Risk.* Washington, DC: American Psychiatric Publishing.

Webster, C., Douglas, K., Eaves, D., & Hart, S. (1995). *HCR-20: Assessing Risk for Violence.* Vancouver: Simon Fraser University.

Mental Status Examination

William F. Doverspike

The Mental Status Examination form provides an outline of the major content categories that are assessed as part of a formal mental status examination. Although many therapists use a checklist approach (in which the clinician simply checks off boxes and squares on a form) in documenting the results of mental status exams, such checklists often fail to capture unique qualities and characteristics of the client. In contrast, a narrative approach (in which the clinician writes a brief narrative description of the client) may not be as quick as a checklist approach, but the narrative approach has the advantage of allowing the therapist to document observations and findings in a more flexible and spontaneous manner. This form encourages a narrative, verbal description of mental status in the therapist's own words while maintaining consistency and organization of the mental status data.

Mental Status Examination*

APPEARANCE

Physical characteristics such as dress, grooming, pupil dilation/contraction, facial expression, perspiration, makeup, body piercing, tattoos, height, and weight.

BEHAVIOR/PSYCHOMOTOR ACTIVITY

Behavior or psychomotor activity includes physical activity and movements such as eye contact, grimacing, excessive eye movement (scanning), posture, and odd gestures. Level of activity through interview can include psychomotor agitation, psychomotor acceleration, psychomotor slowing, or psychomotor retardation. Observations regarding motor behavior can include gait, posture, tremors, and tics.

ATTITUDE TOWARD INTERVIEWER

Attitude toward the interviewer can be discerned by thorough verbal and nonverbal client responses. Attitude can be characterized by descriptors such as friendly, engaging, cooperative, resistant, defensive, withholding, spontaneous, reserved, indifferent, ambivalent, passive, hostile, impatient, passive-aggressive, guarded, suspicious, ingratiating, seductive, or manipulative.

AFFECT AND MOOD

Mood is the client's self-report of the emotional state, which is recorded verbatim, such as euphoric, euthymic, or depressed. Affect refers to the prevailing emotional expression observed by the clinician, such as flat, blunted, constricted, appropriate, variable, or labile (rapidly shifting). Affect is usually described in terms of its content or type, range (variability) and duration, appropriateness, and depth or intensity.

SPEECH AND THOUGHT

Speech is normally described in terms of its rate, volume, amount, complexity, and articulation. Thought content refers to what clients express in terms of specific meaning. Thought process refers to how clients express themselves in terms of logic and organization. Thought process refers to the speed and sequence in which ideas are expressed. Descriptors of thought process can include relevant, connected, logical, coherent, circumstantial, tangential, flight of ideas, loose associations, poverty of thought, perseveration, or confabulation. Obsessions are recurrent, persistent, and involuntary ideas, thoughts, and images that are usually viewed as irrational by others as well as by those experiencing them. Delusions are deeply held false beliefs that cannot be explained on a cultural basis (delusions of reference, persecution, jealousy). Delusions may include bizarre or nonbizarre delusions.

PERCEPTUAL DISTURBANCES

Hallucinations are false sensory impressions or experiences. Illusions are perceptual distortions causing existing stimuli to appear quite different from what they are in reality.

ORIENTATION AND CONSCIOUSNESS

Orientation and consciousness are evaluated by inquiring into the client's awareness of person, place, time, and circumstances along a continuum from alert to comatose. Attention and concentration are based on client's report and clinician's observation.

---

*From the CD-Rom that accompanies the book, *Risk Management: Clinical, Ethical, & Legal Guidlines for Successful Practice*, by William F. Doverspike, 2008, Sarasota, FL: Professional Resource Press. Copyright © 2008 by Professional Resource Press. Reprinted with permission.

MEMORY AND INTELLIGENCE

Memory refers to the ability to recall past experiences. Memory is assessed in terms of remote, recent, and immediate recall. An estimate of client's estimated intelligence can be based on vocabulary, abstraction ability, and general knowledge.

RELIABILITY, JUDGMENT, AND INSIGHT

Reliability refers to a client's credibility and trustworthiness, which are sometimes related to honesty, motivation, and cognitive functioning. When reliability is questionable, it is often useful to seek corroboration of the client's story. Judgment involves making decisions that are constructive and adaptive. Judgment involves "commonsense" reasoning and is often related to impulse control. Insight refers to the client's understanding of his or her problems. Insight may be described in terms such as absent, poor, partial, or good.

CONTRIBUTOR

William F. Doverspike, PhD, is a licensed psychologist and Diplomate in Clinical Psychology, American Board of Professional Psychology (ABPP) and Diplomate in Neuropsychology (ABPN). He teaches graduate courses in psychopathology and professional ethics at Argosy University in Atlanta. Dr. Doverspike is a former President of the Georgia Psychological Association and a current member of the GPA Ethics Committee. He is Editor of the *Georgia Psychologist* magazine and has authored over 100 articles and chapters on a variety of topics ranging from neuropsychology and psychotherapy to professional ethics and spirituality. He currently maintains a private practice in diagnostic consultation and individual psychotherapy at the Atlanta Counseling Center. Dr. Doverspike may be contacted at 6111-C Peachtree Dunwoody Road, Atlanta, Georgia 30328. E-mail: wdoverspike@earthlink.net

Rating of Cognitive and Behavioral Status in Older Adults (R-CABS-OA)

Jeffery B. Allen

The *Rating of Cognitive and Behavioral Status in Older Adults* (R-CABS-OA) is intended to gather cognitive and behavioral symptom information from a variety of sources: Client, Caregiver, and Clinician. While the clinician rates various symptoms/capacities along a four-point Likert Scale according to observations of a given behavior or type of deficit, the client or caregiver provides ratings based on the perceived relative decline from some previous or baseline level. The measure includes 32 items and is divided into six domains: Orientation, Language, Memory, Perceptual/Praxis, Functional Capacity, and Psychosocial. Along with deriving a total score for the measure, mean domain scores are also calculated for the client (self-rating), caregiver, and clinician.

While much of the content of the R-CABS-OA is likely to be familiar to a variety of professionals providing clinical services to older individuals, some terms should be clarified. Within the Orientation domain, temporal orientation refers to the individuals' capacity to identify time of day, date, day of week, season of year, and so forth. Spatial orientation refers to the client's ability to recognize where they are in a building or neighborhood. Context/situation is related to whether the client can identify the purpose of a given situation such as the reason for the current evaluation they are undergoing. Within the Language domain, receptive language and expressive language correspond to the client's capacity to comprehend the speech of others and effectively communicate with speech. Pragmatic language refers to nonverbal aspects of language such as tone of voice, facial expression, and gesturing. While the individual items making up the Perceptual/Praxis section are relatively straightforward, the term Praxis should be defined as it is used in this measure. Praxis refers to the capacity to perform purposeful movements such as copying a geometric design using a pencil, or accurately carrying out multiple step activities such as brushing ones teeth or dressing oneself.

By providing observations based on self, other, or clinician-based ratings, the R-CABS-OA allows for the comparative assessment of symptoms or impairments as experienced by various informants. For example, relatively less-impaired ratings from a client as compared to the clinician may suggest a lack of awareness or insight from the patient's perspective. Alternatively, the client's self-acknowledgement of greater impairment may suggest an element of depression or hopelessness. Along with providing the clinician with an understanding of which domains are relatively more problematic, the opportunity to view qualitative impairment/symptoms across various informant sources may assist the clinician in determining what family/social issues may arise while managing the assessment or treatment of a geriatric client.

Rating of Cognitive and Behavioral Status In Older Adults (R-CABS-OA)

Client/Other Rating Scale	**Clinician Rating of Impairment**
0 = no decline from previous level	0 = no impairment noted
1 = slight decline from previous level	1 = mild impairment noted
2 = moderate decline from previous level	2 = moderate impairment noted
3 = severe decline from previous level	3 = severe impairment noted

	Client Report	*Other Report*	*Clinician Rating*	
Orientation				
1.	____	____	____	Decline/Improvement in temporal orientation
2.	____	____	____	Decline/Improvement in personal orientation
3.	____	____	____	Decline/Improvement in spatial orientation
4.	____	____	____	Decline/Improvement in context/situation orientation
Totals	____	____	____	
Language				
5.	____	____	____	Decline/Improvement in receptive language function
6.	____	____	____	Decline/Improvement in expressive language function
7.	____	____	____	Decline/Improvement in word-finding in conversation
8.	____	____	____	Decline/Improvement in naming objects or people
9.	____	____	____	Decline/Improvement in pragmatic language
Totals	____	____	____	
Memory				
10.	____	____	____	Decline/Improvement in immediate recall (digit span)
11.	____	____	____	Decline/Improvement in long-term recall (after 30 minutes)
12.	____	____	____	Decline/Improvement in remote recall (childhood, etc.)
13.	____	____	____	Decline/Improvement in functional memory (keys)
Totals	____	____	____	
Perceptual/Praxis				
14.	____	____	____	Decline/Improvement in following instructions
15.	____	____	____	Decline/Improvement in ability to perceive objects
16.	____	____	____	Decline/Improvement in ability to draw/construct items
17.	____	____	____	Decline/Improvement in dressing/grooming
Totals	____	____	____	

	Client Report	Other Report	Clinician Rating	

Functional Capacity

	Client Report	Other Report	Clinician Rating	
18.	____	____	____	Decline/Improvement in doing household tasks
19.	____	____	____	Decline/Improvement in managing own money/bills
20.	____	____	____	Decline/Improvement in bathing/grooming
21.	____	____	____	Decline/Improvement in cooking/shopping
22.	____	____	____	Decline/Improvement in remaining safe in the home
23.	____	____	____	Decline/Improvement in getting around/transportation
24.	____	____	____	Decline/Improvement in interacting with others
Totals	____	____	____	

Psychosocial

	Client Report	Other Report	Clinician Rating	
25.	____	____	____	Depression/Sadness
26.	____	____	____	Anxiety/Fear
27.	____	____	____	Suspiciousness/Paranoia
28.	____	____	____	Hallucinations
29.	____	____	____	Delusions
30.	____	____	____	Changes in appetite or sleep(circle)
31.	____	____	____	Irritability or uncooperative (circle)
32.	____	____	____	Motor slowing, rigidity or tremor (circle)
Totals	____	____	____	

MEAN DOMAIN AND TOTAL SCORES ACROSS RATERS

		Client	Other	Clinician
Orientation	(total of items 1-4 divided by 4)	____	____	____
Language	(total of items 5-9 divided by 5)	____	____	____
Memory	(total of items 10-13 divided by 4)	____	____	____
Perceptual/Praxis	(total of items 14-17 divided by 4)	____	____	____
Functional Capacity	(total of items 18-24 divided by 7)	____	____	____
Psychosocial	(total of items 25-32 divided by 8)	____	____	____
TOTAL	(total of all items 1-32 divided by 32)	____	____	____

CONTRIBUTOR

Jeffery B. Allen, PhD, ABPP-CN, is currently a Professor in the School of Professional Psychology at Wright State University in Dayton, Ohio. Dr. Allen's professional experience includes a specialty internship in neuropsychology at Brown University and a rehabilitation focused postdoctoral fellowship at the Rehabilitation Institute of Michigan in Detroit. He is widely published in the areas of neuropsychology, head injuries, and memory in such sources as *Neuropsychologia, Brain Injuries*, and *Archives of Clinical Neuropsychology and Assessment.* His areas of teaching also include physiological psychology and clinical neuropsychology. His research interests include neurobehavioral disorders, quality of life in medical populations, cognitive and neuropsychological assessment, and outcome measurement in rehabilitation. He is Board Certified by the American Board of Professional Psychology in Clinical Neuropsychology and has recently published the text, *A General Practitioner's Guide to Neuropsychological Assessment*, through the American Psychological Association. Dr. Allen can be reached at SOPP, Wright State University, 3640 Colonel Glenn Highway, Dayton, OH 45435-0001. E-mail: jeffery.allen@wright.edu

Treatment Plan Worksheet

William F. Doverspike

The Treatment Plan Worksheet provides a simple way to help clients learn how problems and goals are related. In short-term solution-focused therapy, defining a problem is often considered 90% of the solution. Presenting problems can be reframed into goals that are essentially the opposite of the problems, and goals can be broken down into the component steps that must be taken to achieve them. This worksheet can help therapists transform problems into goals, which can then be translated into the specific objectives needed to attain them.

Treatment Plan Worksheet*

Name: _____ Date: _____

Problem List:

_____

_____

_____

Behavioral Description:

_____

_____

_____

Long-Term Goals:

_____

_____

_____

Short-Term Objectives:

_____

_____

_____

Treatment Plan/Interventions:

_____

_____

_____

Treatment Outcome/Evaluation Criteria/Assessment Measures:

_____

_____

_____

_____

CONTRIBUTOR

William F. Doverspike, PhD, is a licensed psychologist and Diplomate in Clinical Psychology, American Board of Professional Psychology (ABPP) and Diplomate in Neuropsychology (ABPN). He teaches graduate courses in psychopathology and professional ethics at Argosy University in Atlanta. Dr. Doverspike is a former President of the Georgia Psychological Association and a current member of the GPA Ethics Committee. He is Editor of the *Georgia Psychologist* magazine and has authored over 100 articles and chapters on a variety of topics ranging from neuropsychology and psychotherapy to professional ethics and spirituality. He currently maintains a private practice in diagnostic consultation and individual psychotherapy at the Atlanta Counseling Center. Dr. Doverspike may be contacted at 6111-C Peachtree Dunwoody Road, Atlanta, Georgia 30328. E-mail: wdoverspike@earthlink.net

Sleep Disorders*

Most adults need at least 8 hours of sleep every night to be well rested. Not everyone gets the sleep they need. About 40 million people in the U.S. suffer from sleep problems every year.

Not getting enough sleep for a long time can cause health problems. For example, it can make problems like diabetes and high blood pressure worse.

Many things can disturb your sleep.

- Working long hours
- Stress
- A sick child
- Light or noise from traffic or TV
- Feeling too hot or cold
- Wine, beer, or liquor

What are the Different Types of Sleep Problems?

- Insomnia
- Feeling sleepy during the day
- Snoring
- Sleep apnea

Insomnia

Insomnia includes:

- Trouble falling asleep
- Having trouble getting back to sleep
- Waking up too early

Most people will have trouble falling asleep from time to time. It is usually nothing to worry about. Stress, like the loss of a job or a death in the family could cause problems falling asleep. Certain medicines can make it hard to fall asleep. Drinking alcohol or eating too close to bedtime can keep you awake, too.

Insomnia is called chronic (long-term) when it lasts most nights for a few weeks or more. You should see your doctor if this happens. Insomnia is more common in females, people with depression, and in people older than 60.

Treatment

Taking medicine together with some changes to your routine can help most people with insomnia (about 85%). Certain drugs work in the brain to help promote sleep.

---

*This handout was prepared by the U.S. Food and Drug Administration, Office of Women's Health (http://www.fda.gov/WOMENS.getthefacts/sleep.html). It is in the public domain and may be photocopied and distributed without restriciton.

Tips for Better Sleep

- Go to bed and get up at the same times each day.
- Avoid caffeine, nicotine, beer, wine and liquor in the 4 to 6 hours before bedtime.
- Don't exercise within 2 hours of bedtime.
- Don't eat large meals within 2 hours of bedtime.
- Don't nap later than 3 p.m.
- Sleep in a dark, quiet room that isn't too hot or cold for you.
- If you can't fall asleep within 20 minutes, get up and do something quiet.
- Wind down in the 30 minutes before bedtime by doing something relaxing.

Feeling Sleepy During the Day

Feeling tired every now and then is normal. It is not normal for sleepiness to interfere with your daily life. Watch for signs like:

- Slowed thinking
- Trouble paying attention
- Heavy eyelids
- Feeling cranky

Several sleep disorders can make you sleepy during the day. One of these is narcolepsy. People with narcolepsy feel very sleepy even after a full night's sleep.

It is normal to take between 10 and 20 minutes to fall asleep. People who fall asleep in less than 5 minutes may have a serious sleep disorder.

Snoring

Snoring is noisy breathing during sleep. It is caused by vibrating in the throat. Some people can make changes that will stop snoring. These include:

- Losing weight
- Cutting down on smoking and alcohol
- Sleeping on your side instead of on your back

Treatment

You can buy over-the-counter nasal strips to help prevent snoring. You place one over your nose before going to bed to make breathing easier.

Sleep Apnea

Snoring loud and often, together with too much daytime sleepiness, may be signs of sleep apnea. Sleep apnea is a very common sleep disorder. It is also very dangerous. The most common type of sleep apnea happens when your breathing stops during sleep. It can stop for about 10 seconds to as long as a minute. You wake up trying to breathe. This stop-and-start cycle of waking to breathe can repeat hundreds of times a night. The danger is that some time you may not wake up to breathe. If this happens, you can die.

You are likely to feel sleepy during the day if you have this problem. People with sleep apnea tend to be overweight. It is more common among men than women.

Treatment

- The most common treatment is a device that pushes air through the airway. This device is called a CPAP.
- Avoid beer, wine, liquor, tobacco, and sleeping pills.
- Your doctor may also suggest you lose weight.
- In some cases, you may need surgery to make the airway bigger.

Defining and
Detecting Elder Abuse*

What is
Elder Abuse?

Elder Abuse abuse can be defined as mistreatment of an older individual that results in some form of personal harm. It can take many forms including the following:

- *Physical abuse* includes assault, battery, and inappropriate restraint resulting in discomfort, pain, or physical injury.
- *Sexual abuse* results from nonconsensual sexual contact of any kind.
- *Emotional or psychological abuse* is the intended infliction of mental or emotional harm brought about through humiliation, threat, or other verbal or nonverbal behavior.
- *Financial abuse* is the illegal or improper use of an older person's funds, property, or resources.
- *Neglect* is the failure of a caregiver to fulfill his or her caregiving duties.

What is the
Magnitude of the Problem?

Although estimates vary, it is generally believed that 4% to 6% of older individuals in this country are abused. While abuse of any individual (child, spouse, etc.) represents a devastating social problem in our society, the abuse of elders may be especially difficult to detect and recognize. Ultimately, this problem results in significant consequences for the health and quality of life of the elderly, as well as the diminishment of our society as a whole.

How Can
Elder Abuse Be Detected?

Perhaps the most important issue is to be aware of the risk factors for elder abuse that have been identified. These include the following:

- impaired psychological functioning (depression, anxiety, etc.)
- cognitive impairment (dementia, memory deficits, etc.)
- inadequate personal resources (poor housing, poverty, etc.)
- absence of significant others or caregivers
- medical illness or disability

---

*This handout was prepared by the Community Memory Clinic, School of Professional Psychology, Wright State University.

When some concern for the safety of an older individual arises, it is most critical that the elder be interviewed alone by a trained professional. Often, the fear of further isolation/abandonment or retribution may silence the elder if they are interviewed in the presence of the offending relative or caregiver. Many professionals serve in this evaluative role. These include the following:

- physicians
- clinical psychologists
- nurses
- social workers

Often the evaluation of the older individual will include the assessment of cognitive and functional status, as well as the collection of information about their home environment and their treatment by others.

Are There Laws Against Elder Abuse?

All states have laws specifically dealing with elder abuse, neglect, and exploitation. To learn more about your state's laws and reporting requirements, check with your state or local office on aging, Attorney General's office, or adult protective services agency.

Where Can I Find More Information on Elder Abuse?

American Psychological Association, Public Interest Directorate, Office on Aging. (2008). *Elder Abuse and Neglect: In Search of Solutions*. Website: http://www.apa.org/pi/aging/eldabuse.html

Francois, I., Moutel, G., Plu, I., Pfitzenmeyer, P., & Herve, C. (2006). Concerning mistreatment of older people: Clinical and ethical thoughts based on a study of known cases. *Archives of Gerontology and Geriatrics, 42*, 257-263.

Heath, J., Brown, M., Kobylarz, F., & Castano, S. (2005). The prevalence of undiagnosed geriatric health conditions among adult protective service clients. *The Gerontologist, 45*(6), 820-823.

Kemp, B., & Mosqueda, L. (2005). Elder financial abuse: An evaluation framework and supporting evidence. *Journal of the American Geriatrics Society/JAGS, 53*(7), 1123-1127.

Mouton, C., Larme, A., Alford, C., Talamantes, M., McCorkle, R., & Burge, S. (2005). Multiethnic perspectives on elder mistreatment. *Journal of Elder Abuse & Neglect, 17*(2), 21-45.

Introduction to Section IV: Community Interventions

The COMMUNITY INTERVENTIONS section addresses interventions which are targeted at the community level. The first contribution by Beth I. Kinsel addresses baby boomers as caregivers for aging parents. There are significant challenges for adult children who are called upon to assist with the dependency needs of their parents. Dr. Kinsel addresses key factors which affect the caregiving situation including the affective quality of the parent-child relationship, the physical, emotional, and social status of the older parent, and the amount of care needed to maintain the parent in a preferred environment. The goal of this contribution is to provide information for practitioners in order for them to assist Boomer caregivers with their caregiver role. The contribution begins with an overview of caregiving in the United States, followed by a description of the Baby Boomer cohort. Psychosocial aspects of the caregiving experience are addressed, and the ability of Boomers to assess feelings toward their parents is critical to maintaining a productive relationship. Dr. Kinsel promotes a strength perspective which includes empowering people to determine their capacities and potential, focusing on human resilience in the face of adversity, and supporting efforts to work toward health.

The second contribution to this section addresses another important community issue, namely, bullying in schools. Dr. Amy Nitza addresses the problem of bullying in American schools, and identifies a curricular gap in that most school interventions for bullying are designed for elementary and middle school students. This contribution reviews individual, environmental, and contextual factors that support bullying by older adolescents in a high school setting. Individual factors that contribute to bullying and the role of social competence are addressed. Peer influences and the role of school climate are also addressed. The contribution concludes with a comprehensive high school bullying plan, called "The Connectedness is Key Program." The program modules are designed to be relevant to high school students and will provide useful information for practitioners who seek to intervene with bullying in a high school population.

In the third contribution, Patrick Williams addresses the development and marketing of a life coaching practice. Dr. Williams highlights the importance of developing entrepreneurial skills, and provides simple strategies for marketing. He addresses the apprehension experienced by many psychologists when they approach the concept of marketing their skills. He states that the relational and listening skills that psychologists utilize in therapy, can be very helpful in disseminating information about a coaching practice. He provides a series of useful steps for marketing one's practice, utilizes a coaching metaphor, and suggests that clinicians become accustomed to being called "life coach" or "business coach" as opposed to "doctor." The importance of developing a target niche is addressed, and examples of niches are provided in this regard.

Baby Boomers as Caregivers For Aging Parents

Beth I. Kinsel

With the increase in longevity, Baby Boomers will likely face several years caring for their aging parents while at the same time experiencing multiple life course influences in their own lives. The heterogeneity within the Boomer generation (Whitbourne & Willis, 2006) suggests that the caregiving challenges for older Boomers will be different from caregiving challenges for those born nearer the end of the boom. Older Boomers might be retiring and ready to pursue leisure activities, or perhaps continuing to work due to preference or economic necessity. Younger Boomers could still be rearing children, paying for college tuition, and/or on the fast track in their careers. For persons in both groups, finding the time, resources, and energy to assist their parents can be overwhelming. Many adult children faced with the dependency needs of their parents have no idea how to obtain assistance or services. Some take on caregiving responsibilities quite naturally, while others assume the caregiver role with reluctance and trepidation.

Multiple factors affect the caregiving situation. The affective quality of the parent-child relationship; the physical, emotional, and social status of the older parent; the amount of care necessary to maintain the parent in a preferred environment; and racial/ethnic traditions are among the many issues that impact the tenor of the caregiving experience. The focus of this contribution is to provide information for use by practitioners to assist Boomer caregivers to competently perform the caregiver role, with the following objectives: (a) to discuss psychosocial aspects of caregiving common to the Boomer generation; and (b) to delineate interventions and resources the practitioner can utilize in consultation with Boomers related to caregiving demands and activities.

CAREGIVING IN THE UNITED STATES

Despite the increased mobility of American families, growth in the numbers of women in the workforce, and a declining birthrate over the past several decades, families continue to provide the majority of care given to older adults. The primary caregivers in the family are women, representing about 75% of the total family caregiving population (Hooyman & Kiyak, 2008). According to the Family Caregiver Alliance (2006), 29% of all caregivers of older persons are daughters. These women are often labeled the "sandwich generation" as they are likely balancing the care of their children with the care needs of their older parents. In fact, many caregivers will spend about 17 years caring for their children and 18 years providing care to an older parent (Stone & Keigher, 1994).

Advances in the treatment of both acute and chronic illnesses have contributed to increased longevity; thus people are living for longer periods of time, possibly requiring ongoing assistance. Demographers predict that by the year 2030, about 30% of people older than 65 years will need some assistance to continue to live in the community (Hooyman & Kiyak, 2008). Currently approximately 80% of older adults who need supportive care receive it from family, neighbors, or friends informally, rather than from paid caregivers/formal support systems (Hooyman & Kiyak, 2008). Funding for services to support older adults living independently and to complement family care is limited. It is estimated that family caregivers provide care that saves the health care system over $300 billion (Arno, 2006).

For the purpose of this discussion, caregiving denotes both the performance of instrumental tasks (i.e., cooking, shopping) and the provision of emotional support. The range of caregiving tasks falls along a continuum from minimal, such as checking in with the folks one time a week, to total care, whereby the older parent and adult child live together and the child provides the bulk of care the parent needs. The ability of older adults to take care of themselves is generally assessed through their performance of *activities of daily living* (ADLs) and *instrumental activities of daily living* (IADLs) as markers of functional capacity. Among the ADLs are walking, bathing, and eating. Higher order functioning is assessed by how IADLs are performed, which include such things as money management, using the telephone, and shopping for groceries.

There are a variety of reasons adult children become caregivers. Some adult children take on the role of caregiver gradually by assuming one or more of the above-mentioned tasks when the parent needs help. Other children are thrust into the role following a medical incident or time of crisis in the parent's life, suddenly being called upon to provide or coordinate assistance. Care may be given out of obligation; adult children want to repay the parent for all that was done for them when they were young. Another reason adult children take on the caregiver role is that they fear that their parent will be placed in a nursing home if no support is provided. Yet other persons are motivated by guilt related to incidents that happened in the past for which they are trying to compensate. Still others care for their older parents out of love and concern, and it appears to be the natural thing to do.

THE BOOMERS

For this discussion the Baby Boomer cohort is identified as the approximately 80 million individuals born from 1946 to 1964 (Almeida, Serido, & McDonald, 2006). Persons of the "Me" generation/"If it feels good, do it!" mentality are joining the ranks of the aged in record numbers. Noted for being rebellious and touting the benefits of youth, Boomers have historically been cited by society as self-absorbed and rejecting of parental values (Maugans, 1994; Steinhorn, 2006). Further, research reflects that Boomers experience less connectedness or social embeddedness at several levels, including their extended families and communities, as evidenced by low rates of religious and civic participation (Piazza & Charles, 2006). Also perceived as potential deniers of aging, persons in midlife may seek to medicate, erase, or in other ways minimize the realities of growing old. Becoming aware of the changes in their parents with age can signal to Boomers that they, too, are getting older, a realization that may contribute to some discomfort and possibly denial.

A close look at the Boomers reveals a heterogeneous population. The focus of this discussion is the within-group differences that have an effect on the capacity to provide care to aging parents. With the oldest and youngest Boomers being 18-19 years apart, researchers often delineate two or three groups by birth year to capture differences in the experience of social and historical events. Older Boomers are more likely to be experiencing the empty nest, preparing to retire, and anticipating traveling or doing volunteer work. They may have some chronic health problems that impact their functioning. Financially, they tend to be fairly stable (Almeida et al., 2006). Younger Boomers are possibly still caring for children, participating in school and community organizations, maintaining extended family ties, and continuing to work. Further, the potential for financial stress is greater in this group due to providing for young children, for example (Almeida et al., 2006), which could affect the ability to assist with parental care costs.

Additionally, racial/ethnic influences impact Boomer caregivers. First, among the oldest Boomers (born in the late forties), Whites completed college degrees at a rate two times higher than the rate for African Americans and three times higher than completion rates for Latinos (Eggebeen & Sturgeon, 2006). Also in this subgroup, the high school dropout rate among Latinos was 43% and for African Americans about 20%. Less than 10% of Whites in this older group of Boomers did not complete high school. These statistics translate into lower income levels for both African American and Latino Boomers in comparison to Whites. Further, the health of Whites as a group across the lifespan is generally found to be better than the health of African Americans or Latinos. These factors and others influence the amount and types of care adult children are able to provide their older parents.

Despite the various challenges involved, Boomers report having close ties with their parents (Fingerman & Dolbin-MacNab, 2006; Logan & Spitze, 1996) and appear to be open to caregiving. The USC Longitudinal Study of Generations by Gans and Silverstein (2006) revealed that commitment to caring for older parents by Boomers who were born in the decades of the fifties and sixties was higher than that of their parents' commitment to the generation before them. Additionally, an AARP (2001) survey found that about 78% of Boomers born between 1946 and 1956 provided periodic assistance to their parents. Baby Boomers are also more likely to have several siblings who could assist with care than cohorts born prior to or after them (Fingerman & Dolbin-MacNab, 2006). One benefit of larger sibling networks is that Boomers may share the care and move in and out of the primary caregiver role depending on where they are in the life course (Szinovacz & Davey, 2007).

PSYCHOSOCIAL ASPECTS OF CAREGIVING

"By definition, caregiving does not affect your life; it becomes your life. Outside activities disappear. . . ." (McLeod, 1999, p. 81). This statement reflects the extent to which being a primary caregiver can impact one's life. Yet, it is not the tasks or activities involved that contribute to caregiver stress as much as it is the feelings related to the caregiving situation that influence a perception of burden (Hooyman & Kiyak, 2008). The caregiver's feelings toward the parent, the dynamics of the family, the quality of the support network, and the ability to communicate all affect the quality of the adult child-older parent relationship and, in turn, reactions to caregiving.

It is not unusual for adult children to have ambivalent feelings toward their older parents. Children may experience both feelings of closeness and a degree of negativity (Hooyman & Kiyak, 2008; Maugans, 1994). Unresolved issues in the family of origin are likely to recur when the adult child and parent reconnect and spend more time together, or as the older adult becomes dependent on the child. Boomers may extend themselves to their parents to strengthen tenuous ties because they continue to seek parental approval. Despite individuating from the parents, Boomers are still influenced by the level of acceptance they receive from their parents, which can also impact helping behaviors (Maugans, 1994). It may be difficult for the caregiving child to express frustration or anger which can contribute to an undercurrent of tension.

At worst, feelings such as anger, anxiety, hopelessness, helplessness, and sorrow may pervade the relationship (Gallagher-Thompson & Powers, 1997; Silverstone & Hyman, 1989).

Caregivers may become burned out and spiral downward into exhaustion, experiencing sleep problems, apathy, and physical problems such as stomach disorders or aches and pains (Polen & Green, 2001; Silverstone & Hyman, 1989). Some caregivers become clinically depressed and begin to self-medicate with alcohol or by overeating. One study found that persons who are caregivers for their parents were at risk for exhibiting symptoms of depression at a rate twice that for persons not providing parent care (Cannuscio et al., 2002).

Being a caregiver to an older parent can be challenging, but may also bring some unexpected rewards. At its best, the parent-child relationship is characterized by love, warmth, affection, and thankfulness (Hooyman & Kiyak, 2008; Silverstone & Hyman, 1989). Some studies show that caregivers find satisfaction and realize a gain in well-being from their role (Acton & Wright, 2000; Pierce, Lydon, & Yang, 2001), while others reveal increased confidence, self-efficacy, or more closeness to the care recipient (Hooyman & Kiyak, 2008).

The ability of Boomers to assess feelings toward their parents is critical to maintaining the integrity of the relationship (e.g., the adult child and the parent understand that they are working together for the best possible outcome). It is important that adult children determine their views of aging in general and their attitudes toward the aging of their older parents and themselves in particular (Silverstone & Hyman, 1989). Doing so facilitates the caregiver's ability to assess the strengths and weaknesses within the family system and to develop a feasible plan for the provision of care. For example, if a daughter has negative views of growing older, she may react negatively to her aged parent. Further, in struggling with her own age-related changes, said daughter may deny what is happening with her mother or father.

PRACTICE APPROACHES

The role of the practitioner when working with Boomer caregivers requires a general understanding of the psychosocial factors inherent in the caregiving relationship as well as skills and knowledge to address caregiver concerns. Practitioners must be cognizant that each caregiver is on a unique journey that is influenced by family history and dynamics, individual characteristics of both the caregiver and the older parent, and social structural issues, among others. The caregiving journey is a process, and while what needs to be done in a given situation (and perhaps some things that should have been done some time ago) may be quite evident to the practitioner, the caregiver cannot be hurried to take action. It is important to elicit the Boomer's story and validate feelings, providing education and the opportunity to process information. Further, the practitioner will likely work with the Boomer caregiver on an individual level but will also need to address family of origin and nuclear family issues. This suggests approaching caregiving as a family/system issue, with identified strengths in the family providing a framework from which to plan care.

The Strengths Perspective

A primary goal of caregiver consultation is to move the adult child client toward comfort and competence in the caregiver role. Understanding the purpose of caregiving is critical to outcomes. Children may believe that the goal of caregiving is to "take care of Mom or Dad" by doing everything for them, while disregarding their capabilities. This can lead to fostering dependency by the parent, or "helping the helpless" on the road to increased reliance on others. Working out of the strengths perspective (Saleebey, 1996), the practitioner can guide the discussion away from a problem orientation and toward the identification of resources present in the caregiver/family system to assist the older parent to maintain as much autonomy as possible. The strengths perspective supports the creation of an environment that meets the care needs of the parent while enhancing independence.

A guiding premise of the strengths perspective is that each person/family/community is unique, with its own resources and traits. Some of the factors inherent in this approach include empowering people to determine their capacities and potential, acknowledging human resilience in the face of adversity, and working to make possibilities realities rather than attempting to solve problems (Saleebey, 1996). Emphasis is also placed on connectedness, or membership, which supports efforts by the individual, family, or community to work toward health. Using the strengths framework in caregiver consultation emphasizes the positives and enhances hope that changes can be made. Further, with the realization that one is not alone, the Boomer caregiver can begin to draw on other resources to support and supplement individual efforts.

Gain Knowledge About the Aging Service Network

Practitioners who work with Boomer caregivers must become educated about programs and services available to older adults to meet care needs, as well as services targeted specifically to caregivers. Although it may not be possible to be well-informed regarding all resources for older adult families, a basic understanding of the social service network in the community in which one practices will be adequate to answer caregiving questions and make appropriate referrals. Many communities publish or post online a directory of senior service providers; practitioners can familiarize themselves with these references to assist in caregiver consultation.

In general, within the senior service structure there are (a) local organizations funded through cities or counties (or both); (b) nonprofit agencies funded by the government, privately funded, supported by church organizations, and/or grants; and (c) private, for-profit businesses that provide a variety of services. Regional offices known as Area Agencies on Aging administer federal dollars (Older Americans Act and Medicaid) to support older persons living independently in the community. Medicaid dollars from the federal and state government can be used to provide an array of in-home services to low-income older persons (up to approximately 25 hours or more per week in some states) in lieu of nursing home placement.

Funding for older adult services is somewhat limited. Some counties sponsor senior levies that fund in-home care on a smaller scale than do federal programs, providing supportive services for up to 10 hours a week, perhaps. Many of the provider organizations use a sliding fee scale aimed to make services available to as many older people as possible. Homemaking, transportation, home-delivered meals, personal care assistance, and minor home repair are examples of the types of assistance provided. These services complement the support that family members and others give to older persons and are not intended to deliver the total care needed. Such programs have a limited number of dollars but are able to maintain numbers of older persons in their communities at a fraction of the cost of nursing home care. Organizations that might provide supportive services include Councils on Aging and senior citizens centers, for example.

Not only are some caregivers unaware of what services are available, they often do not know that there is little financial help available to cover the cost of care. People may assume that Medicare or other health insurances will pay for in-home care. Unless a parent was hospitalized and follow-up care is ordered by the doctor, most home care is private pay. Likewise, Medicare covers only a small percentage of nursing home care, usually following a hospitalization.

The following discussion delineates issues that are likely to be raised when counseling or consulting with caregiving adult children. This set of issues draws from the caregiving literature and the author's years of practice experience with older adults and their children. Each is briefly discussed and suggestions for related interventions offered. Resources for services and information are included at the end of this contribution.

Status of the Parent-Child Relationship

Before the nuts and bolts of providing care to an older parent can be adequately addressed, it is helpful to assist the adult child client to determine the status of the parent-child relationship. This is important for two reasons: first, it enables the adult child to assess feelings and identify potential areas of conflict between parent and child; and secondly, the clinician and client are then better able to determine ways to collaborate with the parent (and/or other family members), utilizing individual strengths, strengths in the parent-child relationship, and within the family and community to ensure that needs are optimally met.

One way to organize the discussion of relationship status is to determine the role the adult child played in the family of origin. This former role can impact how the older parent will perceive and relate to the child and vice versa (Silverstone & Hyman, 1989). For example, if the child was the family "clown," he or she may not be taken seriously by the parent, even though the child is now a capable adult. In situations in which the parent and child were in conflict in the family home, the adult child who steps in to assist may be perceived as a troublemaker or as antagonistic, despite good intentions. Some older parents continue to view their children as children and have not made a shift to adult-adult status. Also, there are adult children who continue to relate to their parents as dependent children with needs they expect their older parents to meet.

For Boomers who have reached filial maturity (Blenkner, 1965), it will be easier to relate to their parents as adults, accepting them as individuals and forgiving them regarding any difficulties in the relationship, while at the same time being self-aware of negative behaviors. In instances in which conflicts between the older parent and the adult child have not been resolved, or the child continues to be dependent on the parent, the relationship will be more strained. Further, parental expectations for assistance may be unrealistic and/or based on inaccurate appraisals of what the adult child can do. Although research shows that Baby Boomers do things to please their parents (Maugans, 1994), it may be necessary for the child to renegotiate the specifics of the caregiving tasks.

A second area to explore with adult children is how strong a tie they have with their parents. Is the relationship "close"? Has there been emotional distance over the years? It is important for Boomers to identify unresolved issues that could create barriers between them and their parents. In situations in which the family of origin was dysfunctional and/or the parent was the perpetrator of much of the dysfunction, it may be unrealistic for an adult child to expect to comfortably reconnect with the parent. It is not uncommon to hear from adult children that they do not particularly like their parent. What is surprising is that despite such negative feelings, many adult children want to ensure that Mom and Dad receive the best care possible. The practitioner can reassure the Boomer that despite ambivalent feelings it is possible to facilitate an optimal living arrangement for the parent. Achieving this awareness may reduce guilt and enhance the attitude of the adult child regarding the caregiver role.

Facilitate Exploration of Feelings

As with many life issues, adult children may be unaware of their feelings or may deny that any negativity is present. They may ignore feelings, hoping they will just go away on their own. Negative feelings can impede caregiving efforts and contribute to tension between members of the caregiver-parent dyad. Once any unsettling feelings have been identified, the Boomer can work to diminish negativity and build on the more positive dynamics in the relationship. A care recipient is able to pick up on an undercurrent of hostility or anger, which may then sabotage a cooperative relationship.

Identifying feelings places them outside the individual and allows for examination with some detachment. Too often, a caregiver assumes total responsibility for a parent who has never been happy, or who is all too willing to turn over responsibility for everything to someone else. Perhaps the best that can be done for some parents is to ensure that they are safe and adequately clothed and fed. Being happy may never enter into the equation.

The following techniques can assist practitioners in supporting a caregiving Boomer to explore feelings: (a) Provide an opportunity for the adult child to name and own feelings related to the caregiver situation, especially negative feelings; (b) teach the caregiver that "feelings are neither right or wrong, they just are"; (c) reiterate that it is not the feeling that is the problem, it is how one acts or reacts to a given situation; (d) normalize caregiver feelings: "It's not unusual to feel this way under the circumstances"; (e) inform the caregiver that "It's not your job to make your loved one happy"; (f) elicit positives the adult child can enumerate about being a caregiver, as this can contribute to a sense of purpose, well-being, and an appreciation of the parent and his or her life (Hooyman & Kiyak, 2008); and (g) assure the caregiver that knowing feelings can facilitate the identification of strengths of the caregiver dyad, as well as strengths within the larger family/support network (Hooyman & Kiyak, 2008). When the affective quality of the relationship is determined, the Boomer will have an expanded awareness of the climate in which he or she is operating.

Who Is My Parent?

Once the status of the relationship is clarified, the conversation can move toward helping Boomers develop an accurate perception of the parent as a person. Asking how well one knows a parent can stimulate thought and provide a basis for realistic care planning/provision. Adult children will benefit from having as true a picture as possible of their older parent's well-being and lifestyle. Collecting facts related to physical, emotional, and social well-being will facilitate the provision of care and the caregiving relationship. Factors to consider in this dimension are social networks (including family members, friends, and others); how leisure time is spent (activities within and outside the home); medical diagnoses, treatments, and functional capacity; mental status and personality; and business-related information.

It behooves the adult child to be aware of the various persons who are involved in the parent's life. Determining the social network of one's parent provides information about persons who might be of support in times of need. The social network may include family members, friends, neighbors, or persons from organizations to which the parent belongs, such as a church or a social group. By knowing whether Mom has some friends in whom she confides, acquaintances with whom she socializes, and/or people to whom she may provide some support, the adult child can understand the level of connectedness her parent feels to others in her environment. Developing a list of the major players in the parent's life, the Boomer can begin to organize support network information.

Leisure activities enhance well-being and provide pleasure in later life. It is helpful to know whether Dad is active in a senior center or other organizations and how frequently he likes to get out of the house. The pursuit of hobbies or other interests at home also reveals information about the "person" of the parent. Boomer caregivers may find that they enjoy activities also enjoyed by their parent and make plans to pursue some of them together. Finding common ground facilitates the relationship and allows for opportunities for the parent to share stories and the child to develop an appreciation for his or her heritage, perhaps.

Knowing the parent's medical diagnoses enables the caregiver to more knowledgeably collaborate with the loved one regarding issues of health and function. It is important to know what, if any, medications are being taken and for what reason, as many older persons experience side effects from medicines. Keeping a list of medications and dosages will facilitate accurate usage and administration. In instances in which the parent has some cognitive problems, the caregiver may find it necessary to monitor the medication regimen to ensure that meds are being taken as prescribed. Further, depending on the parent's status, the caregiver may also need to accompany the parent to the doctor and consult on areas of concern. It is helpful for Boomers to ask parents if they would prefer some company when it is time to see the doctor.

Mental status and personality factors should also be explored, as normal aging does not alter either one greatly. A review of how the parent handled difficulties and reacted to positive events in the past will provide the adult child with an understanding of present coping capacity. If the parent was an optimist earlier in life, he or she will likely continue to be optimistic in later life. If the parent took a more negative view of the world and events, he or she will tend to be negative with age. Being aware that the basic personality does not change with age allows the adult child to hold realistic expectations of the parent's behavior.

Parents who have a history of mental illness or who become depressed in later life may present additional caregiving challenges. Also, the care of older parents manifesting symptoms of Alzheimer's disease or Parkinson's, or who have other types of neuropsychological impairments, may be more demanding. Practitioners can encourage Boomers to learn as much as they can about the diagnoses and/or acquire education and skills to manage the sometimes-erratic behaviors of their parents.

For adult children who become increasingly involved in caregiving, it is important to learn the business aspects of their older parents' lives. This includes financial status; whether the parent has written a will and where it is located; types of medical insurance coverage the parent has; and whether or not there are provisions for advanced directives and power of attorney, as well as a living will. Additionally, one should learn if there is long-term care insurance or investments to cover the cost of in-home personal care or nursing home placement. Does the parent have funeral arrangements made? Some older parents do not want their children to know their affairs, and it will be important to strategize with the Boomer regarding ways to address this and other sensitive areas with the parent. When couched in terms of planning and soliciting the wishes of the parent regarding care, the concern conveyed by the adult child may allow the parent to be more open than in the past.

Although preparing such a "biography" may seem a daunting task to the Boomer, it will enhance the adult child's awareness of the parent and provides the basis for planning care together. An additional benefit to collecting such information is that the parent and child are communicating generally around "facts" about the parent's life rather than feelings, which provides a safe way to relate and is less emotionally laden.

Teach Communication Skills

For some adult children, initiating a conversation about the parents' need for care is threatening. The older parents may be viewed as strong and independent, as closed to the idea of seeking help, or they may verbalize their expectations that "only a family member" can assist. These factors can contribute to hesitancy on the part of an adult child to raise controversial issues. Conveying respect and warmth will provide reassurance to the parents and facilitate the integrity of the parent-child relationship. Speaking calmly about the status of the relationship provides both parties a basis for understanding each other at times when critical decisions must be made. For example, encouraging the Boomer to state up front that he has a problem with his mother's temper but genuinely wants to help her, clears the air and lets Mom know that her son will make his best effort to assist her to maintain independence. If possible, having such discussions when a parent is not in a crisis is ideal, as it allows for a more open, less intense treatment of the subject.

Although it is not always possible to honor parental requests, providing a forum to discuss such issues conveys to parents that their input and opinions are valued. Adult children must learn that it is not productive to argue with their parents. Even persons with mild to moderate cognitive impairment (such as memory loss) can express their wishes or make choices about care options when given the opportunity. Providing the Boomer with phrases that can redirect a discussion or deescalate an intense exchange will enhance the ability to carry a conversation to a productive resolution.

Educating Boomers about how to maximize conversations with an older parent can enhance communication skills. Techniques (adapted from Edinberg, 1988) that can be used to plan serious discussions include:

1. Choose a time of day to talk when the parent is most alert and not distracted by other activities.
2. Keep language simple and topics to a minimum (to avoid confusion or overwhelming the parent).
3. Use active listening skills. Phrases such as, "You said that you feel so alone since Dad died; you miss him a lot," or "When you asked the doctor about those headaches you've been having you seemed really anxious," assure the parent that he or she has been heard.
4. Use "I" statements: "I think we need to make different plans for the baseball game," or "I feel that you are angry with me," reflect that one is assuming responsibility for one's thoughts or feelings rather than blaming the other.
5. Confrontation: This entails being assertive about the meaning of one's statements such that they cannot be misconstrued and setting limits with one's parent. Being honest about the situation can lead to disagreement but the conversation does not have to escalate into a fight. Following is an example of a response when Mom tells her daughter that she wants to add two more stops to the "short shopping trip": "Mom, when you said you wanted to go shopping this afternoon, you only mentioned the department store. You didn't tell me you wanted to go to the grocery and the hardware store, too. I made arrangements to be out of the office for just 2 hours."

Utilizing counseling sessions or consultation to practice possible conversations with older parents can help the adult child feel better equipped to broach potentially uncomfortable subjects.

A review of any barriers that could inhibit communication between the older parent and adult child is also essential to optimal exchanges. Accommodating the environment to the parent's situation will maximize conversation. For example, checking that the parent has his or her hearing aid and that it is both in the ear and working, having enough lighting to see well, sitting close and maintaining eye contact, and keeping comments brief and to the point to hold attention are all ways to facilitate communication.

Effective planning can occur when the adult child takes a low-key approach to the topic, laying the groundwork for future conversations. Speaking calmly about the status of the relationship provides both parties a basis for understanding one another at a possible future time when critical decisions must be made. Playing the "What-if" game can provide insight into the older parents' thoughts about what types of care they may need as well as how care will be provided, by whom, and when it should be provided. Introducing hypothetical situations allows the parent and child to explore possible options for care.

Subsequent conversations may then focus on specific scenarios. For example, the caregiver might ask: "Dad, what would you do if your cancer comes back and you needed more care than all of us (in the informal support system) can give?" This could open up a conversation about under what circumstances Dad would consider going to a nursing facility, whether he would prefer to receive in-home care regardless of the amount of care required or the cost, or if he would be willing to go to an inpatient hospice. Having such conversations when the parent is relatively stable can facilitate openness and clearer thinking, which might not be possible in the event of a crisis situation.

It is advisable to move the Boomer away from assumptions of parental thoughts about the need for care and toward engagement in meaningful conversation with the parents to solicit their opinions and desires. Too often adult children make decisions based on what they want or think is best for their older parents rather than considering what the parents desire or what might be best for them. For example, some children take a giant leap from a parent's experience of a broken hip to the conclusion that permanent placement in a long-term care facility is required. Although placement may alleviate the anxiety of a child regarding future falls, it could be inappropriate once the parent completes a rehab program.

The practitioner may recognize that the Boomer client and various persons in the family network are having difficulty agreeing as to the best way to care for a parent. Some family members may be very involved in care, and others may not be actively involved but have strong opinions about how care is provided. Also, there may be family members who are in denial about the changes in an older parent. For some families, bringing the major players in the family together for a family conference is beneficial. Silverstone and Hyman (1989) suggest addressing parental needs utilizing eight steps that include:

1. Organize a family meeting.
2. Solicit input from the parents about their situation.
3. Invite persons to the meeting who are concerned and impacted by the parent's need for care, and those who might contribute to the caregiving routine.
4. Allow time for each person to be heard.
5. Determine the primary issues affecting the parent's functioning.
6. Find out who is willing to commit to providing care.
7. Prioritize needs in one's own life so as to be realistic about what one can offer.
8. Achieve consensus or agreement regarding the overall plan of care.

Such a gathering is not appropriate for all families. The practitioner and the Boomer client should discuss the feasibility of having a meeting and strategize about how to handle tense conversations that might be emotionally laden. Laying ground rules for behavior is important. It is also important that the older parent feels included and that his or her opinions are taken into consideration. Not all families are ready or able to have such a conversation. Also, persons who are extremely negative and unlikely to contribute constructively to the group discussion should be excluded (Silverstone & Hyman, 1989).

Promote Self Care

There was life before caregiving and there needs to be balance in life after the adult child becomes a caregiver. Many Boomers are pulled in multiple directions and have multiple demands on their time; if something needs to "give" or remain undone, self-care needs are too often the choice. The practitioner should emphasize that to provide optimal care to the parent, Boomers must also take care of themselves. Over the past few decades, a variety of suggestions for coping with caregiving have been offered by researchers. Because of the diversity among caregivers and their families, not all suggestions will be appropriate to every caregiving situation. Providing a menu from which to select activities that are feasible for the family situation and/or meaningful to a particular caregiver recognizes racial/ethnic, socioeconomic, lifestyle, and other differences.

Assisting the caregiver to identify ways to set boundaries with the parent will enhance feelings of self-efficacy and minimize the perception of being "trapped" in the caregiving role (Edinberg, 1988). Statements such as, "I know that you prefer that I'm here every Saturday, but I'll be taking a class on Saturdays this Spring, so we have to make other plans. Who would you like to ask to be with you?" inform the older parent that his son has other commitments and also includes Dad in the decision as to who might substitute. Once others who could assist have been identified, caregivers can gradually bring them on board to facilitate acceptance of help from someone other than themselves.

It is also important for the Boomer to plan respite for longer periods of time (Hooyman & Kiyak, 2008). Being away for a special weekend or a week or two of vacation facilitates rejuvenation and true relaxation. This provides the caregiver and the parent a much-needed break from each other. It may be necessary for the practitioner to reiterate to the caregiver that any personal funds spent for respite will be well worth the cost. Some family members may pitch in to pay the caregiver's expenses for a vacation, cover the cost of a paid caregiver, or be willing to substitute for the caregiver during this time. Also, most nursing homes have one or two beds available for respite services in the event a caregiver plans to be away for some time. Finances may prohibit some caregivers or families from paying for respite, which necessitates more creativity in seeking help. In these situations extended family members, siblings of the Boomer caregiver, a family friend, or member of the parent's church may be willing and able to assist.

Tips for ongoing self-care include (a) spending time with friends and participating in social activities, (b) engaging in meditation, yoga, or other spiritual practices; (c) maintaining/developing hobbies; (d) exercising regularly; (e) attending a caregiver support group or joining an online caregiver group; (f) journaling to capture feelings and thoughts to obtain clarity; (g) making and keeping personal medical and dental appointments; (h) seeking counseling to resolve unfinished business; (i) hiring a professional care manager – especially those caregivers who live at a distance; (j) hiring persons privately or through an agency to perform more time-consuming tasks; and (k) enrolling the older adult parent in adult day services. Adult day services do not only provide respite for the caregiver; the older parent may benefit greatly from socializing with other people and participating in varied activities.

Enhancing the Support Network

Many caregivers provide care without help from anyone else way beyond the point of good health and/or mental well-being. They may believe that they are the only ones who can properly care for their parents. Older parents may also convince their children that this is true! Sometimes caregivers fear that something could happen while they are not with their parents and want to avoid guilt that might result in this instance. Boomers may so feel the need to be in control that they believe their presence alone can prevent accidents or sudden illness. Managing parental care provides an opportunity for control, especially in the event that there have been disagreements about care planning among siblings. It may seem easier to the caregiver to "just do it myself," thus abandoning plans to engage others after several attempts to arrange care proved unsuccessful.

Encourage the Boomer to ask others for help. Too often when someone says, "Let me know what I can do," a caregiver cannot think of anything that could possibly be done to help. Brainstorm with the Boomer about how to broaden the parental support network. Reaching out to siblings, friends of the parents, neighbors, or the religious organization to which the parent may belong can result in bringing more helpers into the network. Grandchildren are another potential source of help. They may get along better with the older parent than does the adult child. A special relationship with a grandparent can yield positive benefits for grandparent and grandchild as well as the entire support system.

Other people are more inclined to help when they know how long an activity will take or how often they might be called upon to assist. When the caregiver compiles a list of specific chores or tasks that others can do and asks an individual for assistance with only one task, such as taking the parent to the senior center for a weekly bridge game, there may be more success than when others make a general offer of help. By developing a list of persons willing to provide support, the caregiver can organize information about who can and is willing to do what, and when. Keeping such a list minimizes ruminating about whom to call and allows the caregiver to quickly track down needed help.

When the informal support network is stretched, providing all the care it can and that is not enough, it is time for the Boomer caregiver to expand the support network to include formal service providers. Many caregivers resist making the necessary calls. Practitioners can assist Boomers to begin the process of seeking outside help by discussing the types of services and programs available in the community as delineated earlier in this contribution. By being familiar with community resources, practitioners can reassure caregivers, and thus caregiver families, that there is help for their situation.

Boomers may need additional time to process this next step in the caregiving journey. They may feel that they are a failure or that the family support system failed their parent. The situation may have reached a crisis point, at which time there is no longer any question as to whether agency assistance should be arranged. Also, if the older parent's condition has deteriorated to the extent that round-the-clock care is required and is not affordable in the home, a decision for placement in a nursing facility may be required. In this circumstance the caregiver is likely to feel sorrow and grief, as well as some frustration, anxiety, and perhaps depression. Any fears the family may have had about the competency of others to care for the parent could be heightened by the unknown territory of a nursing facility. Again, providing information about long-term care facilities in the community and/or a referral to a care management agency or private care manager will support the Boomer caregiver during this phase of the caregiving journey.

SUMMARY

Baby Boomers generally maintain close ties to their older parents and provide a substantial amount of care to them when needed. Multiple issues impact the quality of the caregiving relationship; among them are feelings of the Boomer about aging generally and the aging of oneself and one's parents, family dynamics, the quality of the support network, and communication. Practitioner's can play a vital role to help Baby Boomers and their families identify and utilize their strengths to maximize the caregiving situation. By providing supportive space to explore the psychosocial aspects of the parent-child relationship, as well as information about available resources, practitioners will empower adult children in their role as caregivers to their aging parents.

CONTRIBUTOR

Beth I. Kinsel, PhD, MGS, is Assistant Professor of Social Work at Wright State University in Dayton, Ohio. She teaches research methods, cultural competence, social gerontology, and human behavior. Her research interests include resilience in later life, mental well-being in older adults, and caregiving. Dr. Kinsel is the director of the gerontology certificate program. As a gerontologist with over 20 years of practice, she worked primarily as a care manager and geriatric community mental health specialist. Dr. Kinsel can be contacted at 270 Millett Hall, 3640 Colonel Glenn Highway, Dayton, OH 45435. E-mail: beth.kinsel@wright.edu

RESOURCES

Cited Resources

AARP. (2001). *In the Middle: A Report on Multicultural Boomers Coping With Family and Aging Issues.* Washington, DC: Author.

Acton, J. G., & Wright, K. (2000). Self-transcendence and family caregivers of adults with dementia. *Journal of Holistic Nursing, 18*, 143-158.

Almeida, D. M., Serido, J., & McDonald, D. (2006). Daily life stressors of early and late baby boomers. In S. K. Whitbourne & S. L. Willis (Eds.), *The Baby Boomers Grow Up: Contemporary Perspectives on Midlife* (pp. 165-183). Mahwah, NJ: Lawrence Erlbaum.

Arno, P. S. (2006). *Prevalence, Hours and Economic Value of Family Caregiving.* Kensington, MD: National Family Caregivers Association and San Francisco, CA: Family Caregiver Alliance.

Blenkner, M. (1965). Social work and family relationships in later life with some thoughts on filial maturity. In E. Shanas & G. Streib (Eds.), *Social Structure and the Family* (pp. 46-61). Englewood Cliffs, NJ: Prentice-Hall.

Cannuscio, C., Jones, C., Kawachi, I., Colditz, G., Berkman, L., & Rimm, E. (2002). Reverberations of family illness: A longitudinal assessment of informal caregiving and mental health status in nurses' health study. *American Journal of Public Health, 92*, 1305-1311.

Edinberg, M. A. (1988). *Talking With Your Aging Parents.* Boston, MA: Shambala Publications.

Eggebeen, D. J., & Sturgeon, S. (2006). Demography of the baby boomers. In S. K. Whitbourne & S. L. Willis (Eds.), *The Baby Boomers Grow Up: Contemporary Perspectives on Midlife* (pp. 3-21). Mahwah, NJ: Lawrence Erlbaum.

Family Caregiver Alliance. (2006). *Women and Caregiving: Facts and Figures.* San Francisco, CA: Author.

Fingerman, K., & Dolbin-MacNab, M. (2006). The baby boomers and their parents: Cohort influences and intergenerational ties. In S. K. Whitbourne & S. L. Willis (Eds.), *The Baby Boomers Grow Up: Contemporary Perspectives on Midlife* (pp. 237-259). Mahwah, NJ: Lawrence Erlbaum.

Gallagher-Thompson, D., & Powers, D. V. (1997). Primary stressors and depressive symptoms in caregivers of dementia patients. *Aging and Mental Health, 1*, 248-255.

Gans, D., & Silverstein, M. (2006). Norms of filial responsibility for aging parents across time and generations. *Journal of Marriage and Family, 68,* 960-976.

Hooyman, N. R., & Kiyak, H. A. (2008). *Social Gerontology: A Multidisciplinary Perspective* (8th ed.). Boston, MA: Pearson Education.

Logan, J. R., & Spitze, G. D. (1996). *Family Ties: Enduring Relations Between Parents and Their Grown Children.* Philadelphia: Temple University Press.

Maugans, J. E. (1994). *Aging Parents, Ambivalent Baby Boomers: A Critical Approach to Gerontology.* Dix Hills, NY: General Hall.

McLeod, B. W. (1999). *Caregiving: The Spiritual Journey of Love, Loss and Renewal.* New York: John Wiley and Sons.

Piazza, J. R., & Charles, S. T. (2006). Mental health among the baby boomers. In S. K. Whitbourne & S. L. Willis (Eds.), *The Baby Boomers Grow Up: Contemporary Perspectives on MidLife* (pp. 111-146). Mahwah, NJ: Lawrence Erlbaum.

Pierce, T., Lydon, J. E., & Yang, S. (2001). Enthusiasm and moral commitment: What sustains family caregivers of those with dementia. *Basic and Applied Social Psychology, 23*(1), 29-41.

Polen, M. R., & Green, C. A. (2001). Caregiving, alcohol use and mental health symptoms among HMO members. *Journal of Community Health, 26*, 285-301.

Saleebey, D. (1996). The strengths perspective in social work practice: Extensions and cautions. *Social Work, 41*, 296-305.

Silverstone, B., & Hyman, H. K. (1989). *You and Your Aging Parent: A Family Guide to Emotional, Physical, and Financial Problems* (3rd ed.). New York: Pantheon.

Steinhorn, L. (2006). *The Greater Generation.* New York: St. Martin's Press.

Stone, R., & Keigher, S. (1994). Toward equitable universal caregiver policy: The potential of financial supports for family caregivers. *Aging and Social Policy, 6*, 57-76.

Szinovacz, M. E., & Davey, A. (2007). Changes in adult child caregiver networks. *Gerontologist, 47*, 280-295.

Whitbourne, S. K., & Willis, S. L. (Eds.). (2006). *The Baby Boomers Grow Up: Contemporary Perspectives on Midlife.* Mahwah, NJ: Lawrence Erlbaum.

Additional Resources:

Administration on Aging website: www.aoa.dhhs.gov

Caregiver's Connection website: www.agingcare.com

ElderCarelink website: www.eldercarelink.com

ElderCare Locator website: www.eldercare.gov   Tel.: (800) 677-1116

Family Caregiver Alliance website: www.caregiver.org

Medicare and Medicaid Tel.: (800) MEDICARE

National Adult Day Services Association website: www.nadsa.org

National Alliance for Caregiving website: www.caregiving.org (Guidance for getting help caring for a loved one at home, caregiver rights and resources, respite care services, and how to advocate on behalf of a loved one)

National Council on Aging website: www.noca.org

National Family Caregivers Association website: www.thefamilycaregiver.org

National Association of Professional Geriatric Care Managers website: www.caremanager.org   Tel.: (520) 881-8008

Bullying Prevention
In High Schools

Amy Nitza

The problem of bullying in American schools has received increased attention in recent years. Bullying has been defined as a subset of aggression that is identified by intentional and repeated acts of aggression that involve an imbalance of power between the perpetrator and the victim (Orpinas & Horne, 2006). This use, or abuse, of power by one child or group of children against another is highlighted by Craig and Pepler (2007), who refer to bullying as a "destructive relationship problem" (p. 86). As such, bullying has destructive consequences for both the children who bully and those who are the victims of such behavior.

Children who bully are developing the ability to manipulate their positions of power (e.g., social status or knowledge of another's vulnerability) to harm others (Craig & Pepler, 2007). When such behavior is used to maintain one's own popularity or social position, this goal may be achieved at the expense of maintaining positive relationships. Ironically, these children may become increasingly disliked over time and have more significant relationship problems later in life (Young, Boye, & Nelson, 2006).

Victims of bullying are at risk for a number of serious social and psychological consequences. These include internalizing problems such as loneliness, anxiety, and psychosomatic symptoms (Kaltiala-Heino et al., 2000; Rigby, 2003; Wolke et al., 2001). Peer and social problems, and school and academic problems are also common (Orpinas & Horne, 2006). In extreme cases, violence can also result. An examination of the characteristics of those responsible for school shootings in recent years found that almost three fourths of them had been responding out of revenge over having been the victims of bullying and harassment (Vossekuil et al., 2002).

As the serious impact of this problem on students and on schools as a whole has been recognized, efforts have been undertaken to determine the origins of such behavior, how it develops, and how it can most effectively be combated or prevented. According to Espelage (2003), bullying can best be understood from a social-ecological perspective; that is, individual characteristics of children interact with characteristics of the environment to create, support, or maintain bullying behavior. Utilizing this framework, a comprehensive bullying prevention program must include some combination of emphasis on promoting individual thoughts, feelings, and behaviors that support healthy relationships, as well as promoting a social environment that is positive, supports students' social and emotional development, and discourages bullying and aggression.

This conceptualization of the problem is supported by reviewing existing programs that have demonstrated evidence of success. In a recent review, the majority of identified programs were school-wide approaches that targeted individual social competence development, restructured the social environment, or both (Horne, Raczynski, & Orpinas, 2008). Based on available evidence, it can be concluded that a comprehensive, school-wide approach to the prevention of bullying should include both of these components.

Another factor that many of the programs identified by Horne, Raczynski, and Orpinas (2008) have in common is that they have generally been designed for use in elementary and middle schools. Little direct discussion of bullying prevention in high schools occurs in the literature. A literature review and examination of known programs reveals that there appear to be no existing bully prevention programs developed specifically for a high school population. It thus appears that when bullying programs are implemented in high schools, existing programs developed for other developmental levels are applied, perhaps with insufficient attention to the specific needs of older adolescents or the ways in which high schools are structured differently from elementary and middle schools.

Many of the factors that contribute to bullying are likely to be similar at the high school level. That is, the social-ecological model of bullying described by Espelage (2003) is likely to be as applicable to high schools as it is to elementary and middle schools. Likewise, social competence and school climate factors can be predicted to be key components of successful interventions in high schools as well. However, both the developmental needs of older adolescents and the structure of the high school setting differ in important ways from those of elementary and middle schools. These developmental and structural differences suggest that an effective bullying prevention program in a high school cannot simply be an elementary or middle school program with a different name. What is known about effective bullying programs may need to be designed and implemented specifically with high schools, and high school students, in mind.

The purpose of this contribution is to review individual and environmental or contextual factors that have been identified as contributing to or supporting bullying and to consider them in the context of older adolescents. The implications of these factors for intervention will be highlighted, and a new program designed specifically to target these factors in older adolescents in a high school setting will be described.

INDIVIDUAL FACTORS THAT CONTRIBUTE TO BULLYING: THE ROLE OF SOCIAL COMPETENCE

As noted previously, bullying can be best understood as a combination of individual characteristics of children interacting with characteristics of the environment (Espelage, 2003). Discussion of the internal characteristics of children that contribute to bullying has largely focused on the role of social skills or social competence. As defined by Orpinas and Horne (2006), social competence refers to "a person's age-appropriate knowledge and skills for functioning peacefully and creatively in his or her community or social environment" (p. 42). Such skills include those used to make positive decisions, solve conflicts without violence, plan for the future, resist negative peer pressure, make friends, and enjoy being around people from different cultures. Social competence has been identified as a protective factor against bullying and aggression (Orpinas & Horne, 2006). As described by Staub (1996): "The conditions and experiences that promote violence in children and youth are, on the whole, the opposite of those that create caring, helping, and altruism" (p. 121). Therefore, an emphasis on the development of social competence in the prevention of bullying is highly appropriate.

Theories of childhood aggression have implicated deficits in one or more areas of social information processing and responding (Crick & Dodge, 1994). These factors, including social processing, decision-making, and responding skills have been used to investigate bullying as a subset of aggression and violent behavior as well. Orpinas & Horne (2006) identified a number of psychological risk factors associated with bullying and aggression. These include the expected outcomes associated with such behavior, the values placed on those outcomes, personal beliefs that support the behavior, an aggressive attributional bias, and a limited range of problem-solving skills. In other words, children who engage in bullying behavior are likely to expect a positive outcome from the bullying and to value that outcome. They are also likely to believe that such behavior is justified, appropriate, or acceptable. Additionally, they may be more likely than other children to attribute the behaviors and intentions of others as aggressive in social situations and to identify few alternate means of responding.

The extent to which these biases in social information processing and decision making represent social skills deficits is a matter of debate. The perception of bullies as children who lack the skills to understand or deal with people in more appropriate ways is perhaps a common one, yet some authors have argued that bullying actually requires a set of social skills that are sophisticated enough to manipulate social power and/or to manage social or group dynamics in some way (Sutton, Smith, & Swettenham, 1999). Particularly in the case of indirect bullying such as social exclusion and other forms of relational aggression, an accurate ability to assess and influence social dynamics is necessary (Young et al., 2006).

It may be that some forms of bullying involve social skills deficits while others involve well-developed social skills combined with a set of beliefs and values that support bullying behavior. However, for both groups it may be that they perceive the relative costs and benefits of bullying behavior positively (Sutton et al., 1999). A recent review of the literature on relational aggression reported that the use of this type of bullying is related to social prominence and peer-perceived popularity (Young et al., 2006). However, the authors differentiate between social prominence and social competence, which includes the ability to maintain positive relationships. They note that children who use relational aggression are ". . . very effective at achieving personal goals in their social relationships, but they may do so at the expense of those relationships" (Young et al., 2006, p. 305).

Espelage (2003) argues that regardless of whether bullying represents social skills deficits or a harmful use of more sophisticated social skills, programs to prevent bullying should emphasize the development of more prosocial and respectful behavior. Similarly, Young et al. (2006) conclude that although little information is available regarding effective prevention and intervention programs specifically for relational aggression, a focus on promoting prosocial skills is likely to decrease the chances that students will interact in threatening and aggressive ways.

An emphasis on prosocial skills may be particularly beneficial in a universal bullying prevention program that promotes social competence for all students. The development of social competence may reduce bullies' reliance on aggressive behavior to accomplish their goals, while also empowering victims to respond to bullying behavior in different ways and to help them learn to avoid the victim role. In addition, an emphasis on social competence may help reduce bullying by empowering bystanders to respond differently. Bystanders, peers who observe other students being bullied, can be deeply affected by observing this process, but may develop a sense of learned helplessness and feel unable to respond (Horne, Bartolomucci, & Newman-Carlson, 2003). Espelage (2003) notes that bystanders tend to possess empathy toward the victims but frequently lack the confidence and skills to intervene. An increased sense of social competence may provide them with the motivation and skills they need to do so. Finally, it is also important to note that the roles of bully, victim, and bystander are not fixed; students may be in each of these different roles at different times. Thus, a universal approach that builds social competence in all students appears particularly important for effective bullying prevention efforts.

This comprehensive approach was adopted by Orpinas & Horne (2006), who have developed a bullying prevention model that targets all students through universal interventions. The development of social competence is a primary component of the model. Specific elements of social competence addressed in the model include (a) awareness of the problem of bullying; (b) emotional development, including learning to recognize and manage their own emotions and to identify the emotions of others; (c) cognitive development, including attributions and problem-solving skills; and (d) a number of specific interpersonal relationship and communication skills. This model does not specify an implementation plan nor does it provide specific interventions. The model also does not discuss high school students specifically. However, each of these components is likely to be highly relevant to high school students and should be considered when developing a high school bullying program.

ENVIRONMENTAL AND CONTEXTUAL FACTORS THAT CONTRIBUTE TO BULLYING

Bullying is a group phenomenon (Espelage, 2003). Regardless of the specific internal social processing or decision-making skills involved in bullying, it is clear that bullying does not occur in isolation. Therefore, any effective intervention program must take into account the social context in which the behavior occurs. In this case, social context refers to both the immediate social structure or peer group that directly surrounds the bullying behavior and the larger cultural and institutional context, including the school (Orpinas & Horne, 2006; Staub, 1996; Sutton et al., 1999).

Peer Influences

Bullying is a social behavior that operates in, and is sustained by, a peer group. This is particulary important in considering bullying in a high school context, as developmentally, the influence of peers is quite strong in high school-age students. The process of identity development occurs in large part through interpersonal and social interactions with peers and the interpersonal feedback individuals receive through that process. Staub (1996) describes the need for a positive identity, connection to peers, and feelings of effectiveness and control as central to development during adolescence.

A large part of this peer interaction occurs in groups. As described by Akos et al. (2007), "In early adolescence, students naturally coalesce into peer groups, which represent students who affiliate with one another based on shared interests, behaviors, and orientations" (p. 53). As peer groups naturally organize and differentiate, group boundaries and norms develop. Conformity to these boundaries and rules then becomes one significant influence on individual behavior (Farmer et al., 2007).

Although peer groups and the interpersonal interactions that happen within them are a natural part of adolescent development, they can have unintended negative consequences. Within peer groups, specific models of acceptable behavior are reinforced. Ronan and Curtis (2008) describe the research on the impact of the negative social influence within peer groups. These negative influences are understood to operate in two separate but related ways: selection and socialization. Selection operates in that peers tend to associate with like-minded peers. In high schools, this selection process often results in cliques and groups in which those with particular styles of social interaction or interpersonal skills migrate toward each other. Once students come together into a group, socialization effects then operate to train, influence, and reinforce specific types of behaviors within the group. Particularly for students with poor social skills and aggressive behavior, this socialization process includes aggressive and coercive problem-solving strategies (Granic & Patterson, 2006) as well as hostile attribution bias (Dodge, Bates, & Pettit, 1990). Thus, students who bully tend to hang out with students who also bully at similar frequencies. These groups of students then tend to increase the frequency of their bullying behavior over the school year (Espelage, 2003).

Group influences not only shape how adolescents perceive and relate to those within their own groups, but also influence how they perceive and relate to those on the outside of their groups. As described by Oppenheimer (2006):

> Within a peer group a hierarchical structure and external attribution processes can be observed. For instance, rejected or disliked children may become a target group or outgroup within the ingroup. Apparently no social group can function without defining either an internal outgroup (e.g. the rejected children) or an external outgroup, which is more likely when the ingroup is cohesive and defined by shared interests and actions. (p. 280)

This devaluation of specific children or groups outside one's own can become another force that supports and sustains bullying behavior.

It appears then that bullying prevention efforts must address both the norms and behaviors that are reinforced within peer groups and the perceptions and relations between groups. This has several important implications. A comprehensive bullying prevention program should connect students from different groups or "cliques" together who might not otherwise connect. Staub (1996) argues that experiential learning through deep and meaningful interactions among members of different social groups is crucial. He maintains that such direct interpersonal experiences are central to reducing devaluation between groups. Through sustained connections with different types of students, socialization can be encouraged that will reinforce more prosocial thoughts and behaviors within groups as well. Natural opportunities for such interactions in high schools are likely to be limited at best and may need to be purposefully structured in order to occur successfully.

School Climate

In addition to the role of the immediate peer group in bullying and aggressive behavior, the overall school climate in which it occurs is also of importance. The development of a positive school climate has been repeatedly identified as a key to prevention and intervention efforts. Orpinas and Horne (2006) reported that a positive climate is clearly related to a reduced problem with bullying and aggression in schools. As described by Oripinas and Horne, in establishing a positive climate, a school's goal should be to "create an environment in which students behave appropriately because they care about each other and because they are engaged in learning, not because they fear being reprimanded" (p. 94).

One important factor in creating a school climate, then, is the sense of connectedness students have toward their school. Students' sense of connectedness contributes to their overall sense of engagement with school, which in turn contributes to a number of important outcomes. Student connection to school has been found to be a salient protective factor against acting-out behaviors in school and a supportive factor in maintaining school attendance and academic achievement (Manning, 2005; Northeast & Islands Regional Educational Laboratory at Brown University, 2001). Similarly, as described by Staub (1996), "Just like bonds to people, bonds to social institutions like school or church diminish aggressiveness" (p. 126). If students feel connected to their school and care about what happens there, they are less likely to tolerate bullying and more likely to intervene.

Relationships with peers have been shown to play a large role in this sense of connection. Students who experience strong positive relationships with peers are more likely to engage in the classroom than those who feel alienated from their peers (Wentzel & Watkins, 2002). Conversely, poor peer relationships and social alienation are risk factors for poor school performance and dropping out of school (Dimmit, 2003; D. S. Kaplan, Peck, & H. B. Kaplan, 1997). Furthermore, students who lack a sense of connectedness to peers and to school are at greater risk for aggressive behavior (Resnick et al., 1997).

Many of the published bullying prevention programs currently in use place an emphasis on school climate in some form. In a recent review of such programs (Horne, Raczynski, & Orpinas, 2008), seven of the nine programs reviewed included interventions intended to improve the social environment as a means of preventing or reducing bullying. None of these programs, however, are designed specifically for high school settings and may not fit easily into the setting and structure of most high schools.

For example, two of the programs that have been widely adopted in schools, the Olweus Bully Prevention Program (Olweus, 1993; Olweus & Limber, 2002) and Bully Busters (Horne et al., 2003; Newman, Horne, & Bartolomucci, 2000), are school-wide programs that emphasize a change in the school climate through interventions at the classroom level. Many of the interventions are delivered by teachers to students in a classroom setting.

At the high school level, this arrangement is likely to be more challenging to implement, and perhaps less effective. The structure of most high schools is such that students don't have the same sustained relationships with teachers that they do in elementary and middle schools. High schools are frequently organized around academic departments in which teachers are content experts who teach the same curriculum to several classes of students each day. Likewise, students participate in several classes per day, each made up of different combinations of teachers and students. Therefore, the school climate in high schools may be shaped and influenced in different ways than in schools in which one teacher is responsible for a single group of students each day.

Social interactions that occur among students themselves play a very large role in the lives of most high school students and in setting the school climate. Such interactions often take place outside the domain of one specific teacher or classroom. Peer relationships and peer groups occur across classrooms and even across grade levels. Classrooms may not be the primary setting that influences the climate within high schools; a successful approach to bullying prevention at the high school level should incorporate these differences into the program model and delivery system.

The importance of addressing the school climate is being increasingly recognized by high schools. This increased attention has resulted in the proliferation of programs such as freshmen academies, smaller learning communities, and other structural changes to improve the overall sense of community within schools. However, such programs are largely oriented toward academic improvements and/or supporting relationships between students and teachers. The relationships that develop among peers, and the sense of being connected to or disconnected from schools that result, are often largely left to chance. However, it is precisely these peer relationships and sense of connectedness that are likely to influence the level of bullying present in high schools. Any successful program should target peer relationships as an important means of prevention and intervention.

DEVELOPING A COMPREHENSIVE HIGH SCHOOL BULLYING PREVENTION PLAN: THE CONNECTEDNESS IS KEY PROGRAM

The research described in the previous section has important implications for the development of a high school bullying prevention and intervention program. First, such a program should build social competence for all students. The relationship between social competence and bullying for high school students is likely to be similar to that of students of younger ages. However, a program to enhance social competence in high school students should be targeted specifically to the relational needs and characteristics of this age group, which are likely to be different from that of younger students. Secondly, such a program should provide opportunities for interpersonal experiences and communication between students and social groups who would not otherwise do so. These should be opportunities for genuine and sustained interactions, as recommended by Staub (1996). Such experiences would provide opportunities for students to learn and practice new ways of interacting and to increase students' overall sense of connectedness, thereby improving the school climate as well.

The Connectedness is Key (CIK) program (Horne, Nitza, et al., 2008) is a bullying prevention and intervention program designed specifically for high school settings. Drawing on the theoretical and empirical literature described above, the CIK program targets reductions in bullying and aggression through two primary goals: the development of a sense of connectedness among students and promotion of the social competence skills necessary to sustain healthy relationships. To accomplish these goals, the program utilizes a peer-led small group format; upperclassmen are trained to cofacilitate small group discussions with freshmen. These discussion groups incorporate structured activities designed to teach, refine, and/or practice specific skills, followed by open discussion and processing to give students the opportunity to implement these skills in the development of peer relationships within the group itself. The program thus utilizes the peer-led group format for addressing both content (i.e., skill building) and process issues (i.e., connectedness and relationship building) in high schools. In doing so, two powerful influences on adolescent behavior serve as guiding principles for the program: group processes and peer relationships.

Use of Group Process

Group-based interventions for adolescents in schools are strongly supported by the literature. Overall, the effectiveness of group counseling with adolescents is well established. For a wide variety of presenting concerns, group interventions are at least comparable, if not superior, to other forms of intervention (Hoag & Burlingame, 1997). Group interventions may even be considered the treatment of choice for many of the concerns facing this population.

The effectiveness of groups with adolescents is due in large part to the fit of groups with their developmental needs. Groups are a natural point of intervention for this population, as peers and social groups play such a large role in the lives of adolescents. Additionally, many of the developmental issues commonly faced by this age group lend themselves well to intervention in a group format. Groups provide the opportunity to experience the universality of their concerns, to feel connected and supported, and to learn through interpersonal experiences. As described by Shechtman, Bar-El, and Hadar (1997):

> There are many advantages to groups for adolescents: They are a natural way for adolescents to relate to each other, they emphasize the learning of life skills, they focus on generalizing behaviors practiced in the group to real-life situations, and they provide multiple feedback and increase self-esteem that comes about through helping others. (pp. 203-204)

Additionally, the group format offers the opportunity for several experiences that are important for adolescents but not as easily provided in individual interventions. These include the opportunity to practice new skills and behaviors, to both give and receive peer support, to learn from the differing ideas and opinions of others, to learn about oneself through feedback from others, and to improve reasoning skills through discussions with peers (Akos et al., 2007). Although the impact of less structured negative peer interaction, or "peer pressure," is well known to parents and educators alike, group interventions for adolescents capitalize on more positive "peer influence" and provide an effective forum for strength-based prevention programs.

As noted by Horne, Stoddard, and Bell (2007), group formats are commonly used in bullying prevention programs. However, such programs may be delivered in a group format with little attention to the group dynamics and process that are often key components of a successful group intervention. Merely putting people together in a group and delivering content is different from utilizing the group itself as an intervention. Students must not only talk about, but experience, the factors that foster healthy relationships. The experiencing comes through activating and utilizing group process. The impact of the CIK program comes not from putting students in groups and having them do activities, but from the opportunities presented by the activities to get students to learn to talk to each other directly and genuinely and to interact with each other in more positive ways.

Use of Peer Influence

In the CIK program, the groups are led by peer mentors. Juniors and seniors who apply to be mentors in the program are screened, selected, and complete a thorough training program in peer mentoring and group leadership. They then co-lead small groups throughout the school year, utilizing the curriculum as described below. This peer-led delivery system is intended to capitalize on the natural influence of peers during adolescence and to reduce peer reinforcement of bullying behavior.

Compared to the literature on group work with adolescents, there is less research on the effectiveness of peer helping programs. However, such programs have been identified as one successful intervention for improving students' connection to school through improving their relationships with each other (Manning, 2005). Such programs come in a variety of forms, including peer counseling, tutoring, mediating, and mentoring. However, they generally have in common the goal of placing students in helping roles with other students, which in turn enhances their own relationship skills. In each case, they provide students with the opportunity to play a proactive role in developing meaningful relationships with other students, thereby connecting them to each other and to the school itself (Manning, 2005).

Within the literature on peer helping programs, references to peer-led groups appear only occasionally. Peer group facilitation programs, like other forms of peer helping, appear to have a positive impact on the self-concept of the students trained as facilitators (Sprinthall, Hall, & Gerler, 1992; Thompson, 1986; Wang, 1987). Initial evidence indicates that such programs have been successful in enhancing personal adjustment of group members as well (Sprinthall et al., 1992; Wang, 1987). At least one study has identified the small group method itself as being responsible for the positive changes in participants (Sprinthall et al., 1992).

Preliminary results from a study of effective peer group leadership indicate that a series of relationship or group process variables are clearly the most meaningful to members (Nitza et al., 2008). Mentor behaviors most frequently described as helpful included listening to members, self-disclosing about their own experiences in high school, and facilitating a safe and welcoming group atmosphere. Conversely, the least frequently listed behaviors were those that dealt with specific program topics or activities. These results suggest that the mentors can effectively be trained to lead groups and that members of such groups find an emphasis on group process and dynamics beneficial. Overall, peer group leadership appears to have a number of potential benefits to group leaders, members, and the school as a whole.

The CIK Program Model

The CIK program contains 17 modules or group sessions. The model emphasizes social competence by addressing prosocial skills and topics in the first section of the program. These skills are referred to as "connects"; that is, skills and topics that promote healthy relationships and therefore help students connect with one another. Then, having covered a range of skills, beliefs, and ideas that promote healthy relationship development, the second set of modules is built to cover a range of problems that occur in peer relationships, or "disconnects," including bullying, relational aggression, and other interpersonal problems. These modules also offer the opportunity to consider how to manage these problems by applying the skills introduced in the first section. Each module in this section is designed to stand alone; schools, or mentor group leaders, are encouraged to select the topics that are of most relevance or interest to their students.

Part One: Connects

The first two modules are introductory sessions that focus on establishing a group climate that will be conducive to the accomplishment of program goals. Module One contains activities to allow students to get to know each other and establish group norms. The goal of Module Two is to introduce students to the overall objectives of the program. It is intended to generate a rationale for the discussions, activities, and skills targeted in the remaining group sessions and, perhaps more importantly, to empower students to want to make their school a better place. The activities in this session are designed to encourage students to reflect on peer relationships and the interpersonal climate of their school and to begin to consider how bullying or relational aggression may be impacting that climate. The goal at this stage is not to prescribe any specific solutions or ideas but rather to encourage students to engage in a genuine conversation about their experiences in a meaningful way.

Module Three focuses on empathy and respect for differences. The goals of the session are to nurture students' capacity for empathy and understanding of each other and to encourage them to respond to each other in an empathic manner. Empathy is crucial to improving interpersonal relationships and the overall school climate; the greater the students' capacity to be empathic with others, the greater their ability to understand the nature of conflicts, to seek common ground, and to find mutually satisfying solutions. Activities in this session are intended to encourage students to share and listen to each others' experiences and to consider how their own values and behaviors impact those around them.

Module Four targets communication skills. Effective communication skills include the ability to communicate ideas and feelings clearly and accurately as well as to hear and actively understand what another person is saying. Both skills are crucial to successful interpersonal relationships. Activities in this module include opportunities to practice sending and receiving verbal messages accurately as well as to practice active listening in genuine conversations.

Module Five focuses on the topic of trust. The need to trust others and to be trusted by them is the foundation of social relationships. Trust is also essential to the success of the program and to the overall reduction of bullying behavior. Students must feel safe enough in their mentoring groups to share their own experiences and discuss situations honestly. Without this foundation, the groups will remain superficial and relationships among students will go no further than they were prior to the group. Similarly, a sense of trust and safety is essential for a school climate that does not condone bullying or relational aggression.

Considering the mentoring groups as models for the larger school community, establishing a group environment that fosters socially respectful interaction and promotes trust is essential. As students explore the concept of trust within their small groups, they will also begin to develop the awareness, skills, and motivation necessary to continue to build meaningful relationships within the school community. Activities in this module serve as demonstrations of the importance of trust. They are intended to serve as prompts for discussion about trust and its effect on the group and the school.

Module Six is entitled "Internal Influences on Behavior." It focuses on the relationship between cognitions and behavior. A common belief among adolescents (and adults as well) is that other people and other events *cause* them to have particular feelings; the corollary is that other people or events *cause* them to behave in a particular way. Such beliefs are problematic in that they remove one from self-blame and from self-control. Many teens who are aggressive toward others blame the victim by claiming that the victim made them do it. Many victims believe they have no choices in a situation, thus allowing themselves to be mistreated. The goal of this module is to reinforce to students that they do, in fact, have some choice over their feelings and behaviors, including how they treat others and how they allow themselves to be treated. The activities in this module utilize principles from cognitive therapy models to highlight how thoughts and self-talk influence feelings and behaviors, and encourage students to explore their own self-talk in specific situations.

Module Seven is entitled "External Influences on Behavior." In order for students to fully understand how they make decisions and choices, particularly social and relational choices, they must explore not only their self-talk and beliefs, but also how they are influenced by others. In high schools, it is common for kids to "go along with the crowd" for a variety of reasons. Frequently friendship, the desire to fit in, striving to be popular, or other forms of peer pressure can influence students to make decisions that they would not otherwise make. Often, these decisions can be made automatically; students may follow the crowd without ever stopping to think about how they have arrived at this decision or the potential consequences of the decision.

The activities in this unit are designed to encourage students to stop and think about the people and social factors that influence their choices. They are intended to make students' social decision making more explicit and therefore more purposeful. In doing so, students may be more able and willing to consider their role in supporting or discouraging bullying and to become more active in taking a stand against it.

Module Eight revisits the topics in the preceding modules to consider what it means to have healthy relationships and what skills and behaviors it takes to develop and maintain such relationships. Both peer friendships and dating relationships are covered. Activities in this module are designed to internalize and reinforce the concepts in previous modules and to apply them through practice in role plays as well as discussion of scenarios and real-life situations. This transitional module also lays the groundwork for consideration of some of the problems that can sabotage healthy relationship development, which is the focus of the second section of the program.

Part Two: Disconnects

The first module in the second section sets the stage for later modules by introducing conflict resolution and problem-solving strategies. The goal of this module is to introduce an overall conflict resolution approach that can then be considered and discussed in each of the modules that address specific types of bullying or relationship problems. The remaining modules cover relational aggression, verbal aggression, physical bullying, cyberbullying, cliques, and harassment and dating violence. The general idea of each module is similar. A specific relational problem is identified and discussed; activities are designed for students to consider their own reactions and behaviors in such situations and to generate alternative choices either individually or as a group. Program directors, or group co-leaders, can thus select the modules that are most relevant to the types of bullying or other relational problems they experience at their own schools. Two of these modules, covering cliques and cyberbullying, are described below as examples.

The module on cliques is designed to highlight and explore the powerful role that peer groups play in students' lives in both positive and negative ways. Even though it is rarely discussed overtly, students are typically highly aware of the different cliques within their school, the characteristics of each clique, and even the unspoken "rules" that tend to guide interactions both within and between cliques. The goal of this module is to make some of the unspoken rules explicit so that students can discuss them openly. The activities in the model are intended to help students explore the role of cliques in their school and to encourage reflection on the impact to individuals when interactions are guided by group stereotypes. In the processing following these activities, students also discuss how they can expand their own social networks beyond their own small peer groups or cliques and contribute to an overall sense of connectedness within their schools.

The module on cyberbullying highlights this increasingly prevalent and dangerous problem. This module is intended to heighten students' awareness about the problem and its consequences. Direct discussion among peers about cyberbullying is important because of the indirect, distant, and even anonymous nature of the behavior itself. By naming it, discussing it and its (often extreme) consequences, as well as reflecting on their own behavior, students will be less likely to be able to engage in the behavior with the same level of disconnectedness and anonymity. Additionally, students may be less likely to be passive bystanders when they become aware of their friends engaging in it. The activities in this module encourage students to discuss the problem openly, to reflect on their own behavior in perpetrating this type of bullying or in standing by or supporting others who do, and to discuss realistic options for intervening when they become aware of the problem.

CONCLUSION

Much is known about the individual and contextual influences on bullying behavior. Several programs have been developed and implemented to address these influences. However, such programs have rarely been designed to meet the needs of high schools specifically. Although the content of such programs is often consistent with the existing literature, the delivery systems for this content do not typically fit well into a high school context.

The CIK program addresses both the individual and contextual influences on bullying while employing a delivery system that is highly relevant to the needs of high school students as well as the structure of the high school setting. The CIK program targets the developmental needs of adolescence by utilizing a group-based, peer-led model that emphasizes not only content and skill development but also relationship development and connectedness among peers. The combined effectiveness of these components addresses the problem of bullying in a theoretically and empirically based, developmentally appropriate format.

CONTRIBUTOR

Amy Nitza, PhD, is an Assistant Professor and Coordinator of the School Counseling Program at Indiana University-Purdue University Fort Wayne (IPFW). Her areas of interest are in family- and group-based interventions with adolescents. She is the producer of the recent DVD "Leading Groups with Adolescents," published by ASGW. Dr. Nitza is a 2008-2009 Fulbright Scholar at the University of Botswana, where she holds appointments to the Department of Educational Foundations and the Centre for the Study of HIV & AIDS. She may be reached at IPFW School of Education, 2101 E. Coliseum Blvd., Fort Wayne, IN 46805. E-mail: nitzaa@ipfw.edu

RESOURCES

Akos, P., Hamm, J. V., Mack, S. G., & Dunaway, M. (2007). Utilizing the developmental influence of peers in middle school groups. *The Journal for Specialists in Group Work, 32*, 51-60.

Craig, W. M., & Pepler, D. J. (2007). Understanding bullying: From research to practice. *Canadian Psychology, (48)*2, 86-93.

Crick, N. R., & Dodge, K. A. (1994). A review and reformulation of social information-processing mechanisms in children's social adjustment. *Psychological Bulletin, 115*, 74-101.

Dimmitt, C. (2003). Transforming school counseling practice through collaboration and the use of data: A study of academic failure in high school. *Professional School Counseling, 6*(5), 340-349.

Dodge, K. A., Bates, J. E., & Pettit, G. S. (1990). Mechanisms in the cycle of violence. *Science, 250*, 1678-1683.

Espelage, D. (2003). Assessment and treatment of bullying. In L. VandeCreek & T. L. Jackson (Eds.), *Innovations in Clinical Practice: Focus on Children & Adolescents* (pp. 83-95). Sarasota, FL: Professional Resource Press.

Farmer, T., Xie, H., Cairns, B., & Hutchins, B. (2007). Social synchrony, peer networks, and aggression in school. In P. Hawley, T. D. Little, & P.C. Rodkin (Eds.), *Aggression and Adaptation: The Bright Side to Bad Behavior*. Mahwah, NJ: Lawrence Earlbaum Associates.

Granic, I., & Patterson, G. R. (2006). Toward a comprehensive model of antisocial development: A dynamic systems approach. *Psychological Review, 113*(1), 101-131.

Hoag, M. J., & Burlingame, G. M. (1997). Evaluating the effectiveness of child and adolescent group treatment: A meta-analytic review. *Journal of Clinical Child Psychology, 26*, 234-246.

Horne, A. M., Bartolomucci, C. L., & Newman-Carlson, D. A. (2003). *Bully Busters: A Teacher's Manual for Helping Bullies, Victims, and Bystanders (Grades K-5)*. Champaign, IL: Research Press.

Horne, A. M., Nitza, A., Dobias, B., Jolliff, D., & Voors, W. (2008). *Connectedness is Key: A High School Bullying Prevention Program*. Manuscript in preparation.

Horne, A. M., Raczynski, K., & Orpinas, P. (2008). A clinical laboratory approach to reducing bullying and aggression in schools and families. In L. L'Abate (Ed.), *Toward a Science of Clinical Psychology: Laboratory Evaluations and Interventions* (pp. 117-131). New York: Nova Science Publishers.

Horne, A. M., Stoddard, J. L., & Bell, C. D. (2007). Group approaches to reducing aggression and bullying in school. *Group Dynamics: Theory, Research, & Practice, 11*, 262-271

Kaltiala-Heino, R., Rimpela, M., Rantanen, P., & Rimpela, A. (2000). Bullying at school: An indicator of adolescents at risk for mental disorders. *Journal of Adolescence, 23*, 661-674.

Kaplan, D. S., Peck, B. M., & Kaplan, H. B. (1997). Decomposing the academic failure-dropout relationship: A longitudinal analysis. *The Journal of Educational Research, 90*(6), 331-343.

Manning, D. (2005). *Connected Students: The Key to School-Initiated Graduation Rate Improvement*. Oroville, WA: Bridges Transitions. Retrieved August 1, 2007 from http://www.bridges.com/marcom/campn/grip/connected_students.pdf

Newman, D. A., Horne, A. M., & Bartolomucci, C. L. (2000). *Bully Busters: A Teacher's Manual for Helping Bullies, Victims, and Bystanders*. Champaign, IL: Research Press.

Nitza, A., Delucia-Waack, J. L., Horne, A. M., & Dobias, B. (2008, March). *Training High School Students in Group Leadership and Mentoring: A Case Study*. Paper presented at the annual conference of the American Counseling Association, Honolulu, HI.

Northeast and Islands Regional Educational Laboratory at Brown University. (2001). Student-centered high schools: Helping schools adapt to the learning needs of adolescents. *Perspectives on Policy and Practice*. Retrieved August 1, 2007 from http://www.alliance.brwon.edu/pubs/perspectives/stdntctrhs.pdf

Olweus, D. (1993). *Bullying at School: What We Know and What We Can Do*. Cambridge, MA: Blackwell Publishers.

Olweus, D., & Limber, S. (2002). *Bullying Prevention Program*. Boulder, CO: Center for the Study and Prevention of Violence, Institute of Behavioral Science, University of Colorado at Boulder.

Oppenheimer, L. (2006). The development of enemy images: A theoretical contribution. *Peace and Conflict, 12*, 269-292.

Orpinas, P., & Horne, A. M. (2006). *Bullying Prevention: Creating a Positive School Climate and Developing Social Competence*. Washington, DC: American Psychological Association.

Resnick, M. D., Bearman, P. S., Blum, R. W., Bauman, K. E., Harris, K. M., Jones, J., et al. (1997). Protecting adolescents from harm – Findings from the National Longitudinal Study on Adolescent Health. *Journal of the American Medical Association, 28*, 823-832.

Rigby, K. (2003). Consequences of bullying in schools. *Canadian Journal of Psychiatry, 48*, 583-590.

Ronan, K. R., & Curtis, N. (2008). Treatment of antisocial youth and families. In L. VandeCreek & J. B. Allen (Eds.), *Innovations in Clinical Practice: Focus on Group, Couples, and Family Therapy* (pp. 5-27). Sarasota, FL: Professional Resource Press.

Shechtman, Z., Bar-El, O., & Hadar, E. (1997). Therapeutic factors in counseling and psychoeducational groups for adolescents: A comparison. *Journal for Specialists in Group Work, 22*, 203-214.

Sprinthall, N. A., Hall, J. S., & Gerler, Jr., E. R. (1992). Peer counseling for middle school students experiencing a divorce: A deliberate psychological education model. *Elementary School Guidance and Counseling, 26*, 279-294.

Staub, E. (1996). Cultural-societal roots of violence: The examples of genocidal violence and of contemporary youth violence in the United States. *American Psychologist, 51*, 117-132.

Sutton, J., Smith, P. K., & Swettenham, J. (1999). Bullying and 'theory of mind': A critique of the 'social skills deficit' view of anti-social behavior. *Social Development, 8*, 117-127.

Thompson, R. A. (1986). Developing a peer group facilitation program on the secondary school level: An investment with multiple returns. *Small Group Behavior, 17*(1), 105-112.

Vossekuil, B., Fein, R., Reddy, M., Borum, R., & Modzeleski, W. (2002). *The Final Report and Findings of the Safe School Initiative: Implications for the Prevention of School Attacks in the United States*. Washington, DC: U.S. Department of Education, Office of Elementary and Secondary Education, Safe and Drug-Free Schools Program, and U.S. Secret Service, National Threat Assessment Center.

Wang, W-h. (1987). The effect of a peer counselor's training program and peer group counseling in a senior high school. *Bulletin of Educational Psychology, 20*, 205-227.

Wentzel, K., & Watkins, D. (2002). Peer relationships and collaborative learning as contexts for academic enablers. *School Psychology Review, 31*, 366-377.

Wolke, D., Woods, S., Bloomfield, L., & Karstadt, L. (2001). Bullying involvement in primary school and common health problems. *Archives of Disease in Childhood, 85,* 197-201.

Young, E. L., Boye, A. E., & Nelson, D. A. (2006). Relational aggression: Understanding, identifying, and responding in schools. *Psychology in the Schools, 43*, 297-312.

Developing a Life Coaching Practice

Patrick Williams

When I started my coaching career, people would often ask, "What sport do you coach?" This is not surprising, given the history of the word *coach* and its tie to athletics. Now, when I say "life coach," people still look at me curiously, but I no longer need to discuss "what sport." Our profession is receiving more and more public awareness and attention.

Coaching and *mentoring* have been common terms in the corporate environment for decades. Executive coaching has always been accepted as a perk or desirable form of consultation and support for high-level management. A new distinction today, however, is mentoring, which is a service provided formally or informally in order to train those employees who might be moving up the corporate ladder internally and who are mentored on the manager's ways. Corporate coaching today is provided both internally (by coaches who work for the company) and externally (by coaches hired by either the company or the managers themselves). Life coaching has now become desirable and accessible to those outside the corporate environment, and many corporate and business leaders understand that, ultimately, it is *all* life coaching.

However, many people in the helping fields are still unaware of what coaching is and how to become a coach. As a way into looking at how one might develop a life coaching practice, it might be useful to first take a look at the history of coaching as a development out of traditional psychology. Psychology and coaching share a similar history, and each can learn much from the other.

THE PSYCHOLOGICAL ROOTS OF LIFE COACHING

Psychological theorists in the early part of the 20th century set the framework for life coaching's "whole and healthy person" view. The shift from seeing clients as ill or pathological toward viewing them as "well and whole" and seeking a richer life is paramount to understanding the evolution of life coaching. Life coaches view clients as whole and brilliant people and focus not on pathology, but on wellness.

Most people would agree that Sigmund Freud (1933/1965, 1982) had a dramatic influence on society's view of mental illness and stimulated a deeper understanding of behavior. Although much of Freud's theory has little applicability to life coaching, he did profess that driving influences in people's lives were not conscious (ego-driven) but unconscious forces –

the id (libido) and the superego (social conscience), which he believed provided rich opportunities for analysis and dream interpretation. It is this emphasis on symbolic thinking that is relevant to and beneficial for life coaching. Life coaches help clients discover their brilliance, which often lies masked or buried in their unconscious mind and can be accessed when they begin to design their lives consciously and purposely.

A few colleagues from Freud's inner circle, including Carl Jung and Alfred Adler, broke away from his theories of neurosis and psychosis, positing theories that were more teleological and optimistic about human potential. Although there remains a significant distinction between therapy approaches and coaching, many of Adler's and Jung's theories are antecedents of modern-day life coaching.

Adler (1927/1998; H. L. Ansbacher & R. R. Ansbacher, 1956), for example, saw himself as more of a personal educator, believing that every person develops a unique life approach that shapes his or her goals, values, habits, and personal drives. He believed that happiness arises from a sense of significance and social connectedness (belonging), not merely from individual objectives and desires. Adler saw each person as the creator and artist of his or her life and frequently involved his clients in goal setting, life planning, and inventing their future – all tenets and approaches in life coaching today.

Similarly, Carl Jung (1933, 1970, 1976; Read, Fordham, & Adler, 1953) believed in the power of connectedness and relationships, as well as a "future orientation" or teleological belief that we create our future through visioning and purposeful living. Many of Jung's writings focused on life after the age of 40. This focus is particularly appropriate for life coaches, because we work primarily with adult learners. Jung often coached adults through a "life review" and encouraged his clients to consciously live their lives by expressing their natural gifts and talents, moving toward greater fulfillment by living life "on purpose."

Jung's theories and approaches also emphasized spirituality and the values expressed as one goes though the process he called individuation – the progression and development of the spiritual self. This is particularly prevalent in the second half of life, a time when life coaches are most likely to experience individuation themselves and support their clients to do the same. Jung also described the importance of myths and rituals, which are increasingly becoming important components of our life coaching clients' lives. I believe therapist-trained coaches are particularly qualified to assist clients in these important stages of adult development.

INFLUENCES OF HUMANISTIC PSYCHOLOGY AND THE HUMAN POTENTIAL MOVEMENT

During this time period, counseling and psychotherapy were starting to be viewed by many as arts more than sciences. The influence of the theories of Maslow (1954/1970, 1962, 1971/1993) and the emergence of humanistic, client-centered approaches (Bugental, 1967; Fadiman & Frager, 1976; Frankl, 1959; Rogers, 1951; among others) saw the client as full of potential and possibility rather than as stricken with neuroses or pathology.

In 1951, Carl Rogers' book *Client-Centered Therapy* defined counseling and therapy as relationships in which the client was assumed to have the ability to change and grow in the context of the clinician-created therapeutic alliance. This alliance evolved from a safe, confidential space granting the client or patient what Rogers called "unconditional positive regard." I believe this shift in perspective was a significant precursor to the development of life coaching.

In the years after World War II, American psychologists began to be influenced by European schools of thought, namely phenomenology and existentialism. These theoretical views laid much of the philosophical foundation for what was to become the Third Force in psychological thought – humanistic psychology. (The early work of Carl Rogers [1951], Kurt Lewin, Prescott Lecky, and, eventually, Abraham Maslow [1954/1970, 1962, 1971/1993] also served as important influences.) Emphasis then shifted to studying the whole person, not just fragmented parts.

Although the philosophies and values of humanistic psychology unified the whole field of psychology, it also polarized the profession. Humanistic psychology arose largely as a reaction against behaviorism's mechanistic view of humanity and was once again concerned with human experience and intrapsychic motivations, as it had been in psychology's earliest years, but these concerns were viewed as nonobservable, nonmeasurable, intervening variables, according to behavioral psychology's precepts.

Abraham Maslow, considered by many to be the father of humanistic psychology, was largely responsible for injecting much-needed credibility and energy into the human potential movement of the 1960s with the publication of his seminal treatise *Toward a Psychology of Being* (1962). In this work, Maslow summarized his research of "self-actualizing people" (a term first coined by Kurt Goldstein) and coined terms such as "full-humanness," "being," and "becoming." This book is largely a continuation of theories he first posited in *Motivation and Personality* (1954/1970). Maslow studied the "healthy personality" of people whom he termed self-actualizers; he researched, questioned, and observed people who were living with a sense of vitality and purpose, and who were constantly seeking to grow psychologically and achieve more of their human potential. It is this key point in history that I believe set the framework for the field of life coaching to emerge in the 1990s. People seeking personal evolution and ways to live more fully do not need psychological counseling; life coaching is a more accurate paradigm for the enhanced outcomes or achievements these clients seek.

Maslow was instrumental in granting value and importance to the idea of personal growth and asserting its necessity for the healthy personality. However, Maslow was not the first to hold these ideas. Many early psychiatrists and psychologists revolted against the orthodox approaches to mental problems and their emphasis on a person's pathological or pathogenic components. The reader has already been introduced to the influential work of Adler and Jung, but Gordon Allport (1937, 1955, 1961), James Bugental (1967), Kurt Goldstein, Karen Horney (1980), Sidney Jourard (1974), Prescott Lecky, Rollo May (1953, 1975, 1979), Carl Rogers (1951), and Fritz Perls also influenced psychology's move toward a wellness perspective that laid much of the groundwork for modern coaching theory, perspective, and techniques.

Third Force Psychology has found its place in mainstream psychology and is represented by an international organization. The first issue of the *Journal of Humanistic Psychology* was published in 1961 and edited by Anthony Sutich. The Association of Humanistic Psychology (AHP) began the following year. Abraham Maslow's ideas were central to the beginnings of both the journal and the association, but the AHP was not organized simply to promote his philosophy. The AHP represents a broad viewpoint, but it emerged as the third major force in psychology (following Freudianism and behaviorism) because of its unitary revolt against mechanistic, deterministic psychology. I believe this philosophical shift took root in a generation that now rejects the idea of sickness and instead seeks wellness, wholeness, and purposeful living. Hence the emergence of life coaching!

INFLUENCES OF MILTON ERICKSON AND SOLUTION-FOCUSED APPROACHES

The work of Milton Erickson (the father of American hypnosis) is a key precursor to the methods used in coaching today. Erickson, an iconoclastic and unique psychiatrist, believed in the inherent ability of individuals to achieve wellness if the reason for an illness could be thwarted (O'Hanlon & Hexum, 1991). Erickson often achieved seemingly "miraculous results" from just a few sessions with a patient. Jay Haley (1986) coined the term "uncommon therapy" to describe Erickson's approach.

Bandler and Grindler (1975), who were students of Erickson, then developed an approach called neurolinguistic programming (NLP), which represents an evolution of much of Ericksonian theory and technique. This approach focuses on outcome for the client and on the powerful use of language and question-asking by the therapist to facilitate transformational change. Linguistics and inquiry are key aspects of the work of a life coach, and much of the heritage of these fundamental coaching facets lies in the early work of Ericksonian practitioners.

More recent psychological approaches that have evolved from Ericksonian and other wellness approaches are the solution-focused therapies. These approaches, which are not insight or depth psychology dependent, are additional powerful influences on modern coaching theory and practices. In addition, Glasser's reality therapy, Ellis's rational emotive therapy, systemic family therapies (Haley, 1986; Madanes, 1981; Satir, 1964, 1976), psychosynthesis (Assagioli, 1965), and many hybrids of these lend themselves to coaching strategies. In all of these approaches, the main focus is not pathology but rather behavioral change through increased awareness and choices to allow for desired future results and solutions to current "problems in living." For example, the work of Bill O'Hanlon (1999; O'Hanlon & Beadle, 1999; O'Hanlon & Hexum, 1991; O'Hanlon & Martin, 1992) emphasizes possibilities and preferencing – an approach that fits well in life coaching relationships. The modern approaches of Steve de Shazer (1985, 1988) and his colleagues, called solution-focused counseling, could just as easily be called coaching. In fact, many of their techniques and approaches for use with difficult clients have been adapted into coaching techniques, such as the miracle question and asking powerful questions that lead to action-oriented steps. And more recently, the growth of Positive Psychology led by Martin Seligman (2002) and colleagues has added much to the credibility of life coaching as applied positive psychology.

Life coaching has, in essence, developed from three streams:

1. helping professions such as psychotherapy and counseling, and related theoretical perspectives as noted above,
2. consulting and organizational development and industrial psychology, and
3. personal development trainings such as Erhard Seminars Training (EST), Lifespring Landmark Forum, and the work of self-help writer and professional speaker Anthony Robbins.

The personal development courses listed above all focus on taking personal action and responsibility for one's life choices. They often include one-to-one coaching as part of their service or recommend it to those who desire sustainable results from the weekend training experience.

Having taken a quick tour of the psychological origins of life coaching, let us now move forward with an examination of what it takes to become a life coach.

BECOMING A LIFE COACH

I believe that therapists are eminently qualified to be life coaches, although I am also clear that many therapists enjoy what they do and have no desire to change their focus. That said, you are well-educated and well-trained, you possess the necessary critical helping skills, and you have many other skills and talents. All of these are essential ingredients for successful life coaches. If I asked you to write out your qualifications, you could draw up a long list. Other than additional training specific to life coaching, you are ready to start today. What might be keeping you from taking the next step?

During my experience coaching and training hundreds of therapists during the past several years, I have discovered what I believe to be the most important ingredient for a successful transition from therapist to life coach. It isn't where you went to college or how you were trained as a therapist. It isn't how successful your therapy practice has been or even how many years you have been a helping professional. The most important indicator of success in transitioning from therapist to life coach is your ability to make a change.

I have seen relatively new therapists transition smoothly into a full-time life coaching practice in a short time, while other experienced professionals struggle to infuse coaching into their practices on even a part-time basis. This journey will require you to think and act differently as a helping professional. I understand it is frightening to let go of the way you have always worked and try something new. This is plain old fear, a common emotion for individuals facing any transition. Whether you are planning to close your therapy practice completely and jump headfirst into life coaching or whether you want to stick your toes in first and try it on a part-time basis, a degree of discomfort is often associated.

As we tell our therapy clients, these fears are likely based on our negative beliefs about the world or about ourselves. If you hold on to these fears, you won't be able to take the risks, seize the opportunities, and develop the positive perspective necessary to function successfully as a life coach. Many therapists share a fear of marketing themselves as a life coach – of managing their coaching practice as a business. You may share this fear, or other fears might occur to you as you read. You can recognize them as the little voice in the back of your head trying to persuade you to put this contribution down and go back to doing what you already know how to do – therapy.

Reclaiming Your Soul: The Joyfulness of Life Coaching

Many therapists and counselors, especially those in private practice, have seen a monumental shift in the profession in the last several decades. Counseling and psychotherapy were, in my opinion, never meant to be part of the medical model, but were seen by many as an art in relating and helping people overcome psychological obstacles in their lives. But somewhere along the line, the therapy profession was included in third-party payment of services by insurance companies. This allowed health insurance to cover psychotherapy if a medical (psychiatric) diagnosis was given to the patient. Most therapists did not even use the term *patient* but instead opted for *client,* lending more credence to the professional view of therapy as being a nonmedical service.

The more we as a profession co-opted to be part of the medical/psychiatric community, the more entangled we became in the managed care system that began infiltrating the profession in the 1980s and became extremely intrusive in the 1990s. Almost every practitioner has seen his or her income drastically reduced and paperwork time increased.

This shift to managed care has caused great chaos, consternation, and burnout among private practitioners, to the point where approximately 10% leave the profession each year and another 10% wish they could! In fact, *Psychotherapy Finances,* in its annual survey of practitioners, states that 23% are taking steps to leave their practice (Williams, 2000). Nineteen percent now list coaching as a service they offer. One might say that coaching was a professional service waiting to happen, and managed care helped it along!

When training therapists about adding coaching to their repertoire, I have both observed and experienced the powerful impact this career transition (whether part-time or full-time) has had. Once clinicians hear about the possibility of working with high-functioning, highly motivated clients who will pay to have a coach, they become filled with excitement and get a joyful expression on their face. After all, most of us never wanted to work with severely depressed or conflicted persons 100% of the time. Didn't you often hope that potential clients would call you because they simply wanted to improve their life? Adding coaching as a new skill set allows you to choose more carefully the clients you see for therapy and attract new clients who are candidates for coaching.

As I describe the coaching relationship and the joyfulness of being someone's personal coach, let me first acknowledge that this joyfulness can also be part of the therapeutic relationship. I have provided counseling or psychotherapy for years, and I know that great joy and gratitude can be gained from assisting a client to overcome severe trauma or emotional struggles. I became a therapist to have a significant positive impact on people's lives and relationships. However, three undeniable factors seem to be at work in the profession of psychotherapy that can lead to a less-than-joyful experience for the therapist.

1. *Length of time in the profession.* Psychotherapy with emotionally fragile people can be draining over the long haul. Therapists give so much of themselves that professional burnout results if they do not self-nurture regularly.

2. *The degree of seriousness of clients' issues.* Therapists who often treat clients with serious and complicated diagnoses are at greater risk of burnout due to the psychic and emotional energy required to deal with such difficult and often irresolvable situations.

3. *Managed care.* Therapists who are trapped in the managed care system have fewer "approved" sessions with their clients and a lesser amount of reimbursement, as well as a reduction in income, more hours of paperwork, and increased liability. This scenario has led to a large percentage of therapists in private practice looking for ways to make a living in cash-only practices and needing to add other income streams to their business. Life coaching is a natural transition that can be added, along with training, speaking, and consulting.

What Makes the Coaching Relationship So Full of Joyful Energy?

Isn't it logical that supporting someone to experience a better life – a more fulfilling and empowered existence – should foster the experience of joy for both the coach and the client? This is a unique quality of the coaching relationship; the energy exchange seems to be less draining on a coach than it often is on a therapist. In fact, if the coaching relationship is draining to you as the coach, you are either working too hard on the client's behalf or the client is not coachable and may instead need therapy.

Many of my colleagues, as well as graduates of my training program who have shifted from therapist to coach, report several factors that have led to a more joyful work experience.

1. *The work schedule.* Coaches can include a mix of face-to-face coaching and phone coaching, and those who do phone coaching can work from home or wherever they happen to be. There are no parking concerns and no need to dress up. Coaches with international clients can even adjust their work hours to accommodate time-zone differences, thereby increasing their market base to global potential. One former therapist says,

   I no longer try to fit into somebody else's system or rules about how something needs to be done. I feel good about that because I can control what I do, and it fits who I am. I can control my schedule so that it fits my personal life, and the balance between work, play, and family is wonderful.

This statement reflects what I have heard from other coaches. You can still be part of your local community and meet people face to face, but your playing field expands to the whole world when you work by phone and e-mail. You still feel very connected with your clients and they with you.

2. *The ability to live and work wherever you desire.* Coaches who work by telephone with occasional in-person sessions can live in desirable places where building a therapy practice would have been difficult (unless one does therapy primarily by phone, which I have serious objections to and which leads to liability concerns as well). I know coaches who live in remote communities, on boats, and even in RVs for periods of time. Telecoaching is not geographically constrained. Some coaches have even exchanged homes with another coach for a month, and their only professional adjustment was to give their clients a different phone number for that period. Our joy of coaching comes in part from the opportunity to live, work, and play anywhere while maintaining a professional presence, as well as an above-average income.

3. *The egalitarian aspect of the coaching relationship.* Psychotherapy and counseling require, or at least assume, a hierarchical aspect to the relationship. Therapy takes on a "doctor-patient" or "expert-client" context and requires strict boundaries and ethics in the relationship outside of the office. In the coaching relationship, the concerns of transference and countertransference are not part of the equation. Although our professional training as therapists certainly makes us sensitive to that construct, we are much freer to be authentic with our clients.

4. *The financial rewards.* Although I realize that money is not the driving factor in all careers, I also believe that as therapists we have been undervalued and underpaid relative to our expertise, training, and effort. So the fact that life coaching can command a higher hourly fee or monthly retainer than therapy and requires no third-party billing is very inviting. To me, remuneration that is appropriate to the value received for the client is very freeing and more in line with other professions, such as accounting, legal services, strategic planning, and public relations. Professions that provide great value and results should command respectable fees.

   I believe that in recent times, professional therapists on average have been making less money and working longer hours. For therapists dependent on third-party payments and managed care rules, hourly fees have dropped and paperwork has increased. Even those who are in a private practice may have trouble commanding fees higher than $100 per hour. Of course, exceptions occur in large metropolitan cities, but this is an average fee. Although some coaching clients may not have the resources to pay more than that, most coaches command fees from $100 to $300 per hour – sometimes more for corporate or executive coaching. In general, coaching is for people who are already successful and who view coaching as a valuable service to assist them in achieving more, making significant changes, and living the life of their dreams.

Total Life Design

If you intend to be a credible coach, live your life as you coach others to live theirs. This does not mean your life must be perfect. Living purposefully means living in full awareness of what can be improved in your life and what you want to maintain or eliminate. This is why I believe it is essential that you also have a personal coach, especially during the beginning of your transition. Even later, when you are successful, having your own coach keeps you focused on your priorities, as well as aware of how your clients may experience the process of coaching. I have had coaches throughout my transitions and have also hired specialists from time to time.

Much of our approach is presented as Total Life Coaching™ (Williams & Thomas, 2005). I coach from a client-centered, whole-person approach, with the knowledge and experience that coaching for improvement in one area of a client's life will undoubtedly affect many other areas since they are all connected.

Here is my own definition of life coaching:

Life coaching is a powerful human relationship where trained coaches assist people to design their future rather than get over their past. Through a typically long-term relationship, coaches aid clients in creating visions and goals for ALL aspects of their lives and creating multiple strategies to support achieving those goals. Coaches recognize the brilliance of each client and their personal power to discover their own solutions when provided with support, accountability, and unconditional positive regard.

Truly effective coaching unleashes the client's individual spirit and deep desires, expands his or her capacity to achieve real change, and can even catalyze personal transformation. This does not occur with simple techniques like goal setting and motivation. It occurs when coaching considers the underlying context for change and facilitates the client's experience of living more on purpose. If you are going to be an effective coach, in a whole-person context, I believe it is essential for you to have done the work yourself. Most coach training programs teach a variety of techniques and strategies for coaching, but many utilize external skills. To be a truly masterful coach, you also must work on changing from within, because the profession of coaching is more about your *beingness* than about skills or techniques.

Many of us have experienced psychotherapy as clients, perhaps as an educational requirement or because we had our own healing work to do. Similarly, I believe masterful coaches must experience coaching on a regular basis and work with a coach on the very issues or desires that will also benefit your clients. For me, that starts with looking at one's life purpose, or life design.

Clients will indeed come to coaching for more mundane reasons than designing their life, but whatever the presenting objective, there is always the possibility of introducing the concept of Total Life Coaching™. For that process, you as the coach must have experienced the power of designing your life and living more on purpose.

Some coaching schools call this concept "coaching from the inside out." I consider it part of a coach's total life design, but whatever you call it, I believe it will help you discover ways to coach your clients about life design and personal fulfillment. In the process, this concept will be useful and perhaps even transformational for you as well. Being able to "walk the talk" as a coach means that you have experienced what you suggest for your clients and that you implement the skills so that your life is a model for your clients. Again, this does not mean that you are living the life of a saint or that you are an enlightened master; it means that you live your life purposefully and are aware of when you get in your own way. You must be committed to modeling how it is to be living a fulfilling life or be on the path to creating a fulfilling life. You generally will attract clients who are one step behind or one step ahead of where you are. Remember, sometimes the student is also the teacher.

With this brief introduction to the origins, benefits, and personal requirements of transitioning into a life coaching practice, we now turn to the hard part for many of us: learning how to build a coaching business. As challenging as it can be at times, we are running businesses and we must be able to look at our practices from that point of view.

DEVELOPING AND MARKETING YOUR LIFE COACHING PRACTICE

As therapists, we were never taught much about building our business. In fact, we do not even call it a business – we call it a practice! Further, most of us were taught that it was even unethical and unprofessional to market or advertise our services. It was not until the late 1980s that we started to run Yellow Pages ads with descriptions of our services, and we certainly never mentioned in conversations at cocktail parties that we could help someone with his or her problem.

As a coach, you are a businessperson providing a unique form of assistance. You can speak about it, advertise it, and enthusiastically let people know you might be able to help them reach their goals. You can even meet in public to discuss how your services might be of use.

Obviously, a crucial component for your transition to life coaching is learning entrepreneurial skills and the simple, powerful development and marketing steps for a successful business. It's only natural for most helping professionals to be uncomfortable with the idea of marketing or selling. The following simple strategies can provide you with new ways to approach marketing as a way of letting people know what you do.

Marketing Versus Selling

Most of us frequently confuse marketing with selling. We probably hear ourselves saying things like:

"I don't like selling."
"I can't take rejection."
"Selling is unprofessional."
"I don't want to appear pushy."
"I became a therapist, not a salesperson."

I understand these fears. They come from your inner gremlin – your self-critic. But you have many options for marketing your business, and it can even be enjoyable and natural. Think of it this way. If you are right-handed and lost the use of your right hand, eventually you would become proficient and comfortable using your left hand. It just takes practice and a willingness to change. And this is a wonderful new opportunity for learning, as well as for repackaging your current skills.

I also believe that the marketing methods you use should be enjoyable (although they may take some practice for you to achieve a good comfort level). Remember that you are not knocking on doors or telemarketing to sell a product that people do not want. Most people will want coaching. The goal is to attract the type of client you want to work with and for whom your services are both valuable and affordable. Isn't that true for the professional services *you* utilize?

Stop Being a Secret!

My basic philosophy is that if you want people to hire you as a coach, you must stop being a secret. The principle of attracting clients is more powerful than the manipulative promotion and selling other sales professionals use, but if you are going to follow the principle of attraction, remember that the word *action* comprises more than half of the word. You will not get clients by just wishing and hoping they will contact you. They need to know you exist, what it is you do, and the benefits they (or those they might refer) might receive by working with you as a coach.

As I have trained professionals to become coaches, I have heard many people talk about their beliefs, myths, and misconceptions about marketing. My training approach is based on five key principles.

1. *Marketing is not selling.* I wish I had thought of it first, but as Peter Drucker, the business and management consultant, said so eloquently: "The purpose of marketing is to make selling unnecessary" (p. 71; Drucker, 2001). I definitely agree. Of course, technically, you are selling. You are selling yourself and your service, but it should be done in a way that does not feel or look like stereotypical high-pressure selling. There is nothing inherently wrong with selling. We all sell and we all buy. Many of us, though, are uncomfortable with types of selling that pressure people into buying something they didn't want. Marketing your coaching services is simply opening a relationship and offering the possibility of coaching being something that could greatly benefit the potential client. It is not meant to be manipulative, seductive, or dishonest. You will need to learn to market yourself until your business grows to the point of being filled mostly by referrals – the ideal position for a self-sustaining business.

2. *Therapists have the necessary marketing skills because we are trained to listen well and communicate clearly, and also because we are good at creating relationships.* This is why marketing gurus of today, especially in service-oriented businesses, say that networking is the key to business success. What is networking? It is developing relationships with people so they know what you do and you know what they do. Networking is the way business is built through cross-referrals or as a way of serving your clients. Coaches who become master networkers and who can refer their clients to other professionals or services that might assist specific concerns will have a thriving business and a reputation as someone who knows whom to call or where to go. C. J. Hayden (2006) says, "Marketing is telling people what you do . . . over and over" (p. 7). So, the keys to success as a new coach come from figuring out what you want to say about your coaching, how to say it, and to whom you want to say it. If you truly love what you do, people will experience your authenticity, and even if they don't want to hire you as a coach, they may know someone who will. In coaching, you are hired more for who you are than for the specifics of what you do. If you are enjoying your life and you coach people so that they can, too, you are very attractive as a coach. People will want some of what you have. They will want you to help them achieve the level of happiness and clarity of vision that you have achieved. All you need to do is guide them to develop their life according to their desired agenda.

3. *Marketing your practice successfully and easily is more likely to occur when you clarify what you do, how you do it, with whom you work best, and so on.* Clarity allows you to focus your efforts, your resources, and your energies. It also allows you to craft a message about your coaching business that will attract clients to you (if you are not a secret). Clarity allows you to create a fulfilling practice, which may or may not be a full practice.

4. *Marketing your coaching business successfully can happen only when you have created the space, time, and energy for this new business paradigm to occur.* This is important. If you want to create a coaching business, you must turn intention into actions, give it energy and time, and be open to the changes in your life this will create.

5. *Be a resource.* As you get to know other coaches, professionals, books, and places where your clients can go for specific help or services, you become increasingly valuable. Keep a good database of international professionals, coaches, and schools. You can often find a helpful direction or resource for your client with a quick phone call or

e-mail. You become a great referral service as well as a great coach. It doesn't take much time or energy if you have the resources and contacts readily available.

First Steps to Marketing Your Practice

In the early stages of developing your coaching business, you can start by getting business cards, creating client folders, and being ready for your first "customer." When you are ready to start coaching (and I hope you have had some formal training), you need to start trying on the metaphoric coach's uniform. Get accustomed to using the phrase *life coach, personal coach,* or *business coach.* The popularity of coaching makes marketing much easier than it used to be. I cannot stress enough, however, that although you may be able to add coaching to your business and learn much from this contribution and other sources, you are not likely to become a masterful life coach without formal coach-specific training, as well as consulting with your own personal coach.

Developing a Target Niche

The current wisdom in marketing today, especially for a service-oriented business, is to develop one to three target niches. As a therapist or counselor, you may have some special expertise or skills that would lend themselves to a specific niche. For example, if you already do marriage or couples counseling, you might consider marketing yourself as a relationship coach. I know many relationship coaches who do couples coaching by phone and attract busy, dual-income couples who want to improve their relationship and often just need the space and time devoted to coaching for transformation to occur.

Another possible niche is family business coaching for a skilled systems-oriented therapist who is knowledgeable about the unique dynamics that arise in family-owned businesses. Associations and specific trainings are available for those who would like to specialize in coaching family businesses. Teen coaching, family coaching, coaching people with ADD, and so on are other obvious niches for skilled therapists.

I know a former career counselor who now has a full-time coaching business with career coaching as a specialty niche. All she really needed to change was the way she described her business. She still gives traditional assessments and job-search "coaching," but now she can do it internationally through faxes and e-mails. When clients complete their career-specific coaching, they often want to retain her as their life coach; the coaching then takes on a more whole-life perspective.

One way to develop a possible niche is to take a look at who comes into your office now. What kinds of clients are you best with? Whom do you enjoy working with the most? On the other hand, many therapists-turned-coaches develop new interests and may not want to do the same type of coaching as the therapy they did. It may also be confusing as to whether you are attracting coachable clients or clients who need therapeutic interventions. This can be one of the most challenging areas in your transition. Confer with your own coach or mentor about this.

Branding versus Niche Development

I have had discussions with many of the trainees in my coach-training business, as well as with therapists I have mentored to become coaches, about the distinction between branding and niche development.

Branding is based on the concept of singularity. It creates in the mind of the prospect the perception that no product on the market is quite like your product. You are your product. The coaching service you provide is your coaching – your style, your personality, your energy, your insight, and your integrity. Branding as a coach implies that you consider your own unique qualities and the unique qualities of the people you really want to coach, and you then give that combination a brand. For example, one coach I know wants to be known as the "life balance coach" and works with "busy professionals on the go who want to achieve balance in work, family, and fun." That is an example of a branding more than a niche. Next, she might think of a niche market where she could find such busy professionals – for example, lawyers, therapists, entrepreneurs, and so on. Can you see how this could be her entrée into coaching? How do you want to be branded?

Ask three friends and three colleagues what they find unique about you and your relationship with them. What do they get from you that is special? You are as unique as a snowflake or a fingerprint. How does that impact whom you coach and how you coach? How might this lead to a *brand?*

No Matter Where You Go, There You Are

Marketing can occur all the time because, as a therapist (and as a coach), it is you whom people hire, and the "you" that you present in public is part of the marketing. Another way to say this is that you are your message. This does not mean you are always selling, but it does mean that informal ways of meeting people or having conversations will eventually lead to the ubiquitous question, "What do you do?" How you answer that question or how you even elicit that question is the simplest, most efficient way to market your coaching business. I and many of my colleagues have actually found clients at the local tennis club, at an informal networking meeting, and on an airplane ride. The latter is actually more common than you think! How many times have you conversed with your seatmate on a plane and asked him or her, "What do you do?" If you ask it of your seatmate, he or she will ask it of you. One of the rules of good networking is to be interested in other people. People love to talk about themselves, and if you are genuinely interested in them – what their business is, what their hobbies are, and what dreams they have – they will most likely ask you what you do. Bingo! You might have a potential client.

Another marketing tip is often called the "elevator speech" or "magic moment." It is a quick response for those inevitable times when someone asks, "What do you do?" I like to refer to it as your "laser intro." A laser intro, as its name suggests, is done quickly and gets right to the point. The point is to let people know what you do so that they might ask more questions about how you do what you do. That leads to further conversation, either right then or at a future time, in which you have an opportunity to share details about how you work as a life coach and how you might be able to support the changes they seek.

The six key components of an effective laser intro or elevator speech include:

1. *Is it clear?* Your response to "What do you do?" must be clear, free of jargon, and easily understood.
2. *Is it concise?* A laser intro should be brief and delivered in 15 seconds or less.
3. *Is it compelling and captivating?* Your message must have a compelling quality – one that begs further inquiry and piques the listener's interest.
4. *Is it conversational?* Your message should be delivered in an informal manner. This takes practice. You must be so natural and automatic with your message that it doesn't sound like a rehearsed speech. A message delivered conversationally will encourage further conversation in your audience.
5. *Is it delivered with confidence?* The more practiced and natural you are and the more confident and passionate you are about what you do, the more attractive your message is to others. Remember that you are your message.
6. *Is the word "coach" in your message?* Somewhere in your message, you must say you are a coach (life coach, business coach, personal coach, relationship coach, parenting

coach, and so on). It is important for you to provide details about your style of coaching so that the listener can judge whether he or she might be interested in your services.

Having two or three laser intros is important so that you can adapt the basic message to your audience while still describing very quickly what you do. Here are a few tried-and-true laser intros I and other coaches have used successfully.

Q: What do you do?
A: I am a personal life coach. You know how people often have that gap between where they are and where they want to be? I work with them on filling the gap and creating the life they really want.

Q: What is it that you do?
A: Pretty much anything I want on any given day! And I teach others to do it, too! Does that sound like something that might interest you?

Q: What do you do?
A: I am a personal life coach. You know how a plumber comes in and snakes out your pipes to get the water flowing freely? What I do is work with people to unclog the personal and business blocks that keep their lives from flowing freely.

After the laser intro gets a person's attention, hopefully he or she will ask something like, "That sounds interesting. How do you do that?" Then the door is open to set a meeting over coffee or, better yet, to grant the person a free 30-minute coaching call so he or she can experience it firsthand. Even if you do not gain a client, the person will, at the very least, be familiar with your style and may become a great referral source for you!

In fact, your goal when you network with people or dialogue about your career is to be open to the possibility that the person may be genuinely interested in what you do and may want to know more. It is at this opportunity that I recommend being a living brochure – don't just talk about what coaching is, demonstrate it. Ask if you can coach the person on something he or she wants to change or a long-term goal. A spot coaching demonstration gives potential clients a taste of coaching, and they may then want the entire menu!

TO LEARN MORE

If you are interested in learning more about becoming a personal or professional coach, please consider these books:

Williams, P., & Davis, D. (2007). *Therapist as Life Coach: An Introduction for Counselors and Other Helping Professionals* (Revised and Expanded Edition). New York: W. W. Norton.

Williams, P., & Menendez, D. (2007). *Becoming a Professional Life Coach: Lessons From the Institute for Life Coach Training.* New York: W. W. Norton.

Williams, P., & Thomas, L. (2005). *Total Life Coaching: 50+ Life Lessons, Skills, and Techniques to Enhance Your Practice and Your Life.* New York: W. W. Norton.

Williams, P., & Anderson, S. (Eds.). (2006). *The Law and Ethics of Coaching: How to Solve and Avoid Difficult Problems in Your Practice.* Hoboken, NJ: John Wiley and Sons.

Drake, D., Brennan, D., & Gortz, K. (Eds.). (2008). *The Philosophy and Practice of Coaching: Insights and Issues for a New Era.* West Sussex, England: Jossey Bass.

Finally, you can contact The Institute for Life Coach Training (888-267-1206 or info@lifecoachtraining.com), which specializes in helping therapists make the transition to coaching.

CONTRIBUTOR

Patrick Williams, EdD, MCC, is a license psychologist and one of the early pioneers of coaching. He began executive coaching in 1990, and in 1998 he founded the Institute for Life Coach Training, an International Coaching Federation (ICF) Accredited Coach Training Program. He speaks internationally on purposeful living, vital aging and new eldering, and the power of the coach approach in empowering and sustaining change. He is the coauthor of *Therapist as Life Coach: Transforming Your Practice*; *Total Life Coaching: 50+ Life Lessons, Skills, and Techniques to Enhance Your Practice and Your Life*; *The Law and Ethics of Coaching: How to Solve and Avoid Difficult Problems in Your Practice*; and *Becoming a Professional Life Coach: Lessons From the Institute for Life Coach Training*. In June 2006, Dr. Williams was awarded the honor of being named the first Global Visionary Fellow by the Foundation of Coaching for his project – Coaching the Global Village – bringing the coaching approach to the underserved through nongovernmental organization (NGO) leaders in developing countries and nonprofit boards. Dr. Williams may be contacted at 17 Lakeside Drive, Palm Coast, FL 32137. E-mail: Pat@LifeCoachTraining.com

RESOURCES

Cited Resources

Adler, A. (1998). *Understanding Human Nature* (C. Brett, Trans.). Center City, MN: Hazelden. (Original work published 1927)

Allport, G. (1937). *Personality: A Psychological Interpretation*. New York: Holt.

Allport, G. (1955). *Becoming: Basic Considerations for a Psychology of Personality*. New Haven, CT: Yale University Press.

Allport, G. (1961). *Pattern and Growth in Personality*. New York: Holt, Rinehart & Winston.

Ansbacher, H. L., & Ansbacher, R. R. (Eds.). (1956). *The Individual Psychology of Alfred Adler: A Systematic Presentation in Selections From His Writings*. New York: Basic.

Assagioli, R. (1965). *Psychosynthesis: A Manual of Principles and Techniques*. New York: Hobbs, Dorman.

Bandler, R., & Grindler, J. (1975). *Patterns of the Hypnotic Techniques of Milton H. Erickson, M.D.* Cupertino, CA: Meta.

Bugental, J. F. T. (1967). *Challenges of Humanistic Psychology*. New York: McGraw-Hill.

de Shazer, S. (1985). *Keys to Solution in Brief Therapy*. New York: Norton.

de Shazer, S. (1988*). Clues: Investigating Solutions in Brief Therapy*. New York: Norton.

Drucker, P. (2001). *The Essential Drucker: In One Volume the Best of Sixty Years of Peter Drucker's Essential Writings on Management*. New York: Harper Collins.

Fadiman, J., & Frager, R. (1976). *Personality and Personal Growth*. Upper Saddle River, NJ: Harper & Row.

Frankl, V. E. (1959). *Man's Search for Meaning*. New York: Pocket.

Freud, S. (1965). *New Introductory Lectures on Psychoanalysis* (J. Strachey, Trans.) New York: Norton. (Original work published 1933)

Freud, S. (1982). *Basic Works of Sigmund Freud* (J. Strachey, Ed. & Trans.). Franklin Center, PA: Franklin Library.

Haley, J. (1986). *Uncommon Therapy: The Psychiatric Techniques of Milton H. Erickson*. New York: Norton.

Hayden, C. J. (2006) *Get Clients Now!* New York: Amacom Books.

Horney, K. (1980). *The Adolescent Diaries of Karen Horney*. New York: Basic.

Jourard, S. M. (1974). *Healthy Personality, an Approach From the Viewpoint of Humanistic Psychology*. New York: Macmillan.

Jung, C. G. (1933). *Modern Man in Search of a Soul*. London: Trubner.

Jung, C. G. (1970). *The Collected Works of C. G. Jung, Volume 10: Civilization in Transition* (G. Adler & R. F. C. Hull, Eds. & Trans.). Princeton, NJ: Princeton University Press.

Jung, C. (1976). *The Portable Jung* (J. Campbell, Ed., R. F. C. Hull, Trans.). New York: Penguin.

Madanes, C. (1981). *Strategic Family Therapy*. San Francisco: Jossey-Bass.

Maslow, A. (1962). *Toward a Psychology of Being*. Princeton, NJ: Van Nostrand.

Maslow, A. (1970). *Motivation and Personality*. New York: Harper. (Original work published 1954)

Maslow, A. (1993). *The Farther Reaches of Human Nature*. New York: Arkana. (Original work published 1971)

May, R. (1953). *Man's Search for Himself*. New York: Norton.

May, R. (1975). *The Courage to Create*. New York: Norton.

May, R. (1979). *Psychology and the Human Dilemma*. New York: Norton.

O'Hanlon, B. (1999). *Do One Thing Different: Ten Simple Ways to Change Your Life*. New York: Morrow.

O'Hanlon, W. B., & Beadle, S., (1999). *A Guide to Possibility Land: Fifty-One Methods for Doing Brief, Respectful Therapy*. New York: Norton.

O'Hanlon, W. H., & Hexum, A. L. (1991). *Uncommon Casebook: The Complete Clinical Work of Milton H. Erickson*. New York: Norton.

O'Hanlon, W. H., & Martin, M. (1992). *Solution-Oriented Hypnosis: An Ericksonian Approach*. New York: Norton.

Read, H., Fordham, M., & Adler, G. (Eds.). (1953). *The Collected Works of C. G. Jung*. New York: Pantheon.

Rogers, C. (1951). *Client-Centered Therapy*. Boston: Houghton Mifflin.

Satir, V. (1964). *Conjoint Family Therapy: A Guide to Therapy and Techniques*. Palo Alto, CA: Science & Behavior.

Satir, V. (1976). *Making Contact*. Millbrae, CA: Celestial Arts.

Seligman, M. (2002) *Authentic Happiness*. New York: Free Press

Williams, P. (2000, July). Practice building: The coaching phenomenon marches on. *Psychotherapy Finances, 26*(315), 1–2.

Williams, P., & Anderson, S. (Eds.). (2006). *The Law and Ethics of Coaching: How to Solve and Avoid Difficult Problems in Your Practice.* Hoboken, NJ: John Wiley and Sons.

Williams, P, & Davis, D. (2007). *Therapist as Life Coach: An Introduction for Counselors and Other Helping Professionals* (Rev. & Expanded Ed.). New York: W. W. Norton.

Williams, P., & Menendez, D. (2007). *Becoming a Professional Life Coach: Lessons From the Institute for Life Coach Training*. New York: W. W. Norton.

Williams, P., & Thomas, L. (2005). *Total Life Coaching: 50+ Life Lessons, Skills, and Techniques to Enhance Your Practice and Your Life*. New York: W. W. Norton

Additional Resources

Berg, I. K. (1994). *Family-Based Services: A Solution-Focused Approach*. New York: Norton.

Biswas-Diener, R., & Dean, B. (2007). *Positive Psychology Coaching: Putting the Science of Happiness to Work for Your Clients*. Hoboken, NJ: Wiley.

Hudson, F. (1999a). *The Adult Years*. San Francisco: Jossey-Bass.

Hudson, F. (1999b). *The Handbook of Coaching: A Comprehensive Resource Guide for Managers, Executives, Consultants, and HR*. San Francisco: Jossey-Bass.

Peterson, C. (2006). *A Primer in Positive Psychology*. New York: Oxford University Press.

Whitmore, J. (1995). *Coaching for Performance*. Sonoma, CA: Nicholas Brealey.

Williams, P. (1980). *Transpersonal Psychology: An Introductory Guidebook*. Greeley, CO: Lutey.

Williams, P. (1997). Telephone coaching for cash draws new client market. *Practice Strategies, 2,* 11.

Williams, P. (1999). The therapist as personal coach: Reclaiming your soul! *The Independent Practitioner, 19*(4), 204–207.

Williams, P. (2000, June). Personal coaching's evolution from therapy, *Consulting Today* [Special issue], 4.

Introduction to Section V:
Selected Topics

The SELECTED TOPICS section includes contributions that do not fit neatly into any other sections of the volume. In the first contribution to this section, Shelley S. Leiphart addresses the emergence of a new discipline combining neuroscience and psychotherapy. She provides a brief history of neuroscience and psychotherapy, and highlights the usefulness of neuroimaging in allowing for the study of all areas of the brain simultaneously. She addresses the importance of having a basic understanding of the brain in order to understand the mechanisms of action involved in psychotropic medication, and provides a useful handout of brain regions and associated functions. She also provides an overview of the neurobiology of memory, implicit and explicit memory, and the process of memory. The contribution ends by addressing empirical support for interventions relating to mood and anxiety disorders.

In the final contribution, Paul J. Hershberger includes a piece on positive psychology and optimal functioning. The positive psychology movement is reviewed, along with definitions of mental health. Benefits and correlates of mental health are addressed, as well as a number of factors in terms of their relationship to happiness. The relationship between optimism, happiness, and good physical health is addressed, as well as approaches to happiness. The contribution ends with a review of interventions that can be used by clinicians, organized around Seligman's concepts of positive emotions, flow, and meaning and purpose.

Combining Neuroscience and Psychotherapy: The Emergence Of a New Discipline

Shelley S. Leiphart

Recent advances in neurological imaging research have begun to highlight the brain regions that have been positively affected by psychotherapy and/or pharmacology with promising findings for the advancement of the field of psychology. The merging of neuroscience and psychotherapy can help to reinforce our current theoretical practices and provide a scientific or medical basis for our work. In this contribution, I wish to offer the reader an overview of the contemporary theories and research findings surrounding the combination of neuroscience and psychotherapy in different psychological disorders and discuss how these findings translate into treatment.

A BRIEF HISTORY OF NEUROSCIENCE AND PSYCHOTHERAPY

The connection between neuroscience and psychotherapy is not a new concept. In fact, Sigmund Freud believed in this connection early on, as he was a neurologist turned psychoanalyst. However, it wasn't until the development of functional imaging that the science of neurological change from psychotherapy could be directly studied and measured. Many in the field of psychotherapy have been reluctant to incorporate the advances of science into their work and have maintained the use of theoretical terminology that cannot be operationalized into scientific research as a way to take a stance against neuroscience and uphold the art of psychotherapy (Rybakowski, 2001). Although their efforts may be viewed as heroic, the other side of the argument believes the field of psychology must pull together toward the discovery of evidence-based treatments in order to remain competitive and not drown in a sea of insurance denials for reimbursement. Pharmacology research has largely begun to address the connection between biology and psychological disorders, but many people are faced with untoward side effects and the potential for lifelong medication usage, aspects that can be undesirable to some. Isn't it the responsibility of the field to explore alternative treatments that could prove to be equally as effective as medication to suit the diverse needs of their clientele?

Neuroscience can be useful not only by validating the strength of our existing therapeutic practices and interventions but also by postulating new directions to expand in, either separately away from or conjointly with our current practices (Cappas, Andres-Hyman, & Davidson, 2005). Although each theory of psychotherapy brings forth its own unique style of intervention and vocabulary, there do seem to be certain common factors that underline the effectiveness of each school of thought, such as the therapeutic relationship and an empathetic environment. Behavioral neuroscience may be yet another factor to unify, rather than divide, the theories through the development of effective skills and interventions.

Neuroimaging

The use of neuroimaging allows for the study of all areas of the brain simultaneously, whereas traditional psychological assessment measures can only look at specific variables independently. Many of the variables involve overlapping functions (e.g., the measurement of processing speed often involves an additional motor component), thus decreasing the ability to tweeze out the specific mechanism of action. Identifying the mechanisms of action for psychotherapy can help to elucidate the differences and similarities between psychotherapy and pharmacology and ultimately serve to identify the best treatment modality based on the presenting symptomology (Linden, 2006).

Researchers can use different types of imaging methods to study and record brain activity depending on their needs and research questions. Positron emission tomography (PET) and single photon emission computed tomography (SPECT) scans are conducted through nuclear medicine and can measure changes in brain metabolism or blood flow, whereas functional magnetic resonance imaging (fMRI) scans do not use radiation and can be used to measure activation patterns during perceptual or cognitive tasks (Linden, 2006). Electroencephalography (EEG) is also less invasive as it measures the electrical activity of the brain through electrodes placed on the scalp (Kalat, 2004).

Why Neuroscience Matters

Why should psychotherapists understand neuroscience and the brain? Having a basic understanding of the brain is essential for the digestion of current research and to understand the mechanisms of action involved in the psychotropic medications our clients are prescribed (Beitman & Viamontes, 2006). We are often asked why we are recommending medication to our clients, and knowledge of neuroscience will facilitate our understanding of the effectiveness of psychotropic drugs and can increase trust in the therapeutic relationship. Furthermore, because research seems to be headed in the direction of discovering the neurobiological correlates of psychotherapy, it is to our advantage to be kept abreast of the latest techniques in order to best meet the needs of our clients.

NEUROANATOMY BASICS

How Do You Pronounce Amygdala Anyway?

It can be confusing or even intimidating to keep all of the brain structures and their functions straight, making digestion of current neuroscience and psychotherapy research difficult. Table 1 (p. 281) will make sense of it all. After viewing Table 1 and you know what the structures are, what does this all mean?

Overview of the Neurobiology of Memory

Currently, the best existing model for memory input, storage, and retrieval is the long-term potentiation (LTP) model (Liggan & Kay, 1999). The LTP model suggests that the stimuli of new experiences can strengthen the neural connections, and that plasticity is the process by which we create and modify those connections in response to the experience (Cappas et al., 2005). Neurogenesis, the birth of new neurons, is an important aspect of improved memory and plasticity to serve as these new connections with which to modify our experiences. It was

---

Table 1: Regions of the Brain and Their Functions

Brain Region	Function
Frontal Lobe	Involved with planning, organization, problem solving, selective attention, and other "higher order" cognitive functions
Prefrontal Cortex	Responds mostly to sensory stimuli that signal the need for movement; important for "higher order" cognitive functions and personality
Dorsolateral Prefrontal Cortex	Motor planning, organization, regulation, working memory
Orbitofrontal Cortex	Involved in decision making
Temporal Lobe	Right side = visual memory; left side = verbal memory; both help in sorting new information
Medial Temporal Lobe	Involved with episodic/declarative memory
Parietal Lobe	Right side = visual spatial processing; left side = understanding of spoken or written language
Occipital Lobe	Processes visual information
Broca's Area	Involved in language processing and speech production
Cingulate Cortex	Part of the limbic system
Insula (insular cortex)	Processes information to produce emotionally relevant contexts for sensory experiences
Hippocampus	Lays down long-term memory
Parahippocampal Gyrus	Important role in memory encoding and retrieval
Amygdala	Generates emotional reactions
Thalamus	Processes sensory information and sends the output to the cerebral cortex
Hypothalamus	Adjusts body chemistry through the regulation of hormones
Locus Coeruleus	Involved with the physiological response to stress and anxiety
Limbic System	Emotion
Basal Ganglia	
Caudate Nucleus	Part of basal ganglia, involved with learning and memory
Putamen	Part of basal ganglia, involved in reinforced learning
Hypothalamic-Pituitary-Adrenal (HPA) Axis	Controls reaction to stress and various body processes such as digestion, immune system, mood, sexuality, and energy usage
Brainstem	Responsible for functions necessary for survival (i.e., breathing, heart rate) and for arousal (being awake and alert)

---

originally believed that humans were born with a finite number of neurons and incapable of neurogenesis (Cappas et al., 2005). How does this relate to the process of therapy? The prefrontal cortex, amygdala, and hippocampus are the structures most closely associated with emotions and memories and are also highly plastic, or changeable. Because therapy typically attempts to bring memories and emotions to the front and center for exploration, therapy seems to be activating the areas of the brain that are most conducive to neurogenesis (Cappas et al., 2005). Therapy's focus on our mental, somatic, and interpersonal lives within the context of psychotherapy can increase plasticity by altering the neuronal firing patterns that will facilitate synaptic growth and form new connections (Siegel, 2006). Some of the basic tenants of therapy facilitate change, so blending neuroscience with psychotherapy doesn't mean we have to start from square one.

Implicit and Explicit Memory

The hippocampus is hypothesized to be involved in long-term memory by serving as the holding station of information for a few weeks before transferring it to certain regions of the cerebral cortex for even longer term memory (Liggan & Kay, 1999). Two distinct systems are involved in memory development and are fundamentally different and separate brain functions, which in turn utilize different neural structures. These systems are referred to as *implicit* and *explicit* memory and have been shown to result in distinct patterns of neuronal activity as evidenced by PET scans and EEGs (Liggan & Kay, 1999). Explicit memory records experiences and stores them for later recall in the temporal lobe structures, primarily the hippocampus (Grosjean, 2005; Liggan & Kay, 1999; Mundo, 2006). Our explicit memories are able to be brought to our conscious awareness through symbols or verbalizations and are labeled as *semantic* or *episodic*. Semantic memories consist of facts or concepts that can be stated (also known as declarative memories), whereas episodic memories capture our historical or autobiographical memories (Rustin & Sekaer, 2004). Specifically, the right hippocampus serves to generate the nonverbal aspects of episodic memory, such as the characteristics of physical spaces, whereas the left hippocampus creates the symbolic semantic memories connected to language (Viamontes & Beitman, 2006).

Conversely, implicit memory is stored unconsciously in the basal ganglia (Liggan & Kay, 1990) and the amygdala (Mundo, 2006) and stems from the emotional experiences and behaviors that are related to our early developmental attachments and overlearned behaviors (i.e., habits). Two different types of implicit memory have also been determined, which is relevant to its use in psychotherapy: *associative* and *procedural* memory. According to Westen (2002), associative memory entails unconscious activation of associated neural networks, such as thoughts, feelings, wishes, and fears, in order to trigger the connections set forth among the networks, also related to priming. Priming is the phenomenon of seeing or hearing words, which increases the likelihood of using them, at least temporarily (Kalat, 2004). Procedural memory, on the other hand, involves the skills we enact unconsciously, which can, in fact, be hampered if consciously focused on (Westen, 2002). For example, we often drive our vehicles or complete activities of daily living without any thought of how we just accomplished the task (which can be a bit unnerving when we drive home from the office and feel as if our car were on autopilot!). But we are able to brush our teeth or read words faster than if we consciously decide what to do next.

Hence, it is hypothesized that, neurodevelopmentally speaking, we are equipped with the capacity for implicit memory at birth, forming emotional and motoric memories, but we do not develop the explicit memory storage banks until early childhood. Because infants have an immaturely developed cerebral cortex, implicit memories at that time are stored in the amygdala and in other regions of the limbic system and basal ganglia (Rustin & Sekaer, 2004). The lack of explicit memory would likely explain the absence of overt memories of our infancy, yet support the fact that infants learn how to shake toys to produce sounds, eat, crawl, and so on.

According to Liggan and Kay (1999), "once learned implicitly, rules may exert a self-perpetuating bias for interpreting later experience in a manner consistent with past experience, regardless of the appropriateness of such an interpretation" (p. 105). Stated simply, these rules can become prosocial or maladaptive patterns that seem to occur without any initiative on the part of the person, and do not always allow for conscious processing prior to the behavior being acted out. Our implicit memory will not only influence how we respond to subsequent situations that are similar to the stored memory, but will also impact our response to ambiguous situations (Grosjean, 2005). Stimuli of the situations are first perceived by the senses, then processed by the brain, and then responded to behaviorally. The information received is responded to in one of three ways: indifference, engagement, or avoidance (Viamontes & Beitman, 2006). We are bombarded with information constantly, much of which does not need to be attended to (e.g., clocks ticking, airplanes flying overhead, conversations in the next room), so we respond with indifference. Other information that is viewed to be important to us is responded to with either engagement or avoidance, and psychotherapy deals primarily with these two (Viamontes & Beitman, 2006).

When looking at the differences between implicit and explicit memory, remember that explicit memory draws upon the conscious awareness or conscious experience of the person. Consciousness is necessary for the explicit encoding of the memory, and there is conscious awareness of remembering the event occurring when the event is later recalled (Rustin & Sekaer, 2004). To explain, we typically do not recall learning how to talk or how to cower in fear; it's just something we *know*. But we can remember the occurrence of learning how to write in the classroom or when we saw the peaks of Yosemite for the first time. We can even remember sitting in Mrs. Smith's kindergarten classroom, picturing her demonstrating how to form letters on the chalkboard.

The Process of Memory

Just how does this process of memory work? Cappas et al. (2005) provided a review of the neuronal processes involved. Long-term memory is said to be associated with regions such as the medial temporal lobe and the prefrontal cortex. Initially, the hippocampus processes the recently learned material, consolidates it, and then organizes it in the cortex. Episodic memory (explicit), also known as autobiographical memory, weaves our personal past experiences with new experiences as we create our life story. Our memories, however, are not perfect accounts of the actual event and can in fact be created differently from the truth based upon the method that is used to retrieve it from memory. Our personality and emotions are connected to our storage and retrieval of the information, so our recall can be affected by our emotional state at the time of the storage or retrieval. Think about a time when your child spilled juice all over the backseat of the car. As you recall this incident while you are in a bad mood, you may reflect on your child as being mischievous or clumsy. Conversely, if you are in a positive mood, you may laugh about it and even miss those childhood days.

Hence, in therapy, it can be possible and rather valuable for the client to recall and integrate painful experiences in such a manner that it can be molded and reframed to signify the positive, or more adaptive, aspects of the situation. It is also beneficial to recall traumatic experiences when in different emotional states or for the therapist to elicit alternative emotional reactions and thoughts.

Information Processing – "Top-Down" and "Bottom-Up"

The amygdala is the key generator of our quick and instinctive, fear-based reactions (Afford, 2007). The cortex, on the other hand, assesses the situation, drawing in outside information, and allows us to think about the experience, though at a slower rate than the amygdala (Afford, 2007). For example, if you see something moving in a bush, the amygdala signals for physical movement and an emotional reaction prior to sending the information to the cortex for additional processing. The cortex then allows you to realize that it was a wind gust that shook the bush. However, when experiences are perceived to be overwhelming, the amygdala holds on to it and doesn't send it for additional processing, as it remains ready for another frightening event. Traumatized clients are thus likely to be holding on to the fear-based reaction, primed to react whenever something related to the trauma is experienced, instead of allowing their mind to fully process each event individually. Without the processing of the original overwhelming event, each subsequent event is likely to be immediately assessed as fear-based without the possibility of safety. Successful psychotherapy is therefore posited to strengthen the cortical control over the amygdala to facilitate "top-down" processing rather than "bottom-up" processing (Afford, 2007).

This "bottom-up" construct is in reference to our "reptilian brain," the subcortical structures that provide us with our core, basic functionalities shared with lower species, such as drives, instincts, and general physical functioning. It is our "higher brain," our cortical structures, that gives us our "top-down" processes that allow for higher order, complex thinking and abstract thought. Psychotherapy is suggested to produce a "top-down" effect, modifying the dysfunction in the subcortical structures in the brain, whereas pharmacology is suggested to provide a reverse effect, working from the subcortical structures inward (Fuchs, 2004). Regardless of the directionality of the effect, success is largely dictated by change in the entire system, rather than the change in specific individual brain regions (Brenner, Roder, & Tschacher, 2006).

PSYCHOLOGIAL THEORIES

Attachment Theory

Attachment theory posits that our early attachment experiences with caregivers are stored unconsciously and give rise to prototypes and rules that set the stage for future relationships. The suggestion that our early attachments and the affective attunement that we do or do not receive can have lifelong effects on our neural development implies that our early affective experiences are deeply, if not permanently, stored in our memory banks implicitly. Attachment relationships with caregivers demonstrate our first experiences with patterns of responsiveness and affective self-regulation (Liggan & Kay, 1999). Because infants are incapable of soothing themselves initially, they seek the guidance and assistance of their caregivers to meet their emotional needs, which in turn facilitates bonding. Failures in early attachment relationships can give rise to poor internal affective modulation and difficulty with self-soothing, which may ultimately lead to an excessive reliance on external sources of regulation. Supportive environments, on the other hand, contribute to regulated stress response systems and balanced cortisol levels, which promotes stronger neurological and central nervous system functioning (Baylis, 2006). Contact with one's support system actually stimulates the release of oxytocin, a neuropeptide linked to relaxation and reduced fearfulness, and facilitates the process of stress modulation and reduction (Baylis, 2006). Negative life events, such as loss, grief, and poor early attachments, have been suggested to be significant determinants of risk and the development of psychopathology (Mundo, 2006).

Interactions between an infant and its caretaker is believed to be a crucial component in the development of the psyche, as this initial internal representation of a relationship fosters a sense of comfort and trust, or lack thereof (Kandel, 1999). In secure attachments, the infant and caretaker can create cyclical patterns of behavior, as they are responsive to the signals, behaviors, and emotional reactions of the other. Responses from the caregiver will reinforce the infant's behaviors, and this will become encoded in the infant's procedural memory banks. Through this process, infants learn that if they cry, for example, their caregiver will arrive and attend to their needs, making them feel secure (Kandel, 1999). Infants with insecure attachments do not experience this symbiotic connection with the caregiver and can therefore experience anxiety when their needs are not met and they are unable to self-soothe. Their procedural (implicit) memory is likely to predict inconsistent outcomes that are mirrored by their caregiver's unreliable pattern of responding.

Psychodynamic Psychotherapy

Psychoanalytic theory was the original, innovative framework for understanding the work-ings of the mind at the beginning of the 20th century. Unfortunately it has had much difficulty maintaining its stronghold by evolving scientifically, because psychoanalysis seems to be much better at creating new ideas than studying them empirically (Kandel, 1999). Freud stated over 100 years ago in 1894 that "biology had not advanced enough to be helpful to psychoanaly-sis," and it was therefore too early to combine the two disciplines in a cohesive manner (Kandel, 1999, p. 507). Although biology has likely surpassed the point to which Freud believed it would need to advance, many psychoanalysts today assume a stronger and opposite stance and state that biology is irrelevant to analysis and protest the blend of the two disciplines. This protest has led to other theories to find empirical validation and stay more current with the latest research. This isn't to say that psychoanalytic theory can't be studied empirically, just that it hasn't to the same extent as other theories, most especially cognitive-behavioral.

Traditional psychodynamic theory emphasizes the role of unconscious processes in the production and continuation of psychopathology. Whether or not one chooses to conceptual-ize cases with the use of the id, ego, and superego concepts, one cannot deny the presence of unconscious processes, especially as it relates to the development of implicit memory.

Object relations theory focuses on the implicit procedures we enact in our thoughts, feel-ings, and behaviors regarding our relationships (Westen, 2002). Usage of the free association technique is asserted on the notion that it will assist the client in making the unconscious conscious, thus bringing those implicit rules to the surface. Neurobiologically speaking, free association will activate the amygdala, the area that connects emotions to our experiences. With the amygdala activated, the client can learn new ways to treat, rethink, and rebuild the emotional and cognitive associations to the trauma (Grosjean, 2005).

Cognitive-Behavioral Therapy (CBT)

Behavioral therapy focuses on the concepts of learning and memory and how they relate to our motor behaviors. Thus, this type of therapy has been shown to involve brain structures such as the amygdala, basal ganglia, and the hippocampus because of their connection to memory (Liggan & Kay, 1999). Cognitive therapy focuses on our patterns of information processing and thought processes and how these cognitions account for our symptomology. Negative cognitions or "cognitive errors" are therefore believed to account for much of the development and maintenance of the pathological symptoms, giving rise to the therapeutic framework. Unlike the behaviors learned implicitly from our attachment relationships, these negative cognitions are quite often part of our conscious awareness, allowing us to evaluate and modify our thought processes. However, it is often argued that the underlying mechanism that initiates the negative cognitions was implicitly learned and should also be brought into awareness in psychotherapy. Cognitive therapy is presumed to stimulate areas of the neocor-tex, specifically the frontal cortex (Liggan & Kay, 1999).

Regardless of the theory used in psychotherapy, certain common factors found across theories can help to produce neurological change. These common factors include (a) a thera-peutic alliance; (b) exposure of clients to their difficulties; (c) a corrective emotional experi-ence; (d) expectations for positive change; and (e) a warm, supportive, empathetic environ-ment (J. D. Frank & J. B. Frank, 1991). The attunement experienced between client and thera-pist as dictated by the development of a supportive environment and therapeutic relationship can promote the calming effects of oxytocin, thus regulating the activity of the hypothalamic-pituitary-adrenal (HPA) axis and the limbic system (Baylis, 2006).

IMAGING, PSYCHOTHERAPY, AND CHANGE – EMPIRICAL SUPPORT

Depression

Clients with depression perceive themselves to be personally defective or at fault even in situations that do not provide any evidence to support these thoughts. The pathology of depression maintains the hyperactivity of the amygdala which can connect negative emotions to emotionally neutral or trivial events, making them appear to be "memorable" and giving them a negative connotation (Viamontes & Beitman, 2006). This may contribute to the perpetual catastrophic thinking of people with depression, as they have a tendency to view many situations inaccurately with emotional intensity, thus continuing their depressive affect and thought processes.

PET studies (Brody, Saxena, Mandelkern, et al., 2001) have shown that subjects with depression had a higher metabolism in the prefrontal cortex, caudate nucleus, and thalamus and lower metabolism in the temporal lobe when compared to the control subjects. Although subjects in this study who were treated with paroxetine had a greater decrease in their symptoms of depression than those treated with interpersonal psychotherapy (IPP), both treatments were successful. Normalization of the metabolism in the prefrontal cortex and temporal lobe occurred in both treatment groups. Other PET studies showed that subjects with depression revealed a decrease in the basal activity of the dorsolateral prefrontal cortex and, on other occasions, increased activity in the ventrolateral prefrontal cortex (Etkin et al., 2005). Brody, Saxena, Schwartz, et al. (2001) and Martin et al. (2001) compared the effects of IPP with either the serotonin-norepinephrine reuptake inhibitor (SNRI) venlafaxine or the selective serotonin reuptake inhibitor (SSRI) paroxetine and found that both modes of treatment reversed the abnormalities found in the prefrontal cortex. In a separate study, Brody, Saxena, Mandelkern, et al. (2001) found that anxiety, sadness, and psychomotor retardation were the symptoms related to depression that were most strongly correlated with metabolic change in the ventral frontal lobe following either IPP or paroxetine.

Hollon and colleagues (1992) studied the effects of cognitive therapy and imipramine hydrochloride in subjects with depression. Subjects received cognitive therapy over a 12-week session and focused on identifying and modifying negative beliefs and maladaptive information processing in order to reduce symptoms. Although neuroimaging was not used in the measurement of change in this study, it is important to note that there was no significant difference in the level of symptom reduction found between those receiving pharmacology and those receiving cognitive therapy. A meta-analysis (see DeRubeis et al., 1999, for a review) of four comparative studies did not support the assumption that pharmacology was superior to CBT in severely depressed outpatients, and there appeared to be no such trend for pharmacology to produce more rapid early change than CBT either.

Depression severity has been consistently correlated with regional blood flow and glucose metabolism in the amygdala and can even remain elevated during periods that are asymptomatic (Drevets, 1998). The amygdala has also been linked to plasma cortisol levels during depressive episodes, and the failure of pharmacology treatment to stabilize cortisol levels can place people at an increased risk for relapse (Drevets, 1998).

Even though some studies show activation in some brain regions and others do not, support for differentiation of treatment methods as they pertain to the top-down versus bottom-up mechanisms in use with depression was expressed in research from Goldapple et al. (2004). Their findings suggested that successful cognitive-behavioral treatment affected the medial frontal lobe and the cingulate cortex (top-down), whereas pharmacology affected the limbic-subcortial structures of the brainstem, insula, and subgenual cingulate (bottom-up). As such, Goldapple and colleagues (2004) stated that CBT should therefore focus on modifying dysfunctional cognitions which would lead to a reduction of vegetative symptoms, and pharmacology should follow the opposite route.

Anxiety Disorders

Posttraumatic Stress Disorder

Clients with anxiety tend to perceive danger in situations that are not dangerous. But persons with posttraumatic stress disorder (PTSD) developed their anxiety symptoms following their involvement with a traumatic event. Remnants of the trauma often remain in the person's mind, contributing to the misperception of danger. Numerous areas of the brain are associated with anxiety, including cortical regions such as the frontal, temporal, and occipital cortices, along with subcortical regions such as the amygdala, hippocampus, hypothalamus, thalamus, and locus coeruleus (Kraly, 2006). During traumatic events, large amounts of stress hormones can be secreted, which, along with activation of the amygdala, can temporarily cease the functioning of the hippocampus, leading to disintegrated elements of perception, behavior, and emotional reactions (Siegel, 2006). The amygdala is responsible to the arousal of the autonomic nervous system after perceiving a threatening or fearful situation (Kandel, 1999). Provocation of PTSD symptoms through the presentation of trauma-related stimuli yielded increased activation in the right amygdala, while lowered activation in medial prefrontal areas was noted during traumatic event recall (Linden, 2006).

Although all experiences seem to be learned implicitly and thus processed through subcortical structures like the basal ganglia, our nontraumatic experiences are believed to stem from the declarative domain and function from the hippocampus, flowing outward to the association and prefrontal cortices, and incorporating our conscious and symbolic memories (Mundo, 2006). Traumatic experiences, by contrast, appear to be a part of the nondeclarative domain and function from the amygdala, encompassing the unconscious, emotional aspects of our memories (Mundo, 2006). Thus, during periods of stress and trauma, the amygdala has been shown to be hyperactive and overstimulated, whereas the hippocampus may be less active than normal, which can cause the memory to be stored with intense emotional and autonomic elements, rather than a more accurate, declarative memory (Grosjean, 2005; Mundo, 2006).

Generalized Anxiety Disorder

Generalized anxiety disorder (GAD) is hypothesized to stem from various neurobiological functions. Hyperactivity of the anterior cingulate gyrus (ACG) is linked to the ruminating thoughts and worries associated with GAD. The ACG's function is to strengthen and filter the information communicated between the amygdala and the prefrontal cortex (Wehrenberg & Prinz, 2007). The amygdala attaches the emotional component to an event; the prefrontal cortex assesses the validity of this emotional response by applying detailed information from the hippocampus and proceeds to send modulating information back to the amygdala (Wehrenberg & Prinz, 2007). To understand this more clearly, I'll give the following example: Imagine you are waiting for a friend to arrive from out of town, and she is late. You have tried to call her cell phone, but she is not answering. Immediately, the amygdala produces a sense of urgency and worry, and you start thinking about all of the catastrophes that could have happened to your friend. The hippocampus and the prefrontal cortex assess the situation and determine that her plane may be delayed, her phone could be turned off, or she may have stopped for gas and isn't near her phone. These realistic possibilities then communicate to the amygdala to calm down and decrease its emotional excitation.

Low levels of serotonin can aggravate the hyperactivity of the anterior cingulated gyrus, which can facilitate an increase in worrying and ruminating thoughts (Wehrenberg & Prinz, 2007). Serotonin may be one of the mediators in behaviorally learned changes in stimulus response whether through pharmacology or psychotherapy. GABA is another important neurotransmitter involved in the maintenance of worry as it may not fully allow for the relaxation of neurons and consequently lead to an increase in the firing of neurons in the basal ganglia (Wehrenberg & Prinz, 2007). The heightened activity in the basal ganglia can also be a factor in clients' subjective feeling that they are immobile or incapable of acting in an emergency situation, even though they are perfectly capable of handling the situation.

The HPA is activated under stress and secretes glucocorticoids, an essential survival feature in the short term, but one that can cause hippocampal atrophy after prolonged exposure (Kandel, 1999; Kraly, 2006). The reduced hippocampus can cause the amygdala to transmit fear that is not proportional to the information received from the thalamus and cortices (Kraly, 2006). Although the atrophy can be reversed upon removal of the stress, memory impairment can occur, especially with declarative (explicit) memory (Kandel, 1999).

Anxiety can elicit excessive unconscious activity in the amygdala, but this can be normalized through psychotherapeutic techniques or possibly by utilizing the processes of top-down inhibitory areas of the frontal cortex (Etkin et al., 2005). As such, Etkin et al. posit that neuroimaging could then differentiate between unconscious and conscious processes and help to identify which changes in the brain are contributing to, if not responsible for, the improvements in behavior.

Panic Disorder

Panic Disorder involves a series of intense episodes of extreme anxiety known as panic attacks combined with behavioral change or unending worry about the potential for having other attacks (American Psychiatric Association [APA], 2000). It has been suggested that cortical sites such as the medial prefrontal cortex are central in the modulation of anxiety and panic responses, as these sites are involved with higher order sensory information processing (Gorman et al., 2000). Psychotherapy treatments such as CBT are hypothesized to work from a bottom-up approach starting from the amygdala to decondition the learned contextual fear response and decrease cognitive errors, and later strengthening the medial prefrontal cortex in its ability to inhibit the amygdala (Gorman et al., 2000).

Obsessive Compulsive Disorder

Obsessive Compulsive Disorder (OCD) is characterized by recurrent, unwanted thoughts, referred to as obsessions, and ritualized, repetitive acts, known as compulsions, the latter of which are often used to rid oneself of the anxiety associated with the obsession. It has been suggested that the basal ganglia, limbic, thalamic, and cortical brain regions are involved in the development and perpetuation of OCD symptoms (Baxter et al., 1992). Baxter and colleagues (1992) studied the neurobiological effects of behavioral therapy and fluoxetine hydrochloride on subjects with OCD using PET imaging. Subjects who received behavioral therapy participated in 8 to 12 sessions consisting of individualized exposure and response-prevention techniques. PET imaging results posttreatment revealed changes in the glucose metabolic rates of the right head of the caudate nucleus following successful treatment with either fluoxetine or behavioral therapy. Similar findings were noted in Linden (2006).

Neuroimaging studies of OCD have researched the basal brain metabolism or basal cerebral blood flow of subjects following the use of medication (SSRI) or psychotherapy. Successful treatment, regardless of the modality, was often found to have restored the brain to a condition resembling normal control subjects, which suggested that, in at least some cases, psychotherapy and medication affected similar brain areas (Etkin et al., 2005). PET scans have also revealed an increase in basal glucose metabolism in the caudate nucleus following either fluoxetine or exposure psychotherapy. Similarly, successful treatment with CBT showed a reduction in the glucose metabolism in the orbitofrontal cortex, caudate nucleus, and thalamus (Kraly, 2006). Both SSRIs and behavioral therapy have been shown to affect similar subcortical regions of the brain (Allen, 2003). Exposure to OCD symptom provocative stimuli by Rauch et al. (1994) led to increased regional cerebral blood flow in the right caudate nucleus, left anterior cingulate cortex, and the bilateral orbitofrontal cortex, which is consistent with the brain regions affected by successful treatment.

Specific Phobias

Specific phobias have been revered as the "easier" disorders to study because their symptoms can be easily replicated in a laboratory, and their symptoms are often more uniform across subjects (Linden, 2006).

Social Phobia. Tillfors et al. (2001) used PET scans to measure the neuronal activation of subjects with social phobia who were asked to give a prepared speech while in the scanner and in the presence of others. Their results showed a larger increase in regional blood flow in the amygdala and the hippocampus when compared to others who just gave the speech alone. Futhermore, Tillfors and colleagues (2001) found decreased activity in the medial temporal lobe and the amygdala following treatment with either citalopram or cognitive-behavioral therapy. Furmark et al. (2002) also reported decreases in amygdala and hippocampal activity following similar treatment groups. The activity of the amygdala can also yield outwardly expressed behavioral gestures, as adults have shown greater activity when presented with angry faces, and children often misclassify angry expressions (Etkin et al., 2005). Hypoactivation of cortical areas that are critical in the processing of negative facial expressions in combination with heightened amygdala activity is suggestive of greater "bottom-up" responding to threatening or frightening situations (Etkin et al., 2005).

Both psychotherapy and pharmacology have been shown to produce comparable changes in blood flow to the amygdala and hippocampus in persons with social phobia as their symptoms reduce (Kraly, 2006). Cognitive-behavioral therapy and pharmacology (i.e., paroxetine and venlafaxine) have proven to be effective, as CBT seems to facilitate the shift from bottom-up processing to top-down processing. This shift helps clients to move their attention away from threatening stimuli and accurately assess the situation, thus dampening the activity of the amygdala. Pharmacology, on the other hand, seems to facilitate bottom-up processing by decreasing the excitation of the amygdala, allowing for an assessment of the situation. The top-down versus bottom-up effect is also noted in psychotherapeutic and psychopharmacological treatments for depression.

Spider Phobia. Spider phobia is one of the most prevalent forms of specific phobias in which people experience lasting and intense fear when faced with spiders, either real or imaginary, and create behaviors to avoid spiders at all costs (APA, 2000). Paquette et al. (2003) examined the neurobiological effects of cognitive-behavioral psychotherapy in persons with spider phobia using functional magnetic resonance imaging (fMRI). The CBT techniques utilized consisted of gradual exposure to spiders by way of guided mastery with pictured and live spiders and education about cognitive errors and misbeliefs. fMRI data from this study prior to receiving CBT treatment revealed significant activation in the dorsolateral prefrontal cortex, the parahippocampal gyrus, and the visual associative areas for subjects with spider phobia. Neither the dorsolateral prefrontal cortex nor the parahippocampal gyrus was shown to be activated in the control group prior to CBT treatment. The prefrontal activation is surmised to be related to the use of cognitive strategies to self-regulate the fear and anxiety produced, a top-down process (Johanson et al., 1998; Paquette et al., 2003). Additionally, contextual fear memory appears to involve the hippocampus; thus, activation in the parahippocampal gyrus is likely related to the activation of the fear conditioned response (Paquette et al., 2003). Activation of the visual associative areas was suggested to be related to increased visual attention to the spider stimuli, which may consequently lead to sustained anxiety reactions. Following CBT treatment, fMRI findings showed no significant activation in the dorsolateral prefrontal cortex or the parahippocampal gyrus for the subjects with spider phobia, making their activation more similar to normal controls (Paquette et al., 2003). Paquette and colleagues (2003) suggested that this finding means that psychotherapy, such as CBT, has the potential to modify dysfunctional neural circuitry and "rewire" the brain by deconditioning the conditioned contextual fear response and reducing cognitive errors and catastrophic thinking.

IMPLICATIONS FOR PSYCHOTHERAPY

Many naysayers of psychotherapy try to suggest that therapy is simply a conversation between two people to exchange words and ideas. They do not believe there is a "science" or an "art" to psychotherapy and therefore that it cannot yield any real physiological or neurological change. On the contrary, psychotherapy is very much an attachment relationship that is highly capable of producing such change through emotional regulation and the restructuring of patterns existing in our implicit memory (Amini et al., 1996). Furthermore, despite the advances in the use of pharmacology in the treatment of various disorders, psychotherapy has continued to play a significant role in treatment, and the combination of psychotherapy and pharmacology has even led to better outcomes than the use of either modality in isolation for certain disorders (Etkin et al., 2005). Therapy, regardless of orientation, can instruct the cortical structures to gain control of the subcortical limbic system structures by increasing our ability to apply logic and reason to our emotional reactions (Baylis, 2006). For example, the orbitofrontal lobes are involved in the activation of the sympathetic and parasympathetic functions of the autonomic nervous system, and therapy can assist in the regulation of our responses to perceived stresses and challenges (Baylis, 2006).

A supportive and empathetic therapeutic relationship and environment can establish the emotional and neurological context that is favorable to the effects of plasticity and neuronal development (Cozolino, 2002). This relationship provides protection, safeguarding, and the support needed to be able to tolerate stress and work through traumatic experiences. Stress releases glucocorticoids into the body, which has been shown to reduce hippocampal volume over time, as stated above. Because this atrophy can be reversed, effective stress management can then increase the hippocampal volume and improve memory and emotional regulation.

Siegel (2006) posited that our brain is capable of observing others and mirroring their perceived behaviors and emotional expressions while integrating them into its repertoire of internal states. Both verbal and nonverbal actions on the part of the therapist are observed in therapy and can be perceived both accurately and inaccurately by the client, but nevertheless they become part of a mirrored neuronal system. Thus, as therapists, our changes in bodily state may serve as the path to empathetic attunement and prosocial interpersonal skills for our clients. Our use of empathy may ultimately increase neural activation in our clients and enhance their level of self-regulation. Thinking back to attachment theory, clients' interactions with their caregivers set the stage for their initial development of self-soothing and self-regulation. Now, the therapist essentially serves in the caregiver role and can create the positive patterns of attachment, empathy, and emotional attunement. Additionally, a therapist's own shifts in brain or body state, often referred to as "countertransference," may provide insight into the fluid or static inner experiences of our clients.

Psychotherapy should therefore be designed to identify and highlight these implicitly learned attachment patterns to allow for conscious recognition and processing in order to facilitate new learning and change (Liggan & Kay, 1999). This framework thus allows for the therapist and client to work conjointly in the development of new behaviors and relationship behaviors to be acted out explicitly and repeatedly until the behaviors become habits and implicitly stored. Psychotherapy is hypothesized to involve both implicit and explicit memory and knowledge by stimulating the communication between the two systems to increase the integration and modification of emotions, cognitions, sensations, and behaviors (Mundo, 2006).

Gabbard (2000) suggested through a model of temperament and character traits that psychotherapy and medication may target different variables and may therefore complement each other when used in combination. The four dimensions of temperament – novelty seeking, harm avoidance, reward dependence, and persistence – are linked to the dopamine, serotonin, and noradrenaline neurotransmitters according to this model (Gabbard, 2000) and are thus more likely to be influenced by pharmacology. On the other side, the character variables of self-directedness, cooperativeness, and self-transcendence are linked to environmental influences and may be more responsive to the therapeutic techniques of psychotherapy.

The use of CBT techniques in the successful treatment of anxiety disorders and depression to produce neurobiological change was well cited in the literature above. These interventions, such as identifying cognitive errors, can reduce depressive and anxious cognitions by activation of more positive and realistic thoughts and switching from automatic thoughts to deliberate and effortful thinking (Folensbee, 2007). Applying neuroscience, these shifts would lead to an increased activation of our frontal lobes and explicit memory systems such that the implicit memory systems involving maladaptive cognitions and emotions would become disrupted (Folensbee, 2007). Thus, the maladaptive arousal states activated by the amygdala can be reduced and rewired into more prosocial and nondepressive or nonanxious states. The bottom-up processes dictated by the pathological states would then be thwarted by the newly integrated thoughts that are relying on logic and reason, rather than instinct and unconscious drives, producing top-down processing of environmental stimuli.

Change can also be produced by having the client engage in simple or more familiar tasks that rely on the lower levels, or more primitive aspects of the brain. Encouraging clients to take walks, read, spend time with friends, or watch movies does require much effort, but it can activate the development of positive neural networks, affect, and arousal at the subcortical level. Therapy then can focus on the higher order, cortical processes. Similarly, the use of relaxation techniques can also help to reduce the anxiety and increase the production of oxytocin and the development of calm and balanced neural networks by gaining control over the amygdala.

With respect to PTSD, when we ask our clients to recall traumatic events, the memory is often laden with powerful emotions and imagery and without emphasis on the lesser affectively charged components. Although developing a narrative of the traumatic event within a therapeutic environment can be highly beneficial in the rewriting of the story, difficulties can arise in the synthesizing and categorization of the event into a cohesive story. This difficulty is likely due to a shrunken hippocampus, reduced activation of the left hemisphere, and decreased activity in the prefrontal cortex, anterior cingulated gyrus, and in Broca's area, as evidenced by neuroimaging findings (Peres, Mercante, & Nasello, 2005).

Reduced activity in Broca's area can also affect the client's ability to verbally convey the details of the trauma. Through the process of narrative therapy, it is necessary to uncover the other aspects of the traumatic event, such as experiences that occurred before and after, and coping mechanisms to assist in the rewriting of a complete story and to help reduce the strong emotional connections. Erasing the traumatic memories is an active learning process to rewrite the trauma and build stronger, healthier neural connections. By providing interventions early after the onset of PTSD, therapy may help prevent the consolidation of traumatic memories and may prevent the development of a more serious disorder (Baer, 2006).

CONCLUSION

Although many of these studies cited above suggest that psychotherapy and pharmacology can produce similar effects in their neurobiological changes, it does not mean that their mechanisms of action are the same. Rather, it does raise questions as to the combined or separate uses of each modality, depending upon the presentation of the disorder at hand. Some clients benefit greatly from the use of pharmacology, while others experience untoward side effects or have difficulty complying with dosage instructions. Psychotherapy may then prove to be an acceptable and comparable alternative to thwart the negative effect but still produce neurological change.

It is possible, and hopeful, that in future research, distinct differences in the treatment of brain abnormalities may be noted between the two modalities of psychotherapy and pharmacology. Etkin et al. (2005) suggested that we may eventually be able to differentiate between the brain regions that are contributing to the symptom reduction and improvement and those that are involved with the mechanisms of specific types of psychotherapy. Should this occur, the science of psychotherapy may be able to move in the direction of being able to "prescribe" for specific interventions to occur for the most effective treatment of disorders.

CONTRIBUTOR

Shelley S. Leiphart, PsyD, is currently a neuropsychology fellow at the New Mexico Veterans Affairs Health Care System in Albuquerque, New Mexico. She is a recent graduate of Wright State University's School of Professional Psychology. Her training is in clinical psychology with special interests in traumatic brain injuries and dementia. Dr. Leiphart may be contacted via e-mail: Shelley.Leiphart@gmail.com

RESOURCES

Afford, P. (2007). Get your head around the thing inside it. *International Journal of Psychotherapy, 11*(1), 5-14.

Allen, J. R. (2003). Biological underpinnings of treatment approaches. *Transactional Analysis Journal, 33*(1), 23-31.

American Psychiatric Association. (2000). *Diagnostic and Statistical Manual of Mental Disorders* (4th ed. text rev.). Washington, DC: American Psychiatric Association.

Baer, M. (2006). Neuropsychotherapy. *Annals of the American Psychotherapy Association, 9*(1), 28-29.

Amini, F., Lewis, T., Lannon, R. & Louie, A. (1996). Affect, attachment, memory: Contributions toward psychobiologic integration. *Psychiatry, 59,* 213-239.

Baxter Jr., L. R., Schwartz, J. M., Bergman, K. S., Szuba, M. P., Guze, B. H., Mazziotta, J. C., et al. (1992). Caudate glucose metabolic rate changes with both drug and behavior therapy for obsessive-compulsive disorder. *Archives of General Psychiatry, 49,* 681-689.

Baylis, P. J. (2006). The neurobiology of affective interventions: A cross-theoretical model. *Clinical Social Work Journal, 34*(1), 61-81.

Beitman, B. D., & Viamontes, G. I. (2006). The neurobiology of psychotherapy. *Psychiatric Annals, 36*(4), 214-220.

Brenner, H. D., Roder, V., & Tschacher, W. (2006). Editorial: The significance of psychotherapy in the age of neuroscience. *Schizophrenia Bulletin, 32*(1), S10-S11.

Brody, A. L., Saxena, S., Mandelkern, M. A., Fairbanks, L. A., Ho, M. L., & Baxter Jr., L. R. (2001). Brain metabolic changes associated with symptom factor improvement in major depressive disorder. *Biological Psychiatry, 50,* 171-178.

Brody, A. L., Saxena, S., Schwartz, J. M., Stoessel, P., Gillies, L. A., Fairbanks, L. A., et al. (2001). Regional brain metabolic changes in patients with major depression treated with either paroxetine or interpersonal therapy: Preliminary findings. *Archives of General Psychiatry, 58*(7), 631-640.

Cappas, N. M., Andres-Hyman, R., & Davidson, L. (2005). What psychotherapists can begin to learn from neuroscience: Seven principles of a brain-based psychotherapy. *Psychotherapy: Theory, Research, Practice, Training, 42*(3), 374-383.

Cozolino, L. J. (2002). *The Neuroscience of Psychotherapy.* New York: W.W. Norton.

DeRubeis, R. J., Gelfand, L. A., Tang, T. Z., & Simons, A. D. (1999). Medications versus cognitive behavior therapy for severely depressed outpatients: Mega-analysis of four randomized comparisons. *American Journal of Psychiatry, 156,* 1007-1013.

Drevets, W. C. (1998). Functional neuroimaging studies of depression: The anatomy of melancholia. *Annual Review of Medicine, 49,* 341-361.

Etkin, A., Phil, M., Pittenger, C., Polan, H. J., & Kandel, E. R. (2005). Toward a neurobiology of psychotherapy: Basic science and clinical applications. *Journal of Neuropsychiatry and Clinical Neuroscience, 17*(2), 145-158.

Folensbee, R.W. (2007). *The Neuroscience of Psychological Therapies.* New York: Cambridge University Press.

Frank, J. D., & Frank, J. B. (1991). *Persuasion and Healing: A Comparative Study of Psychotherapy* (3rd ed.). Baltimore, MD: Johns Hopkins University.

Fuchs, T. (2004). Neurobiology and psychotherapy: An emerging dialogue. *Current Opinions in Psychiatry, 17,* 479-485.

Furmark, T., Tillfors, M., Marteinsdottir, I., Fischer, H., Pissiota, A., Langstrom, B., et al. (2002). Common changes in cerebral blood flow in patients with social phobia treated with citalopram or cognitive-behavioral therapy. *Archives of General Psychiatry, 59*(5), 425-433.

Gabbard, G. O. (2000). A neurobiologically informed perspective on psychotherapy. *British Journal of Psychiatry, 177,* 117-122.

Goldapple, K., Segal, Z., Garson, C., Lau, M., Bieling, P., Kennedy, S., et al. (2004). Modulation of cortical-limbic pathways in major depression: Treatment-specific effects of cognitive-behavioral therapy. *Archives of General Psychiatry, 61,* 34-41.

Gorman, J. M., Kent, J. M., Sullivan, G. M., & Coplan, J. D. (2000). Neuroanatomical hypothesis of panic disorder, revised. *American Journal of Psychiatry, 157*(4), 493-505.

Grosjean, B. (2005). From synapse to psychotherapy: The fascinating evolution of neuroscience. *American Journal of Psychotherapy, 59*(3), 181-197.

Hollon, S. D., DeRubeis, R. J., Evans, M. D., Wiemer, M. J., Garvey, M. J., Grove, W. M., et al. (1992). Cognitive therapy and pharmacotherapy for depression. *Archives of General Psychiatry, 49,* 774-781.

Johanson, A., Gustafson, L., Passant, U., Risberg, J., Smith, G., Warkentin, S., & Tucker, D., (1998). Brain function in spider phobia. *Psychiatry Research, 84,* 101-111.

Kalat, J. W. (2004). *Biological Psychology* (8th ed.). Belmont, CA: Wadsworth/Thomas Learning.

Kandel, E. R., (1999). Biology and the future of psychoanalysis: A new intellectual framework for psychiatry revisited. *American Journal of Psychiatry, 156*(4), 505-524.

Kraly, F. S. (2006). *Brain Science and Psychological Disorders.* New York: W.W. Norton.

Liggan, D. Y., & Kay, J. (1999). Some neurobiological aspects of psychotherapy: A review. *Journal of Psychotherapy Practice and Research, 8*(2), 103-114.

Linden, D. E. J. (2006). How psychotherapy changes the brain – the contribution of functional neuroimaging. *Molecular Psychiatry, 11,* 528-538.

Martin, S. D., Martin, E., Rai, S. S., Richardson, M. A., & Royall, R. (2001). Brain blood flow changes in depressed patients treated with interpersonal psychotherapy or venlafaxine hydrochloride: Preliminary findings. *Archives of General Psychiatry, 58*(7), 641-648.

Mundo, E. (2006). Neurobiology of dynamic psychotherapy: An integration possible? *Journal of the American Academy of Psychoanalysis and Dynamic Psychiatry, 34*(4), 679-691.

Paquette, V., Levesque, J., Mensour, B., Leroux, J., Beaudoin, G., Bourgouin, P., et al. (2003). Change the mind and you change the brain: Effects of cognitive-behavioral therapy on the neural correlates of spider phobia. *Neuroimage, 18,* 401-409.

Peres, J., Mercante, J., & Nasello, A. G. (2005). Psychological dynamics affecting traumatic memories: Implications in psychotherapy. *Psychology and Psychotherapy: Theory, Research, and Practice, 78,* 431-447.

Rauch, S. L., Jenike, M. A., Alpert, N. M., Baer, L., Breiter, H. C., Savage, C. R., et al. (1994). Regional cerebral blood flow measured during symptom provocation in obsessive-compulsive disorder using oxygen 15-labeled carbon dioxide and positron emission tomography. *Archives of General Psychiatry, 51,* 62-70.

Rustin, J. R., & Sekaer, C. (2004). From the neuroscience of memory to psychoanalytic interaction: Clinical implications. *Psychoanalytic Psychology, 21*(1), 70-82.

Rybakowski, J. (2001). Neurobiological aspects of theory and practice of psychotherapy. *Archives of Psychiatry and Psychotherapy, 3*(4), 79-87.

Siegel, D. J. (2006). An interpersonal neurobiology approach to psychotherapy. *Psychiatric Annals, 36*(4), 248-256.

Tillfors, M., Furmark, T., Marteinsdottir, I., Fischer, H., Pissiota, A., Langstrom, B., et al. (2001). Cerebral blood flow in subjects with social phobia during stressful speaking tasks: A PET study. *American Journal of Psychiatry, 158*(8), 1220-1226.

Viamontes, G. I., & Beitman, B. D. (2006). Neural substrates of psychotherapeutic change. *Psychiatric Annals, 36*(4), 225-236.

Wehrenberg, M., & Prinz, S. (2007). *The Anxious Brain.* New York: W.W. Norton.

Westen, D. (2002). Implications of developments in cognitive neuroscience for psychoanalytic psychotherapy. *Harvard Review of Psychiatry, 10,* 369-373.

Well Above 70: Positive Psychology and Optimal Functioning

Paul J. Hershberger

The term "mental health" is most commonly used with reference to the presence or absence of mental disorder or mental illness, whether this is explicit or implicit. This may, in part, reflect how it tends to be easier to define mental illness than mental health. The current mission statement of the National Institute of *Mental Health* [italics added] (NIMH) is "to reduce the burden of mental illness and behavioral disorders through research on mind, brain, and behavior" (NIMH, 2007), and the NIMH accordingly funds research related to mental disorders.

Mental health clinicians primarily work with individuals, couples, families, or groups who are experiencing problems that in some way meet diagnostic criteria for a mental disorder using the *Diagnostic and Statistical Manual of Mental Disorders* (4th ed.; *DSM-IV*; American Psychiatric Association [APA], 1994). When formally recording such a diagnosis, Axis V reflects the assessment made by a clinician on the Global Assessment of Functioning (GAF) scale, a rating of an individual's psychological, social, and occupational functioning. Although the scale ranges from 1 to 100, 70 is effectively the ceiling utilized for current functioning in the clinical setting, as this rating is the highest in the category of "mild symptoms." The current contribution, however, concerns itself with functioning "well above 70." The GAF scale description of 91 to 100 reads, "superior functioning in a wide range of activities, life's problems never seem to get out of hand, is sought out by others because of his or her many positive qualities" (APA, 1994, p. 32). Positive psychology addresses those aspects of human life that facilitate functioning "well above 70."

DEFINING MENTAL HEALTH

Sigmund Freud is reported to have defined mental health as the ability to love and to work, although the veracity of this quote is questioned. Nonetheless, it is a good starting point for a functional definition of mental health. Many other theorists and philosophers have made substantial contributions to our understanding of what constitutes a good life, such as Erikson's (1963) description of successful resolution of psychosocial challenges or Maslow's (1970) depiction of self-actualization. In the middle of the 20th century, Marie Jahoda (1958) published *Current Concepts of Positive Mental Health*, contending that mental health included (a) acceptance of oneself; (b) accurate perception of reality; (c) autonomy (freedom from social pressures); (d) enviromental mastery; (e) growth, development, becoming; and (f) integration of personality. Vaillant (2003) has described six models of positive mental health, which include "above normal," positive psychology, maturity, emotional or social intelligence, subjective well-being, and resilience. The World Health Organization's (2004) definition of mental health is "a state of well-being in which the individual realizes his or her own abilitites, can cope with the normal stresses of life, can work productively and fruitfully, and is able to make a contribution to his or her community" (p. 12).

Recognizing that mental health is more than the absence of mental illness, a two-continua model of mental illness and mental health has been advocated (Keys, 2007; Tudor, 1996). Keyes (2007) has reported data indicating that the correlation of mental illness (defined in his research as symptoms of major depressive disorder, generalized anxiety disorder, panic disorder, and alcohol dependence) and mental health was -.53, which means that less than 30% of the variance in mental health can be attributed to the presence or absence of mental disorder. Distinct from mental illness, the absence of mental health is described as languishing, while optimal functioning is characterized as flourishing. Flourishing is defined by 13 dimensions grouped in three categories (Keyes, 2007):

1. Positive Emotions (positive affect, avowed quality of life),
2. Positive Psychological Functioning (self-acceptance, personal growth, purpose in life, environmental mastery, autonomy, positive relations with others), and
3. Positive Social Functioning (social acceptance, social actualization, social contribution, social coherence, social integration).

Categorizing individuals using the presense or absence of mental illness and three demarcations for mental health (languishing, moderately mentally healthy, and flourishing), Keyes reports that 7% of people have a mental illness and are languishing, 14.5% have a mental illness but are moderately mentally healthy, 3% have a mental illness but are flourishing, 9.5% have no mental illness but are languishing, 50.8% have no mental illness and are moderately mentally healthy, and 16.8% have no mental illness and are flourishing (Keyes, 2007). These data suggest that successfully treating mental disorders does not automatically result in flourishing, and that there is much potential to help more people flourish in life, especially those without a mental disorder. Positive psychology has much to offer with respect to helping people achieve optimal functioning, flourish, and live well above 70.

WHAT IS POSITIVE PSYCHOLOGY?

The positive psychology movement was named by Martin E. P. Seligman as a specific initiative during his presidency of the American Psychological Association in 1998. Prior to this, however, and throughout the history of psychology, there have been many theorists, investigators, and clinicians interested in positive aspects of human functioning, such as counseling psychology's emphasis on individual strengths and assets (e.g., Lopez et al., 2006), Ed Diener's (1984, 2000) work on well-being, and the late C. R. Snyder's (1994) interest in hope. What was initiated by Seligman a decade ago was a much more concerted and coordinated effort to learn more about how to better develop the good life.

Peterson (2006) defines positive psychology as the "scientific study of what goes right in life, from birth to death and at all stops in between" (p. 4). His book, *A Primer in Positive Psychology*, represents an excellent introduction to and overview of positive psychology. It is beyond the scope of this contributiion to attempt a comprehensive review of the field of positive psychology, but examples of some of the work that has been and is being done can give a flavor of the variety of topics in this burgeoning field. In order to provide a foundation for positive psychological interventions that can be utilized by clinicians, the following areas will be considered: benefits and correlates of happiness and well-being, Seligman's perspective on authentic happiness, and character strengths.

Benefits and Correlates of Mental Health

Being satisfied and content with life is a state preferable to being unhappy or discontent. "I just want to be happy" is a phrase heard by many health professionals. The authors of the Declaration of Independence asserted that the pursuit of happiness is one of the unalienable rights, along with life and liberty. Note that happiness was regarded as something to be pursued, not a given. To be happy and engaged with life and to find life meaningful and purposeful contribute in a substantial way to overall quality of life.

From the perspective of the aforementioned two-factor model, mental health improves quality of life and function in the presence or absence of a mental disorder. Although mental illness is extremely costly to workplace productivity, mental health enhances productivity. Positive affectivity, that is, the tendency to experience positive moods, is associated with greater job satisfaction (Watson, 2002).

Although many if not most people would agree with the assertion that money doesn't buy happiness, consumer behavior in Western cultures would suggest otherwise. Studies of the correlation between economic status and life satisfaction make it clear that a change in financial status that moves a person out of poverty is associated with a sustained increase in satisfaction. However, further increases in wealth have a very small correlation with happiness (Myers, 2000). One of the reasons for this is that humans typically adapt to change, whether positive or negative. The thrill of *the new car* today wanes as the vehicle gradually is just *the car*. The phrase "hedonic treadmill" has been used to describe the elusive pursuit of a sustained increase in happiness through material acquisitions (Diener, 2000). This may be one important reason why many individuals are not "flourishing."

Peterson (2006) has reviewed a number of other factors with respect to their relationship to happiness. Perhaps surprisingly, some of the factors that have very low correlations with happiness (defined as .2 or less) include educational level, having children, social class, ethnicity, and physical attractiveness. Factors that have moderate correlations with life satisfaction (defined as .2 - .5) include being married, having more friends, and reporting spirituality to be important. Large correlations with happiness (.5 or greater) are found with being employed, having a sense of gratitude, and being optimistic. The personality factors of conscientiousness and extraversion have moderate correlations with happiness, while neuroticism has a moderate but negative correlation with life satisfaction.

One of the consistent patterns in the research that has identified correlates of happiness, well-being, life satisfaction, and quality of life is that good relationships are perhaps the most important factor. Peterson's (2006) summary of positive psychology is that other people matter. As will be seen, there is a social flavor to many of the positive psychology interventions, even if it simply involves telling others about a good experience.

With respect to cognitive functioning, negative emotional states tend to narrow attention, a phenomenon that certainly has adaptive features. For example, anxiety narrows attention onto the perceived threat so that one's behavioral focus can be on problem solving in order to reduce that threat. Positive emotional states tend to broaden attention. Fredrickson's (2001) "broaden and build" theory of positive emotions describes how positive emotions enhance creativity, expand other cognitive functions, help undo the effects of negative emotion, and in turn contribute to the building of future resources (such as interpersonal relationships).

There is an extensive scientific literature linking optimism and happiness to better physical health. Positive emotions and an optimistic outlook have been associated with healthier behaviors, better relationships (which tend to be correlated with better health), and better adjustment to a variety of illnesses (Taylor & Sherman, 2004). Data exist suggesting that happiness is associated with greater longevity. For example, in a retrospective study of nuns that involved analysis of autobiographies written when vows were originally taken approximately 6 decades earlier, those in the highest quartile of the expression of positive emotions in the autobiographies lived approximately 7 years longer than those in the lowest quartile in the expression of positive emotions (Danner, Snowdon, & Friesen, 2001). Similarly, positive attitudes toward aging among middle-aged and older adults were associated with living approximately 7 years longer over a 23-year period (Levy et al., 2002). There is a corresponding literature that denotes how negative affectivity and neuroticism are associated with poorer physical health (Goodwin & Friedman, 2006; Salovey et al., 2000). With respect to optimal function, the phrase "well above 70" has an intended double meaning. In addition to the reference to the GAF score described earlier, persons with better mental health are statistically more likely to have good health above age 70 and live well past the age of 70. It should be noted that an important link between emotions and health appears to be healthy behaviors, in that happy people tend to behave in healthier ways.

Approaches to Happiness

Martin Seligman (2002) describes three primary contributors to overall life satisfaction, which he refers to as authentic happiness. First is the experience of positive emotions. These include positive emotions about the past (e.g., gratitude), present (e.g., joy), and future (e.g., hope). Second is the experience of engagement or flow in one's life. Csikszentmihalyi (1990) asserts that flow experiences are most likely to occur in one's work, and involve challenge that isn't so great that it exceeds one's capabilities. In flow states a person typically loses awareness of the passage of time. It is hypothesized that flow experiences function as "happiness capital" in that they seem to contribute to future well-being. The third main contributor to life satisfaction from Seligman's perspective is a sense of meaning and purpose in life, which typically involves commitment to features of life or endeavors larger than oneself. An online inventory is available (without charge but with required registration) which measures the extent to which an individual is deriving benefit from each of these three dimensions (www.authentichappiness.sas.upenn.edu).*

Peterson (2006) reports that Seligman has more recently considered yet another route to happiness, the pursuit of victory. This reflects the observation that some people derive satisfaction in life from winning at their goal pursuits. Whether or not this indeed represents another important contributor to life satisfaction is currently being studied.

Character Strengths

One of the noteworthy accomplishments in positive psychology to date has been the book *Character Strengths and Virtues: A Handbook and Classification* (Peterson & Seligman, 2004). This "manual of the sanities" (or un*DSM*) was developed to be a parallel volume to the *DSM*, in that it is a classification for features of the good life. Twenty-four human strengths are grouped under six broad categories of virtues:

- wisdom and knowledge (creativity, curiosity, open-mindedness, love of learning, perspective)
- courage (bravery, persistence, integrity, vitality)
- humanity (love, kindness, social intelligence)
- justice (citizenship, fairness, leadership)
- temperance (forgiveness, humility, prudence, self-regulation)
- transcendence (appreciation of beauty and excellence, gratitude, hope, humor, spirituality)

---

* Although all websites cited in this contribution were correct at the time of publication, they are subject to change at any time.

In order for a human strength to be included in the manual, a number of criteria had to be met, some of which were that the strength is widely valued across cultures, that the behavioral expression of the strength does not diminish others, that the expression of the strength is fulfilling, that the strength is traitlike, and that the strength is measurable. The book devotes an entire chapter to each strength, describing the strength and its history, how it is measured, how it is developed, and interventions to develop the strength, if known. A brief overview of the strengths, including definitions of each, may be found at the www.viastrengths.org website.

The endeavor to classify strengths has included the development of tools to measure the strengths. The VIA (Values In Action) Inventory of Strengths (VIA-IS) consists of 240 items measuring the degree to which respondents agree that a description pertaining to one of the strengths applies to them. Most individuals can complete the inventory in approximately 30 minutes. Test feedback gives respondents a list of the 24 strengths, in the order in which the strengths are characteristic of them. Typically emphasized are the top five strengths, frequently described as "signature strengths." There is also a VIA Strength Survey for Children which is best suited for use by teenagers. Furthermore, there is a VIA Structured Interview, although this measurement approach does not quantify the strengths. The VIA-IS may be completed online at www.viastrengths.org or at www.authentichappiness.sas.upenn.edu, both without charge but with required registration.

Hundreds of thousands of individuals have completed the VIA-IS, resulting in an extensive collection of data regarding the 24 character strengths. For example, the strengths found to be most strongly correlated with life satisfaction have been zest, gratitude, hope, and love (Park, Peterson, & Seligman, 2004).

REVIEW OF INTERVENTIONS

This review of possible interventions that can be used by clinicians will be organized around Seligman's three approaches to happiness, that is, positive emotions, flow, and meaning and purpose. Interventions that less clearly fall under these categories will be reviewed as a miscellaneous group. The interventions described here have been taken either from resources cited at the end of this contribution, the author's training in Authentic Happiness Coaching (a program conducted by Drs. Martin Seligman and Ben Dean), the author's own ideas/practices, or a combination of these sources.

Positive Emotions

Past

Although the phrase "attitude of gratitude" is a cliché, having a perspective of thankfulness is a component of having a positive view of the past (as well as the present). "Tell me about something for which you are thankful" represents the most basic manner in which a clinician might have a client take a perspective of gratitude.

A more intensive gratitude intervention has been referred to as "Three Good Things." The specific instruction is as follows: "For one week, each night before you go to bed, write down three things for which you are thankful." One might additionally ask the individual to also indicate why the good thing happened in order gain perspective on perceived causal factors.

Writing a gratitude letter is another intervention that emphasizes thankfulness. The instruction here is: "Think of someone whom you have not properly thanked for something good that he or she has done for you. Write that person a thank-you letter." Building on this, the individual can be encouraged to make an appointment with that individual, if possible, and read the letter to him or her in person. Simply sending the letter is certainly an alternative, albeit less engaging and personal.

Present

"How are you well today?" Such a question can be used as an initial greeting or at another time in a session with a client. The question calls for the respondent to identify some aspect of health or function that is good. Similarly, one can ask a client to specifically describe something that is going very well in life. Attention to detail enhances the experience. This often is not the primary perspective brought to a clinician's office, so the exercise requires individuals to take an alternative and/or broader view of their lives.

Clients can be asked to write a story that depicts them at their best. Similarly, in a group setting participants can be requested to do positive introductions in which they describe themselves at their best, rather than introducing themselves with descriptions of common demographic variables. In either case, the emphasis is on paying attention to one's positive qualities and strengths.

In the day-to-day busyness of life, persons often look for shortcuts, intending to be more efficient with time. In order to foster positive emotions in the present, one can spend more time with something that is enjoyable. The idea is to find "longcuts," that is, activities that one can intentionally spend more time doing. This could involve taking a longer route when walking on a pleasant day, or simply devoting more time to a valued activity or with a valued person.

Whether or not a pleasant activity is planned, is an intentional longcut, or just spontaneously occurs, individuals can be encouraged to *savor* such events (Bryant & Veroff, 2006). Savoring involves paying attention to the details of the activity or experience, utilizing as many of the senses as possible. Savoring can be enhanced by taking mental photographs of the experience and/or by obtaining actual souvenirs. Furthermore, telling others about the pleasant activity creates an opportunity to reexperience the positive emotion associated with that circumstance.

Future

Generating more positive emotions about one's imagined future can be done by reconceptualizing past experiences. This may involve reflection on how one adapted to a negative circumstance or outcome. "Tell me about an experience in your life in which some door closed on you, but you later found another door that was open to you." This is not to suggest that there is always a "silver lining," but rather that one of the important ways that people cope with adversity is to find opportunities. Such recognition is one pathway to fostering hope.

More formally, one can encourage and direct a client in attribution retraining, that is, learning to make attributions of negative outcomes in a manner that results in the individual being more hopeful about the future. In brief, in the face of a negative outcome, a pessimistic explanation involves attributing the cause of the experience to factors that are always present (enduring) and which affect everything in one's life (pervasive). On the other hand, an optimistic attribution involves explaining the outcome using factors that are temporary (not always) and specific (not everything) to the particular event. To illustrate, upon discovering that one's checking account is overdrawn, a pessimistic attribution might be "I can't do anything right," whereas an optimistic attribution could be "the one time I forgot to record a check is the one time my account is overdrawn." Books that can be recommended to clients for such attribution training include *Learned Optimism* (Seligman, 1998) and *The Resilience Factor* (Reivich & Shatte, 2002).

Flow

Many individuals have certain activities in which they can become thoroughly engaged and absorbed and thereby experience flow. This is particularly true for activities that involve some challenge which they are capable of meeting. Unfortunately, the current emphasis on multitasking in many work settings can inhibit flow experiences. An intervention in this context might involve identifying an activity that has "flow" potential, and then finding a way to protect blocks of time for that activity in which distractions are minimized or eliminated. Although this intervention may involve the individual speaking with a work supervisor or work team, it nonetheless has potential to enhance one's work experience if supported by others. Outside of the work setting, clients can similarly be encouraged to find and protect time for engagement in activities that have potential for the experience of flow.

Interventions that make use of the identification, expression, or development of one's character strengths will be discussed here. It has been hypothesized that there is potential to experience flow when one is expressing one's strengths in a meaningful or significant endeavor, although it should be understood that other benefits can come as well from the behavioral expression of character strengths.

Simply identifying one's signature strengths may be interesting and affect one's perspective of self, but the expression of strengths has much more potential. One very basic but important intervention is to have clients select one of their character strengths to intentionally express in a new way. (If an individual is unable or unwilling to complete the VIA Inventory of Strengths to identify signature strengths, the clinician can ask the individual to identify one of the best aspects of his or her personality and explore how that characteristic can be expressed in new or more intensive ways.) One might focus on the work setting as a place to intentionally express one or more strengths, given that the work setting is most commonly where individuals experience flow.

Another way to utilize character strengths is to identify a strength that is not one of that individual's signature strengths, but nonetheless a strength that the individual would like to further develop. One might choose to develop one of the strengths most closely related to life satisfaction (i.e., love, zest, gratitude, optimism). Another option would be to focus on the strength of self-control or self-regulation, a resource that is associated with numerous functional benefits, but which has been found to be the least endorsed among the 24 strengths (Peterson, 2006). In any case, the development of a strength is to be intentional (i.e., lots of thought) with an emphasis on practicing the strength in a social context. Brief suggestions for developing each of the strengths may be found in Peterson's (2006) *A Primer in Positive Psychology* (pp. 159-162).

Meaning and Purpose

Most individuals experience a sense of satisfaction and meaning when being kind to others and/or helping others. The concept of "planned acts of kindness" simply involves identifying specific and intentional behaviors that express kindness and, of course, implementing such plans. One variant of this concept is to give the "gift of time" in which one actually devotes time to doing something for another or spending time with another person, as an alterative to purchasing a gift or card.

In the consumer realm, meaning can be fostered in gift-giving with the option of giving to a charity in honor of the recipient, emphasizing a charity that carries meaning for the person being honored or which in some fashion might reflect one of the character strengths of the person being honored. For one's self, consumerism can have added meaning when money is spent on something that has potential to add to the flow or sense of purpose in one's life (as an alternative to some thing that temporarily creates positive emotion but to which one readily adapts).

With respect to character strengths, a "meaning" intervention might involve discovering a new way to express a strength that involves serving something larger than oneself. Ideally this would be a new activity and would be done with intentional emphasis on the strength being expressed (e.g., "I am expressing my strength of fairness through writing this letter on behalf of a person being treated unfairly in my community").

Clinicians often avoid the realm of spirituality unless they explicitly represent a particular belief system or work from a particular religious or spiritual framework. Without any identification of or acknowledgement of one's own belief system, a clinician can encourage clients to further explore their spirituality and the expression thereof as a means to support the meaning/purpose in their life.

Miscellaneous

There are a number of research efforts that fall under the large umbrella of positive psychology that have obvious applied implications. Three of these will be mentioned here: the positivity/negativity ratio in interpersonal interactions, capitalization, and satisficing/maximizing.

Positivity/Negativity

Gottman's (1994) work describing the ratio of positive to negative interactions with married couples is well known. Positive interactions are characterized by expressions of support, appreciation, and encouragement, whereas negative interactions include sarcasm, cynicism, and disapproval. In essence, he has found that a 5:1 ratio of positive to negative comments predicts that the couple is less likely to divorce. Similarly, Fredrickson and Losada (2005) studied teams in the workplace. Flourishing teams (defined by performance appraisals, productivity, and customer satisfaction) had a positive to negative ratio in their interactions of 3:1. With their nonlinear dynamics systems approach, they further assert that the upper limit of positive to negative interactions before a relationship begins to suffer is approximately 12:1. That is, some conflict and negative feedback is useful in relationships, but clearly should be a small proportion of all interactions.

Clients (whether individual, couples, or families) can be encouraged to work toward a more desirable positivity/negativity ratio in their personal, occupational, and/or community relationships. This involves the practice of supportive, complimentary, and kind comments/behaviors with others, while decreasing the expression of sarcastic, disapproving, or denigrating comments/behaviors.

The proposal of a "strengths date" represents an opportunity for a couple to experience positive interaction. Such a date involves planning and spending time in an activity or activities that allows both individuals to express one or more of their signature strengths.

Capitalization

Also in the interpersonal realm, Gable and colleagues (2004) have studied the process of sharing of good news along with how persons respond to the sharing of good news. Gable defines capitalization as the process of informing another person about the occurrence of a personal positive event and thereby deriving additional benefits from it. The additional benefits include reexperiencing the positive emotions associated with the experience each time the story is shared, and further solidifying the experience in memory with each retelling. With regard to responding to the sharing of good news, Gable characterizes responses using the combinations of the active-passive and constructive-destructive dimensions:

- Active-destructive: pointing out the downsides of the positive event
- Passive-destructive: no indication of caring; disinterest; little eye contact
- Passive-constructive: silently supportive; little emotional expression
- Active-constructive: enthusiastic response; asking open-ended questions to hear more; expression of positive emotion

Gable reports that among dating couples, a pattern of active-constructive responding to good news was a better predictor of relationship longevity than was how the couples managed conflict, long considered a good predictor of the health of a relationship.

The obvious applications of this work involve encouraging clients to share good news with others (some will need in-session practice to allay their fear that sharing good news constitutes "bragging") and to respond in an active-constructive fashion when others share good news with them. Clinicians themselves may choose to model the active-constructive response when a client shares good news, unless such a response is contraindicated with a given client.

Maximizing/Satisficing

Acknowledging the many benefits that can come with having choices in life, Schwartz (2004) has studied the problems that can ensue when there are too many choices. He uses the terms maximizing and satisficing to describe the poles of a continuum of how an individual may approach a choice. Maximizing involves striving for the best possible outcome, whereas satisficing consists of obtaining an outcome that is "good enough" with respect to desired criteria. Persons who tend to maximize feel obligated to do exhaustive searches to find the best, and in the process create high expectations about their choice. Unfortunately, maximizers are found to experience less happiness, less optimism, less satisfaction with life, lower self-esteem, more regret, more perfectionism, and more depression. Swartz encourages selective maximizing so that persons can be satisfied with "good enough" more of the time.

High-achieving and perfectionistic clients may particularly benefit from learning to satisfice more and maximize selectively. One specific way to teach satisficing is to identify something that the client is planning to purchase. Have the client identify desired qualities of the product. Then have the client agree to do a limited (not exhaustive) search for a product that meets the desired qualities, making the purchase without ensuring that the product chosen was necessarily the best quality or best deal.

INTERVENTION RESEARCH

Internet

Via the Internet, Seligman et al. (2005) conducted a random-assignment, placebo-controlled study with 471 volunteer participants. The five positive psychology interventions tested were (a) three good things, (b) taking the VIA-IS and receiving feedback, (c) using a different character strength (based on VIA-IS feedback) in a new way each day for 1 week, (d) gratitude letter and visit, and (e) writing a story about themselves at their best. The placebo condition involved writing about their earliest memories every night for 1 week. The time frame for the interventions was 1 week. Participants completed depression and happiness inventories prior to the intervention and at subsequent selected intervals.

All groups were happier at the conclusion of the 1-week intervention interval, including the placebo control group. One week later, the placebo control group, the VIA-IS and feedback group, and the "you at your best" story group were back to baseline. Those doing the gratitude visit were happier for 1 month but then were no different from the control group. Those in the "three good things" and "using your strengths" groups were happier and less depressed at the 1-, 3-, and 6-month follow-up intervals.

Although the actual intervention period was for only 1 week, it is noteworthy that the two intervention groups that exhibited sustained benefits involved activities that could readily be continued. In fact, further analysis indicated that those in these groups who indeed continued the activities were the ones who were most likely to experience sustained increase in happiness.

Positive Psychotherapy

Because positive psychology interventions have been discovered to decrease depressive symptoms as well as increase happiness, two therapy studies have been conducted with depressed clients in which the treatment consisted of positive psychology interventions (Seligman, Rashid, & Parks, 2006).

The first study involved six-session group positive psychotherapy with mildly to moderately depressed students. Each session focused on an intervention and related homework, with review of the exercise at the subsequent session. The exercises included in the intervention were using signature strengths, three good things, writing a positive obituary, gratitude visit, active-constructive responding, and savoring. One year after the conclusion of treatment, participants scored in the nondepressed range of depressive symptoms, whereas the no-treatment controls still scored in the mild to moderate range of depression.

The second study involved individual positive psychotherapy with participants who were more seriously depressed. Therapy was conducted over 12 weeks and involved up to 14 sessions, again with each session focused on a positive psychology intervention, homework practice, and follow-up of the practice that had been done between sessions. The Seligman et al. article (2006) includes a table with session-by-session descriptions of the treatment protocol. Clients were randomized to positive psychotherapy or treatment as usual (eclectic psychotherapy). Positive psychotherapy clients were also compared to a nonrandomized matched group receiving treatment as usual and antidepressant medication. At posttreatment, positive psychotherapy clients were doing better on all outcome measures than either comparison group.

Although both of these studies are preliminary, the results suggest that positive psychotherapy interventions may benefit clinical as well as nonclinical populations. At this point there is no apparent contraindication to utilizing positive psychology interventions in the context of other psychotherapeutic interventions, especially with depressed clients.

PRACTICE APPLICATIONS

Given the current environment in which mental health primarily refers to mental disorder or illness, it may be that the most obvious and available arena for utilizing positive psychology interventions is with individuals in clinical practices, that is, persons with global assessment of functioning (GAF) scores below 70. The early research described previously with positive psychotherapy shows promise in this regard, that is, to help persons' GAF scores move up toward 70. However, the aim of the interventions isn't to simply get persons to a GAF of 70, but rather to help individuals function well above 70. From the perspective of the two-continua model of mental illness and mental health (Keys, 2007; Tudor, 1996), it may be that positive psychology interventions are beneficial with respect to both treating mental illness and promoting mental health (i.e., flourishing). It is reasonable to regard positive psychology interventions as adjunctive or complementary to other treatment approaches with clinical populations.

Although it is yet to be studied, there is promise for positive psychology interventions in medical settings as well as mental health settings. As noted earlier, happiness and optimism tend to be associated with better physical health, so that better physical health outcomes may be supported though positive psychology interventions. Furthermore, persons with medical problems are at higher risk for mental health problems (and the converse is true as well) so that these individuals may benefit from intervention from both the medical and mental health perspectives.

Aside from the clinical arena, positive psychology interventions are well suited to coaching of various types, organizational consultation, and educational endeavors. In these realms, the goals of intervention typically involve more effective functioning, whether personal, interpersonal, occupational, avocational, recreational, educational, or the like. Being well above 70 has numerous advantages for all of these domains. Positive psychology is beginning to provide relevant tools that are useful for fostering optimal function.

Positive psychology interventions have shown promise in the preliminary research that has been conducted to date, but there is a long way to go until proven methods exist which can reliably move individuals to GAF scores well above 70. Nonetheless, the positive psychology literature, both with respect to understanding life satisfaction and helping people attain a better quality of life, does already provide the clinician with direction for the client whose request is "I just want to be happy."

RESOURCES FOR CLINICIANS

Those interested in reading an introduction to positive psychology are directed to *A Primer in Positive Psychology* (Peterson, 2006) or *Authentic Happiness* (Seligman, 2002). The Peterson (2006) book provides the more recent overview while the Seligman (2002) book is the original presentation of Seligman's perspective on positive psychology. Practitioners who primarily do coaching may prefer *Positive Psychology Coaching: Putting the Science of Happiness to Work for Your Clients* (Biswas-Diener & Dean, 2007) as an introductory text. Two books that contain edited chapters on particular aspects of positive psychology are *Positive Psychology in Practice* (Linley & Joseph, 2004) and *Handbook of Positive Psychology* (Snyder & Lopez, 2002), although neither resource contains many specific recommendations for clinicians. *Character Strengths and Virtues: A Handbook and Classification* (Peterson & Seligman, 2004) is the primary reference for clinicians seeking detailed information on specific character strengths.

The Happiness Hypothesis: Finding Modern Truth in Ancient Wisdom (Haidt, 2006) takes a more philosophical look at happiness and life satisfaction. *The Paradox of Choice: Why More is Less* (Schwartz, 2004) describes the background and research in the concepts of maximizing and satisficing. Gilbert's (2006) *Stumbling on Happiness* is an engaging and mind-provoking discussion of how human beings are very poor predictors of what will make them happy, and includes ideas on how to avoid making some predictable errors.

The most comprehensive Internet resource for information about positive psychology and links to other resources is the web page for Seligman's Positive Psychology Center at the University of Pennsylvania (www.ppc.sas.upenn.edu). This site contains links to the other Internet addresses included earlier in this contribution.

CONTRIBUTOR

Paul J. Hershberger, PhD, ABPP, is currently Professor of Family Medicine and Director of Behavioral Science for the Dayton Community Family Medicine Residency Program in the Department of Family Medicine, Wright State University Boonshoft School of Medicine. Previously he served as a staff psychologist at the Dayton Veterans Affairs Medical Center, primarily working in clinical health psychology. His ongoing attention to health promotion sparked a more recent interest in positive psychology, and in May 2004, he completed the Authentic Happiness Coaching Program. Dr. Hershberger may be contacted at 2345 Philadelphia Drive, Dayton, OH 45406. E-mail: paul.hershberger@wright.edu

RESOURCES

American Psychiatric Association. (1994*). Diagnostic and Statistical Manual of Mental Disorders* (4th ed.). Washington, DC: Author.

Biswas-Diener, R., & Dean, B. (2007). *Positive Psychology Coaching: Putting the Science of Happiness to Work for Your Clients.* Hoboken, NJ: John Wiley & Sons.

Bryant, F. B., & Veroff, J. (2006). *Savoring: A New Model of Positive Experience.* Mahwah, NJ: Lawrence Erlbaum.

Csikszentmihalyi, M. (1990). *Flow: The Psychology of Optimal Experience.* New York: Harper & Row.

Danner, D. D., Snowdon, D., & Friesen, W. V. (2001). Positive emotions in early life and longevity: Findings from the nun study. *Journal of Personality and Social Psychology, 80,* 804-813.

Diener, E. (1984). Subjective well-being. *Psychological Bulletin, 95,* 542-575.

Diener, E. (2000). Subjective well-being: The science of happiness and a proposal for a national index. *American Psychologist, 55,* 34-43.

Duckworth, A. L., Steen, T. A., & Seligman, M. E. P. (2005). Positive psychology in clinical practice. *Annual Review of Clinical Psychology, 1,* 629-651.

Erikson, E. H. (1963). *Childhood and Society.* New York: Norton.

Fredrickson, B. L. (2001). The role of positive emotions in positive psychology: The broaden and build theory of positive emotions. *American Psychologist, 56,* 218-226.

Fredrickson, B. L., & Losada, M. F. (2005). Positive affect and the complex dynamics of human flourishing. *American Psychologist, 60,* 678-686.

Gable, S. L., Reis, H. T., Impett, E. A., & Asher, E. R. (2004). What do you do when things go right? The intrapersonal and interpersonal benefits of sharing positive events. *Journal of Personality and Social Psychology, 87,* 228-245.

Gilbert, D. (2006). *Stumbling on Happiness.* New York: Knopf.

Goodwin, R. D., & Friedman, H. S. (2006). Health status and the five-factor personality traits in a nationally representative sample. *Journal of Health Psychology, 11,* 643-654.

Gottman, J. (1994). *Why Marriages Succeed or Fail: And How You Can Make Yours Last.* New York: Fireside.

Haidt, J. (2006). *The Happiness Hypothesis: Finding Modern Truth in Ancient Wisdom.* New York: Basic Books.

Jahoda, M. (1958). *Current Concepts of Positive Mental Health.* New York: Basic.

Keyes, C. L. M. (2007). Promoting and protecting mental health as flourishing. *American Psychologist, 62,* 95-108.

Levy, B. R., Slade, M. D., Kunkel, S. R., & Kasl, S. V. (2002). Longevity increased by positive self-perceptions of aging. *Journal of Personality and Social Psychology, 83,* 261-270.

Linley, P. A., & Joseph, S. (Eds.). (2004). *Positive Psychology in Practice.* New York: Wiley.

Lopez, S. J., Magyar-Moe, J. L., Petersen, S. E., Ryder, J. A., Krieshok, T. S., O'Byrne, K. K., Lichtenberg, J. W., & Fry, N. A. (2006). Counseling psychology's focus on positive aspects of human functioning. *The Counseling Psychologist, 34,* 205-227.

Maslow, A. H. (1970*). Motivation and Personality* (2nd ed.). New York: Harper and Row.

Myers, D. G. (2000). The funds, friends, and faith of happy people. *American Psychologist, 55,* 56-67.

National Institute of Mental Health. (2007). Mission statement. Retrieved December 21, 2007, from http://www.nimh.nih.gov/

Park, N., Peterson, C., & Seligman, M. E. P. (2004). Strengths of character and well-being. *Journal of Social and Clinical Psychology, 23,* 603-619.

Peterson, C. (2006). *A Primer in Positive Psychology.* New York: Oxford University Press.

Peterson, C., & Seligman, M. E. P. (2004). *Character Strengths and Virtues: A Handbook and Classification.* New York: Oxford University Press.

Reivich, K., & Shatte, A. (2002). *The Resilience Factor.* New York: Broadway Books.

Salovey, P., Rothman, A. J., Detweiler, J. B., & Steward, W. T. (2000). Emotional states and physical health. *American Psychologist, 55,* 110-121.

Schwartz, B. (2004). *The Paradox of Choice: Why More is Less.* New York: HarperCollins.

Seligman, M. E. P. (1998). *Learned Optimism: How to Change Your Mind and Your Life.* New York: Pocket Books.

Seligman, M. E. P. (2002). *Authentic Happiness.* New York: Free Press.

Seligman, M. E. P., Rashid, T., & Parks, A. C. (2006). Positive psychotherapy. *American Psychologist, 61,* 774-788.

Seligman, M. E. P., Steen, T. A., Park, N., & Peterson, C. (2005). Positive psychology progress: Empirical validation of interventions. *American Psychologist, 60,* 410-421.

Snyder, C. R. (1994). *The Psychology of Hope: You Can Get There From Here.* New York: Free Press.

Snyder, C. R., & Lopez, S. J. (2002*). Handbook of Positive Psychology.* New York: Oxford University Press.

Taylor, S. E., & Sherman, D. K. (2004). Positive psychology and health psychology: A fruitful liaison. In P. A. Linley & S. Joseph (Eds.), *Positive Psychology in Practice* (pp. 305-319). New York: Wiley.

Tudor, K. (1996). *Mental Health Promotion: Paradigms and Practice.* New York: Routledge.

Vaillant, G. E. (2003). Mental health. *American Journal of Psychiatry, 160,* 1373-1384.

Watson, D. (2002). Positive affectivity: The disposition to experience pleasurable emotional states. In C. R. Snyder & S. J. Lopez (Eds.), *Handbook of Positive Psychology* (pp. 106-199). New York: Oxford University Press.

World Health Organization. (2004). *Promoting Mental Health: Concepts, Emerging Evidence, Practice (summary report).* Geneva, Switzerland: Author.

Subject Index

Continuing Education
Available for Home Study

The most recent volumes of *Innovations in Clinical Practice* are available as formal home-study continuing education programs. This best-selling, comprehensive source of practical clinical information is complemented by examination modules which may be used to earn continuing education credits.

Credits may be obtained by successfully completing examinations based on those contributions in each volume which have been selected by the editorial advisory board. Each of these contributions explores a timely topic designed to enhance your clinical skills and provides the knowledge necessary for effective practice. After studying these selections, a multiple-choice examination is completed and returned to the Professional Resource Exchange for scoring. Upon passing the examination (80% of test items answered correctly), your credits will be recorded and you will receive a copy of your official transcript.

At the time of publication of this volume, continuing education modules are available for Volumes 18 through 20 of *Innovations in Clinical Practice: A Source Book*. Each module contains examination materials for 20 credits (equivalent to 20 hours of continuing education activity). Twelve-credit programs are available for *Innovations in Clinical Practice: Focus on Children and Adolescents* and *Innovations in Clinical Practice: Focus on Violence Treatment and Prevention*. Fourteen-credit programs are available for *Innovations in Clinical Practice: Focus on Adults* and *Innovations in Clinical Practice: Focus on Health and Wellness*. An 18-credit program is available for *Innovations in Clinical Practice: Focus on Group, Couples, & Family Therapy*, and a 20-credit program is available for *Innovations in Clinical Practice: Focus on Sexual Health*. *Innovations in Clinical Practice: A 21st Century Sourcebook (Vol. 1)* also contains 20 credits.

The *Innovations in Clinical Practice* Continuing Education (CE) Programs are one of the most efficient ways to stay current on new clinical techniques and obtain formal credit for your study. If your professional associations and state boards do not currently require formal CE activities, you may still wish to consider these programs as an excellent means of receiving feedback on your professional development. These self-study programs are . . .

- *Relevant* - selections are packed with information pertinent to your practice.
- *Inexpensive* - typically less than half the cost of obtaining credits through workshops and these expenses may still be tax deductible as a professional expense.
- *Convenient* - study at your own pace in the comfort of your home or office.
- *Useful* - the volumes will always be available as a practical reference and resource for day-to-day use in your professional practice.
- *Effective* - as a means of staying up to date and obtaining feedback on your knowledge acquisition and professional development. In most states with continuing education requirements, credits earned from American Psychological Association (APA) approved sponsors are automatically approved for licensure renewal. Consult your profession's state board for their policies regarding the status of programs offered by APA approved sponsors.

Specific learning objectives, faculty credentials, and program instructions are available upon request.

The Professional Resource Exchange, Inc. is approved by the American Psychological Association to sponsor continuing education for psychologists. The Professional Resource Exchange, Inc. maintains responsibility for these programs and their content. We are also recognized by the National Board for Certified Counselors to offer continuing education for National Certified Counselors. We adhere to NBCC Continuing Education Guidelines (Provider #5474). Florida Continuing Education Provider (BAP #349). Florida CE Broker Provider #50-2943. This program also meets the qualifications for continuing education credit for MFCCs and/or LCSWs as required by the California Board of Behavioral Sciences (PCE # 816).

To receive additional information on these CE programs, please see next page. ⟶

Do You Want More Information?

Yes! Please Send Me . . .

❏   Information on the other volumes in the *Innovations in Clinical Practice* series (Tables of Contents for all volumes and ordering information).

❏   Information on your home-study continuing education programs.

❏   Your latest catalog.

Name: _____
(Please Print)

Address: _____

Address: _____

City/State/Zip: _____
Is this ❏ home or ❏ work?

Telephone: (_____) _____ Fax: (_____) _____

E-Mail: _____

My Primary Profession Is: _____

For Fastest Response . . .

Fax to Our 24 Hour FAX Line at **1-941-343-9201**

OR

E-mail to **orders@prpress.com**

OR

Visit Our Website: **http://www.prpress.com**

Or Mail This Form To . . .

Professional Resource Press
PO Box 15560 • Sarasota FL 34277-1560